The Handbook of Clinical Trials and Other Research

Alan Earl-Slater

Executive Advisory Panel

Ann Bowling	Anna Donald
Malini Haria	Warwick Hunt
David Kernick	Jane Sharp

Tom Walley

RADCLIFFE MEDICAL PRESS

Radcliffe Medical Press Ltd
18 Marcham Road
Abingdon
Oxon OX14 1AA
United Kingdom

www.radcliffe-oxford.com
The Radcliffe Medical Press electronic catalogue and online ordering facility.
Direct sales to anywhere in the world

British Library Cataloguing in Publication Data

A catalogue record for this book is available from the British Library.

ISBN 1 85775 485 9

Typeset by Advance Typesetting Ltd, Oxon
Printed and bound by TJ International Ltd, Padstow, Cornwall

Preface

Anyone involved in healthcare over the last five years will have noticed that we are fast approaching a situation where we want 'evidence-based everything'. Rightly or wrongly, clinical trials are being seen as the best possible source of evidence.

Despite the increasing volume of information, years of experience continue to show that there is a pressing need for a book on clinical trials that seeks to blend terminology with clarity, and which is sprinkled with a healthy dose of contemporary examples to which busy people can relate.

The objectives of this handbook are as follows:

- to introduce terms used in clinical research

- to extend the range of terms used in the discipline

- to make the terminology more accessible and clear

- to contribute to the standardisation of the terminology

- to improve understanding of the meaning of the terms

- to provide a collection of contemporary examples to which readers can relate

- to indicate some references that you can follow up

- to offer insight into contemporary issues, arrangements and developments in the governance of research, whether or not that research is a clinical trial.

And yet there is more, much more, that needs to be appreciated and understood beyond research terminology and methodology. For example, there are various issues surrounding the management of research, emerging laws and policies, and the impact of research on thinking, knowledge and practice. This book seeks to give a glimpse into some of the issues beyond research terminology and methodology.

This handbook reflects many of the terms used in clinical research in general and in clinical trials in particular. It is written as a refresher for those who already know something about clinical research, and as an introduction for the many who are novices to the topic. Overall, this book aims to be a useful adjunct for anyone involved in clinical research, whether as patients, purchasers, providers, sponsors, advisers or analysts.

Each definition in this handbook is important in its own right. When you add elements together you can develop a more powerful critique of a clinical trial. Many of the terms in this book are cross-referenced. For example, the term **Definitive clinical trial** is cross-referenced to **Clinical trial, Comparing research methods, Duhem's irrefutability theory, Falsificationism, Lakatosian research programme, Mega-trial, Primary question, Problems with regard to putting evidence into practice** and **Research questions and research methods**. One reason for cross-referencing in this way is to indicate terms in other parts of the book that relate to the defined term. The cross-reference may signal a different method (e.g. a parallel trial is methodologically different to a cross-over trial). The cross-referencing is also designed to capture terms that raise issues with the defined term.

Some references are included at the end of most terms. These give you an example of the term under discussion or direct you to some further reading on the topic. Anyone following up the references will gain a deeper and wider insight into the issue under consideration. Most of the references are quite recent and come from the major journals. This is to make your life a little easier, it is hoped, by identifying readily available references.

Whilst this book uses many examples drawn from the published literature, this does not mean that anyone in my advisory panel or myself endorses or agrees with any of the conclusions in the studies quoted.

How can you use this handbook? Below are some ideas.

- If you come across a term that may be used in clinical research and you need clarification on its meaning, refer to this book.

- If you want to learn some of the tools of the trade of clinical research, refer to this book.

- If you want to use clinical research terminology in your own work, check with this book that you are using the correct terms.

- Gain in one resource some insight into issues, arrangements and developments in research governance, whether or not that research is a clinical trial.

- Participate – contact me if there is a term that you think could be included in the next edition of the book, or if you have good examples of a term that you think a wider audience would appreciate.

This is important. If you would like more details on statistics, ethics, epidemiology, health economics, evidence-based healthcare, health service organisation or outcomes research, the following books are recommended.

- Altman D (1977) *Practical Statistics for Medical Research*. Chapman and Hall, London.

- Matthews JNS (2000) *An Introduction to Randomised Controlled Clinical Trials*. Arnold Texts in Statistics, Edward Arnold, London.

- Boyd KM, Higgs R and Pinching AJ (1997) *The New Dictionary of Medical Ethics*. BMA Books, London.

- Last JM (1995) *A Dictionary of Epidemiology*. Oxford University Press, Oxford.

- Earl-Slater A (1999) *Dictionary of Health Economics*. Radcliffe Medical Press, Oxford.

- Li Wan Po A (1998) *Dictionary of Evidence-Based Medicine*. Radcliffe Medical Press, Oxford.

- Fulop N, Allen R, Clarke A and Black N (2001) *Studying the Organisation and Delivery of Health Services: research methods*. Routledge, London.

- Bowling A (1995) *Measuring Health*. Open University Press, Buckingham.

- Bowling A (1997) *Measuring Disease*. Open University Press, Buckingham.

There are thousands of clinical trials currently taking place – too many to catalogue in one book. Information about particular clinical trials may be found by checking the following sources:

- the Internet (e.g. see http://www.controlled-trials.com, http://hiru.mcmaster. ca/cochrane, http://www.cochrane.org, http://www.nrr.org, http://clinicaltrials. gov, http://www.evidence-basedmedicine.com.

- NHS sources (e.g. see *National Research Register*, a CD collection of research available from the NHS Executive or on the Internet (http://www.doh.gov.uk/ research/nrr.htm)

- your local or regional clinical trial ethics committees

- your local primary care group, trust or board, hospital or health authority

- your regional drug information office

- trial sponsors

- international organisations.

To become more expert in clinical trials, you also have to look at some of the literature on such trials that can be found in the above sources (e.g. National Research Register (NRR), Cochrane Collaboration, Food and Drug Administration, *British Medical Journal*, clinicaltrials.gov. The *Evidence-Based Medicine* website (www.evidence-basedmedicine.com) is certainly worth looking at for summary reports of published research and analysis. You should also speak to those involved in trials (e.g. the NRR has contact names and addresses of trialists), read actual trial reports (where these are available, ask the trial sponsors), meet up with colleagues to discuss a particular clinical trial, and gain insight from your own and others' experiences. Ask the speaker questions when you hear a presentation on a trial in a meeting, workshop, continuing education and training meeting, seminar or conference. Ask your clinical practice if they will discuss a clinical trial. You can join or set up discussion groups. Find out what training courses or workshops you can attend. Discuss issues with your family, friends and colleagues. Write to your local newspaper asking what interest the paper takes in local clinical trials. Write to magazines and radio stations asking what interest they have in clinical trials.

The terms in this handbook can be used in many other settings beyond healthcare – for example, trials in education, social care, law and order, materials testing in manufacturing, agriculture (e.g. crop trials) and veterinary practice.

I am grateful for the sincere enthusiasm, hospitality, insight, expertise and friendship received from many of those with whom I have worked. These people, from international organisations, industry, academia, government, healthcare, research councils and the private and voluntary sectors, have shared their knowledge and advice freely with me, and none of them refused to respond to my continued thirst for understanding and my relentless quest for clarification. In the course of writing this book I have been in contact with over 300 people across the world. They have personally been thanked for their help, enthusiasm, support and kindness.

Some will be named and thanked publicly. These people reviewed and became advisers on what I was writing, and their insight and clarity were of great value. They are true professionals with a genuine sense of purpose and passion.

Alan Earl-Slater
alaneslater@hotmail.com
May 2002

Expert Advisory Panel

Although I retain full responsibility for the actual contents of this book as now published, a very special 'Thank You' is due to the members of the Expert Advisory Panel.

- **Professor Ann Bowling**, Professor of Health Services Research, Department of Primary Care and Population Sciences, University College Medical School, London.

- **Dr Anna Donald**, Managing Director, Bazian Limited, London.

- **Ms Malini Haria**, Associate Editor, Drug and Therapeutics Bulletin, The Consumers' Association, London.

- **Dr Warwick Hunt**, Head of Clinical Governance and Quality Development, Northamptonshire Health Authority, Northampton.

- **Dr David Kernick**, General Practitioner, St Thomas' Health Centre, Exeter.

- **Ms Jane Sharp**, Director of Medicines Information, Pharmacy Department, Northwick Park NHS Hospital, Harrow.

- **Professor Tom Walley**, Department of Pharmacology and Therapeutics, University of Liverpool, Liverpool.

This book is dedicated to Maria

A

Absolute benefit

The absolute benefit is the benefit gained from a particular intervention for example, lowered cholesterol, alleviation of pain, or life saved. *See* **Absolute benefit increase**; **Health**; **Quality of life**.

Absolute benefit increase

The absolute benefit increase (ABI) is the difference in event rates.

$$ABI = \text{experimental event rate} - \text{control event rate}$$

Suppose evidence from a recently published clinical trial shows that a new regimen for dealing with acute myocardial infarction increases the likelihood of certain patients being alive after 30 days compared with patients on the usual care regimen. Out of 100 patients on the new regimen, 93 individuals are alive at 30 days, whereas out of 100 patients who received usual care, only 86 individuals are alive at 30 days.

Using the above data:

$$ABI = 93/100 - 86/100 = 7\%$$

This means that the new regimen for dealing with acute myocardial infarction has an absolute benefit increase of 7% over the usual care regimen.

This measure is to be used when the outcomes in the experimental regimen are better than the outcomes in the control regimen. *See* **Absolute benefit**; **Absolute risk reduction**; **Relative benefit increase**.

Absolute risk

The absolute risk is a measure of the risk of an event occurring in a group.

Suppose a clinical trial on stroke prevention in high-risk patients provides the following results (*see* Table 1).

Table I Absolute risk

	Outcome		
	Stroke occurs	Stroke does not occur	Total
New care	a (100)	b (200)	a + b = 300
Usual care	c (120)	d (180)	c + d = 300
Total	a + c = 220	b + d = 380	a + b + c + d = 600

In the new care regimen 100 high-risk patients had a stroke and 200 did not. In the usual care regimen 120 patients had a stroke and 180 did not.

Referring to Table 1, the absolute risk (AR) of stroke in the new care group is:

$$AR_{newcare} = \frac{a}{a + b}$$

Using the data in Table 1, we have:

$$AR_{newcare} = \frac{100}{100 + 200} = \frac{100}{300} = 0.33$$

This means that the absolute risk of a patient having a stroke in the new care group is 33%.

The absolute risk of stroke occurring in the usual care group is as follows:

$$AR_{usualcare} = \frac{c}{c + d}$$

Using the data in Table 1, we have:

$$AR_{usualcare} = \frac{120}{120 + 180} = \frac{120}{300} = 0.40$$

This means that the absolute risk of a patient having a stroke in the usual care group is 40%. *See* **Absolute risk reduction; Incidence; Likelihood ratio; Odds; Odds ratio; Relative risk; Relative risk reduction.**

Absolute risk increase

The absolute risk increase (ARI) is a measure of the absolute difference in risk of an event in the experimental group of patients compared with the other groups of patients (controls). This measure is to be used when the risk in the experimental group exceeds that in the control group.

If the absolute risk in the experimental group is 10% and the absolute risk in the control group is 6%, then the absolute risk increase is 4% (i.e. 10 – 6). In general, then:

$$ARI = \text{experimental event rate} - \text{control event rate}$$

This measure does not give any impression of the relative risk between the regimens in the trial. *See* **Absolute benefit increase; Absolute risk; Absolute risk reduction; Number needed to harm; Relative risk; Relative risk reduction**.

Absolute risk reduction

When the absolute risk in the control group is higher than that in the new regimen, the difference is called the absolute risk reduction.

Looking at the right-hand column of Table 2, the absolute risk reduction (ARR) is as follows:

$$ARR = X - Y$$

More generally, the absolute risk reduction (ARR) is calculated as follows:

$$ARR = \text{control event rate} - \text{experimental event rate}$$

Recent examples where absolute risk reductions have been assessed include the following:

- paediatric cystic fibrosis patients receiving care at home compared with care in the hospital setting
- different medication options in *Helicobacter pylori* eradication
- different options when treating patients with dementia and looking at the reduction in risk of the patient being institutionalised.

Suppose that your primary care group (PCG) and hospital have been involved in a clinical trial on stroke prevention in high-risk patients. Table 2 shows some results of that trial.

Table 2 Absolute risk reduction

	Outcome			
	Stroke occurs	*Stroke does not occur*	*Total*	*Risk of events*
New regimen	a (100)	b (200)	a + b = 300	$Y = a/(a + b) = 100/300 = 1/3$
Usual care	c (120)	d (180)	c + d = 300	$X = c/(c + d) = 120/300 = 2/5$
Total	a + c = 220	b + d = 380	a + b + c + d = 600	

Using the data in Table 2, we have:

$$\text{ARR} = \frac{2}{5} - \frac{1}{3} = 0.067 \text{ or } 6.7\%$$

This means that the new care regimen reduces the absolute risk of stroke by 6.7% compared with the existing programme.

While it is a useful measure of the results of clinical trials in itself, the ARR can also be used to determine how many people need to be treated in order to avoid one event (e.g. to answer questions such as how many need to be treated in order to avoid one having a stroke). *See* **Absolute benefit increase; Absolute risk; Absolute risk increase; Likelihood ratio; Number needed to treat; Odds; Odds ratio; Relative risk; Relative risk reduction**.

Acceptable risk

An acceptable risk is one for which the benefits of a choice are thought to outweigh the dangers. For example, when reviewing an application for a market licence for a new drug, the assessors use risk–benefit calculus to help to determine whether the known benefits of the medication outweigh the risks.

In general, what is thought to be an acceptable risk is conditioned by scientific data, independence of judgement, the present situation of the decision-maker, experience, and social, moral and economic issues.

Wider still, what is deemed to be an acceptable risk in, for example, food production depends on these factors and on politics. *See* **Bayesian analysis; Committee on the Safety of Medicines; Medicines Control Agency**.

Acceptance area

Suppose you make a statement that taking anti-obesity medication has no effect in reducing the patient's weight after one year. It is quite easy to make such statements. What is interesting is whether or not, in the face of the evidence, the statement can be accepted.

The acceptance area is the set of results that leads us to accept the statement, sometimes also called the acceptance region.

Your statement can be written as follows:

$$H_o: x_{t-1} = x_t$$

where x_{t-1} is the patient's weight one year ago at time $t-1$, and x_t is the patient's weight today. Once the results of the trial are available, an analysis can be performed to test your statement. The patient may be heavier, lighter or of the same weight as last year. Therefore we need an upper limit and a lower limit to our acceptance area. Any results that fall within the acceptance area mean that, on the basis of the evidence, your statement or hypothesis need not be rejected. Any results that fall outside the acceptance area mean that your statement or hypothesis is not accepted. Figure 1 provides an illustration.

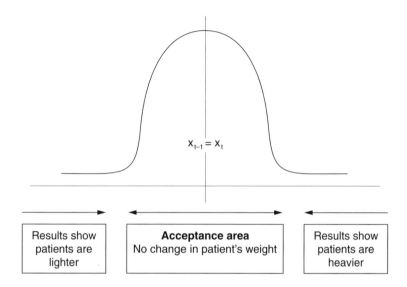

$$x_{t-1} = x_t$$

| Results show patients are lighter | **Acceptance area** No change in patient's weight | Results show patients are heavier |

Figure 1 Acceptance area (two tail example).

Suppose that a colleague in the primary care group makes a statement claiming that, as far as she understands, patients with relapsing remitting multiple sclerosis do not improve as a result of a one-year integrated welfare–physiotherapy–health medication package.

Once the results of the trial are available, an analysis can be performed to test the statement of no improvement. In this case we use one rejection region – that is, one tail (*see* Figure 2). Why is this? The statement of 'no improvement' allows us to accept results that show 'no change' or 'worse'!

If the results fall outside the acceptance area, then on the basis of this evidence, your colleague's statement or hypothesis cannot be accepted. Figure 2 provides an illustration.

The size of the acceptance area, the numbers involved and the shape of the curve all depend on the specifics of the trial, the distribution of the data and the assumptions therein. You also need to know what is meant by the terms used, such as the patients were 'no better', 'worse' or showed 'no improvement'. *See* **Clinical significance; Confidence interval; Duhem's irrefutability theory; Falsificationism; Hypothesis testing; Lakatosian research programme; Null hypothesis; One-tailed test; Protocol; *P*-value; Statistical significance; Statistical test diagram; Statistical tests: ten ways to cheat with statistical tests; Subgroup analysis; Two-tailed test.**

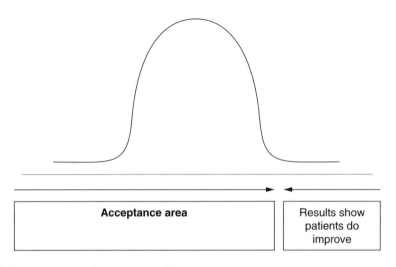

Figure 2 Acceptance area (one tail example).

Accountability

Accountability arises when a person or a group of people are answerable or have to give account to another person or group of people for an action, task or decision that they have taken or were supposed to have taken.

Accountability is concerned with who is accountable:

- to whom

- for what

- where

- when

- why

- how

- for how long.

There are two constructs in accountability, namely the form of accountability and the line of accountability. The *form* could be managerial, legal, ethical, clinical, financial, regulatory or professional accountability. The *lines* could involve any collection from patients, doctors, clinical trial sponsors, clinical trial managers, host institutions, the regulators, the ethics committee and the legal system. *See* **Audit; Clinical trial steering committee; Data-monitoring committee; Declaration of Helsinki; Due process; Multicentre research ethics committee; Principal investigator; Research governance in the NHS; Transparency.**

○ Medical Research Council (1998) *Guidelines for Good Clinical Practice in Clinical Trials.* Medical Research Council, London.

○ Smith S (2000) Accountability: for whom the bell tolls. *Br J Gen Pract.* **50**: 426–7.

Acquiescence response

When people are more likely to agree to something they are said to exhibit an acquiescence response – that is, they are more likely to say 'yes'.

This is a sometimes subtle but always interesting term for clinical trials, because it can affect the following:

- inviting people (e.g. patients, clinicians) to take part in a trial

- the questions used to elicit and measure outcomes

- the questions used to establish the merits and applicability of trial results to clinical practice.

There is no robust evidence indicating how prevalent or important the acquiescence response is. *See* **Closed question; Consent; Deferred consent; Leading question; Open question; Outcomes pyramid; Qualitative analysis; Research question; Types of research questions.**

Action research

Over the last 50 years 'action research' has been described and defined in various ways by different people, e.g. Kurt Lewin, Stephen Corey and David Hopkins to name a few. In 1994, for example, Emily Calhoun suggested that it was 'a fancy way of saying let's study what's happening and decide how to make it a better place'.

Action research is a family of methodologies which jointly pursues action (or change) and research (or understanding) at the same time. It seeks to be a virtuous spiral of action and of research. The spiral involves cycles. As Figure 3 shows, each cycle involves reconnaissance, planning, action and reflection. In the later cycles, action research continuously refines the methods, data and interpretation in the light of the evidence and understanding developed in the earlier cycles.

- *Reconnaissance.* An exploratory stance is adopted, where specification and understanding of the problem are developed.

- *Plan.* Plans are made for some form of intervention strategy.

- *Action.* After negotiation and discussion with interested parties, the intervention is carried out.

- *Reflection and revision.* Evaluation of the intervention and re-evaluation of the initial problem.

Before, during and after each intervention observations are made, and information is collected and analysed. Action research generally involves a 'look, think, act' process. It is therefore intended to foster a deeper understanding of a given situation, starting with conceptualising and particularising the problem, and moving through

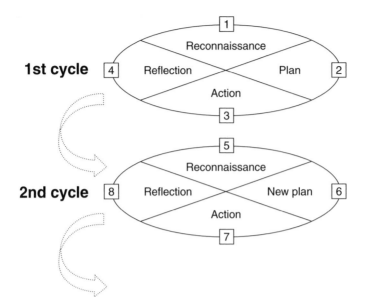

Figure 3 An action research spiral.

several actions, reflections, refinements and evaluations. It also makes us think about the contexts we are working in, how they affect our judgements and our interpretations upon which those judgements are based. The spiral process repeats itself until the desired improvements to practice are achieved.

Action research:

- is an *emergent* process that takes shape as understanding increases

- is an *iterative* process that converges towards a better understanding of practice and change

- is *pragmatic* in terms of action and of research

- is *participative* (among other reasons, change is usually easier to achieve when those affected by the change are involved in each cycle)

- is *reflective*

- is *'evidence based'*

- often *blends qualitative and quantitative* research and action.

Action research has the potential to generate genuine and sustained improvements in practice because it can offer:

- greater feelings of ownership of action and of analysis

- pragmatic insight into real life issues, ambitions, constraints and solutions

- new opportunities to reflect on and assess work
- scope and structure to explore and test new ideas, methods and materials
- possibilities to assess how effective the new approaches were in context
- positive and constructive opportunities to share feedback with friends and colleagues
- a basis for formulating and acting on the evidence and analysis.

In healthcare, action research has been used in:

- enhancing patient information leaflets
- reviving recruitment into research programmes
- restoring asthmatics' compliance with their medication regimen
- adapting clinical research management programmes
- transforming cancer patients' care paths
- reducing medication errors
- enhancing pastoral and moral support services for families in a children's hospital
- developing physiotherapy services for the elderly and newly disabled
- improving training and induction programmes for new members of ethics committees
- managing patient and practitioner change from one medicine to another
- developing nurse-led disease management clinics
- refining dispensing pharmacists' interaction and involvement with patients, nurses and doctors in repeat prescribing programmes.

Action research has also been used in areas such as law and order and social care, and is, currently, a popular approach in the field of education. *See* **Audit**; **Benchmarking**; **Caldicott Guardians**; **Clinical trial**; **Comparing research methods**; **Declaration of Helsinki**; **Documentary analysis**; **Exploratory data analysis**; **Primary question**; **Problems with regard to putting evidence into practice**; **Qualitative research checklist**; **Research governance in the NHS**; **Triangulation**.

○ Bowling A (1987) *Research Methods in Health: investigating health and health services.* Open University Press, Buckingham.

○ Earl-Slater A (2002) The superiority of action research. *Br J Clin Gov.* In press.

○ Stringer ET (1996) *Action Research: a handbook for practitioners.* Sage Publications, London.

Active control

The term 'active' means an intervention that is capable of producing a treatment effect. When you want to look at a new regimen of drug, then a clinical trial can be run comparing this with an active control – a control intervention that is by definition active. *See* **Active control clinical trial; Active control equivalence trial; Control; Placebo.**

Active control clinical trial

An active control clinical trial is an experiment that compares one active treatment with another active treatment.

For example:

- in a trial of women with heavy menstrual bleeding, Cooper and colleagues addressed the question of whether or not transcervical resection of the endometrium is better than medical management for relieving menstrual symptoms

- Kaplan and colleagues used a sophisticated trial including active controls, placebo and combination intervention. In particular, they examined loperamide–simethicone versus loperamide alone, simethicone alone, and placebo, in the treatment of acute diarrhoea with gas-related abdominal discomfort

- Lamy and colleagues used an active control in their trial of the oxygen-carrying compound diaspirin cross-linked haemoglobin and blood transfusion after cardiac surgery

- Leff reported on a trial designed to determine the relative efficacy of three regimens in treating acute episodes of depression and in preventing relapse over a 2-year period. Couples (e.g. a man and his partner) in which the depressed person was living with a 'critical' partner were randomly allocated as couples to one of the three regimens, namely medication, cognitive therapy or marital therapy. One question for you to consider is why we did not have combinations of these regimens in the trial, as we would have in practice. Another question to consider when you encounter active control trials is the reasoning behind the choice of control.

Figure 4 provides an example.

Some clinical trials include more than one active control. For example, Saklayen identifies a study in which antihypertensive and lipid-lowering treatment is used to prevent a heart attack, where over 40 000 high-risk patients with hypertension are treated with a thiazide or calcium-channel blocker or an ACE inhibitor or an alpha-blocker. The final results from the study are due around 2002.

Was the most appropriate control used, and was the most appropriate dose as employed in practice used? These are two important questions, because some active control studies have used an active control that was not very common in clinical practice.

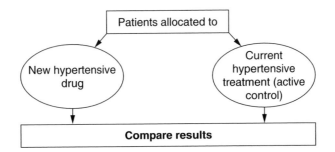

Figure 4 Active control trial.

Some trials have included active controls and placebos as comparator groups. For example, patients with heartburn were allocated to either omeprazole, cisapride or placebo in a trial published by Hatlebakk and colleagues. *See* **Active control; Active control equivalence trial; Combination trial; Factorial trial; Placebo.**

- ○ Cooper KG, Parkin DE, Garratt AM *et al.* (1999) Two-year follow-up of women randomised to medical management or transcervical resection of the endometrium for heavy menstrual loss: clinical and quality of life outcomes. *Br J Obstet Gynaecol.* **106**: 258–65.

- ○ Hatlebakk JG, Hyggen A, Madsen PH *et al.* (1999) Heartburn treatment in primary care: randomised double blind study for 8 weeks. *BMJ.* **319**: 550–3.

- ○ Kaplan MA, Prior MJ, Ash RR *et al.* (1999) Loperamide-simethicone vs. loperamide alone, simethicone alone, and placebo in the treatment of acute diarrhoea with gas-related abdominal discomfort. *Arch Fam Med.* **8**: 243–8.

- ○ Lamy ML, Daily EK, Brichant JF *et al.* (2000) Randomized trial of diaspirin cross-linked hemoglobin solution as an alternative to blood transfusion after cardiac surgery. *Anesthesiology.* **92**: 646–56.

Active control equivalence trial

An active control equivalence trial is an experiment that aims to demonstrate that one active treatment is equivalent to another. Equivalence is usually in terms of safety, efficacy, quality or bioavailability.

For example, Farnier and colleagues studied the efficacy of atrovastatin compared with simvastatin in patients with hypercholesterolaemia.

In some new trials the results have been reported in terms of primary outcomes (e.g. an equal low number of heart attacks). Figure 5 illustrates this.

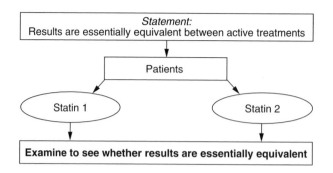

Figure 5 Active control equivalence trial.

See **Active control; Active control clinical trial; Baseline; Clinical trial; Control; Equivalence trial; Non-inferiority trial; Outcomes pyramid; Placebo; Primary outcome; Superiority trial; Surrogate endpoint.**

○ Farnier M, Portal JJ and Maigret P (2000) Efficacy of atrovastatin compared with simvastatin in patients with hypercholesterolemia. *J Cardiovasc Pharmacol Ther.* **5**: 27–32.

Acute

An acute event is a sudden or rapid onset of a clinical condition. *See* **Adaptive–adoptive trial; Chronic.**

Adaptive–adoptive trial

An adaptive–adoptive trial is an experiment in which the intervention given to one patient is dependent on the reactions of earlier patients to that treatment.

One form is as follows.

• If treatment of earlier patients was successful in terms of the outcomes that were achieved, then the next patient is allocated to that regimen.

• If treatment of earlier patients was unsuccessful with regard to one particular treatment, then the next patient is allocated to another regimen.

Figure 6 illustrates this.

The aim of an adaptive–adoptive trial is to reduce the proportion of treatment failures.

Adaptive–adoptive trials are more common in acute disease and surgery, where outcomes are seen relatively quickly. They have also been used in community care, when redesigning hospital patient discharge protocols, and in laboratory research.

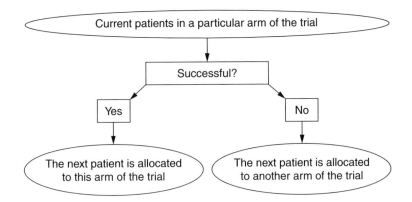

Figure 6 Adaptive–adoptive trial.

Although the adaptive–adoptive system maximises the number of patients on the successful arm of the trial, the following issues need attention.

- You need to know what is meant by success.

- You need to be able to see it quite quickly.

- You need to be able to measure it quite quickly.

- What should you do if a patient is successful on some measures of outcomes but not on other measures?

See **Acute; Bernoulli trial; Cross-over trial; Factorial trial; Open-label trial; Play-the-winner rule; Primary outcome; Randomised controlled trial; Sequential trial; Two-armed bandit allocation.**

○ Birkett JJ (1985) Adaptive allocation in randomised controlled trials. *Control Clin Trials*. **6**: 146–55.

○ Chalmers I (1999) Why transition from alternation to randomisation in clinical trials? *BMJ*. **319**: 1372.

○ Rosenberger WF (1999) Randomized play-the-winner clinical trials. Review and recommendations. *Control Clin Trials*. **20**: 328–42.

Additive effect

In general, the additive effect in a clinical trial is the combined sum of effects from more than one intervention.

For example:

- Dempsy and colleagues looked at the additive bronchoprotective and broncho-dilator effects with single doses of salmeterol and montelukast in asthmatic patients who were suboptimally controlled on inhaled corticosteroids

- Fisher and colleagues addressed the question of whether or not adding tamoxifen to lumpectomy and radiation therapy prevented cancer in ipsilateral and contra-lateral breasts

- adding dorzolamide 2% twice daily to timolol maleate solution 0.5% twice daily when treating exfoliation glaucoma or primary open-angle glaucoma.

Suppose that three interventions are provided to a patient who is currently on kidney dialysis in a clinical trial:

- T is the kidney transplant

- D the kidney-transplant anti-rejection medicine

- E is an appropriate patient education video.

If T results in t, D in d and E in e, and the effects are simply additive, then the final effect of the three interventions will be t + d + e.
  However some issues arise.

- If the effects are of different importance, weights can be assigned to the outcomes to reflect the degree of importance of each effect. For example, the success of the kidney-transplant anti-rejection drug may be much more important than the success of the patient education video.

- The net effect may be misleading. For example, it could be zero (0.5 + 1 − 1.5), although the individual effects are not zero. This is why it is important to see the raw numbers and their sum.

- Can various outcomes be lumped together in one sum? *See* **Adjunctive therapy; Combination trial; Confounding factor; Multiplicative effect; Primary outcome; Primary question; Synergy.**

○ Dempsy OJ, Wilson AM, Sims EJ *et al*. (2000) Additive bronchoprotective and bronchodilator effects with single doses of salmeterol and montelukast in asthmatic patients receiving inhaled corticosteroids. *Chest*. **117**: 950–3.

○ Fisher LB, Dignam J, Wolmark N *et al*. (1999) Tamoxifen in treatment of intraductal breast cancer. National Surgical Adjuvant Breast and Bowel Project B-24: randomised controlled trial. *Lancet*. **353**: 1993–2000.

○ Konstas AG, Maltezos A, Bufidis T *et al*. (2000) Twenty-four-hour control of intraocular pressure with dorzolamide and timolol maleate in exfoliation and primary open-angle glaucoma. *Eye*. **14**: 73–7.

Adjunctive therapy

Adjunctive therapy is an intervention that is given in addition to another intervention. For example, in clinical trials:

- acamprosate as an adjunct to patient counselling in the maintenance of abstinence in the treatment of detoxified alcoholics

- orlistat as an adjunct to a mildly hypocaloric diet in the management of obesity

- external-beam irradiation as an adjunctive treatment in patients with failing dialysis shunts.

Adjunctive therapy is usually given in the expectation that the combined effects will generally be greater than the effects of giving the interventions separately. Sometimes adjunctive therapy is called adjuvant therapy. *See* **Additive effect; Adjuvant therapy; Co-intervention; Combination trial; Confounding factor; Factorial trial; Multiplicative effect; Outcomes pyramid**.

○ Cohen GS, Freeman H, Ringold MA *et al.* (2000) External beam irradiation as an adjunctive treatment in failing dialysis shunts. *J Vasc Interv Radiol.* **11**: 321–6.

○ Spitler LE, Grossbard ML, Ernstoff MS *et al.* (2000) Adjuvant therapy of stage III and IV malignant melanoma using granlocyte-macrophage colony-stimulating factor. *J Clin Oncol.* **18**: 1614–21.

Adjusting for baseline

At the start of a clinical trial, particular details of each patient are recorded. These are termed baseline data. For example, in an anti-obesity trial you may have baseline data on patients' body weight, body mass index, hip-to-waist ratio, high-density lipoprotein, low-density lipoprotein, age, gender, ethnicity, dietary intake, energy intake, energy expenditure, energy storage and exercise record.

The results at any point during the trial or follow-up should then take into account the baseline data. This is called adjusting for baseline (*see* Figure 7).

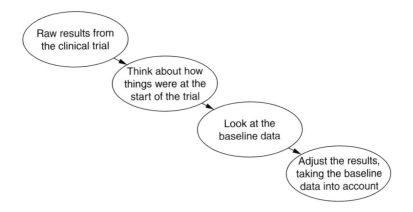

Figure 7 Adjusting for baseline.

Two examples are given below.

- In a trial to determine whether the integration of medical and social services with case management programmes improves outcomes and reduces costs in frail elderly people living in the community, Barnabei and colleagues adjusted for baseline values of gender, marital status, living status, financial status, physical and cognitive function, medical conditions and medications used.

- Sullivan and Bybee reported on a randomised controlled trial with 2-year follow-up to determine whether intervention by paraprofessional advocates reduced abuse and helped women to meet their needs and goals. The trial provides unadjusted and adjusted results. The authors adjusted for baseline levels of physical violence, psychological abuse, depression, quality of life and social support.

One simple approach is to subtract the baseline measure from the outcome measure in order to obtain a net figure. How one actually adjusts the data will depend on issues such as the specifics of the research protocol and statistical advice. *See* **Baseline; Baseline balance**.

- Barnabie R, Landi F, Gambassi G *et al.* (1998) Randomised controlled trial of impact of model of integrated care and case management for older people living in the community. *BMJ*. **316**: 1348–51.

- Sullivan CM and Bybee DI (1999) Reducing violence using community-based advocacy for women with abusive partners. *J Consult Clin Psychol*. **67**: 43–53.

Adjuvant therapy
Another term for adjunctive therapy. *See* **Adjunctive therapy**.

Advantages of evidence from clinical trials
As a source of evidence, clinical trials have both advantages and disadvantages.

Table 3 provides a summary of the key advantages of evidence from clinical trials.

Table 3 Top ten advantages of securing and using evidence from clinical trials

1 The patients are carefully chosen.
2 The patients are carefully monitored.
3 Specific measures of outcome are used.
4 The clinical and statistical importance of outcomes can be identified and discussed.
5 The care path that the patient follows is identified and analysed.
6 Trials can give direction to future research ideas and questions.
7 The data from the trial provide a starting point for discussing the care of patients in practice (e.g. how the trial compares with national or local protocols).
8 The clinical trial can be used as the basis of a model to simulate what happens or could happen in local practice (e.g. in a primary care group).
9 Trials can be used to identify what information is missing in local practice and how that information can be gathered for local practice.
10 Different trials or contrasting evidence provide the ideal opportunity for discussing the best possible care packages for particular patients in the locality.

These should be carefully considered:

- at the design stage of the trial
- when writing up
- when circulating the results of the trial
- when making decisions partly on the basis of trial evidence.

As a small exercise, turn each of the ten advantages into a question. For example, Advantage 1, 'The patients are carefully chosen', turns into Question 1, 'How are the patients actually chosen?' Once you have turned Table 3 into a set of ten questions, work with a colleague and look at the trial literature on one product, and see how many questions you can answer. *See* **Disadvantages of evidence from clinical trials; Entry criteria; Exclusion criteria; Primary question; Problems with regard to putting evidence into practice; Questions to ask before getting involved in a clinical trial; Systematic review.**

○ Earl-Slater A (2001) Critical appraisal of clinical trials: advantages and disadvantages of evidence from clinical trials. *J Clin Govern.* **6**: 136–9.

○ Earl-Slater A (2001) Critical appraisal of clinical trials: barriers to putting trial evidence into clinical practice. *J Clin Govern.* **6**: 279–82.

○ Rosser WM (1999) Application of evidence from randomised controlled trials to general practice. *Lancet.* **353**: 661–4.

Adverse drug reaction

In any clinical trial involving medication there will always be the possibility of a patient experiencing an adverse drug reaction, and the same is true of clinical practice. An adverse drug reaction is an unfavourable and undesirable outcome of the consumption of a drug. Examples of adverse drug reactions (ADR) include nausea, vomiting, fatigue, oedema, rhinitis, tachycardia, photosensitivity, hypersensitivity, organ failure and fatality.

An adverse drug reaction may to some degree be *predictable*. For example:

- hypotension in patients taking anti-hypertensive drugs
- sedation in patients taking carbamazepine.

Some adverse drug reactions may be *temporary*. For example:

- nausea due to the patient getting used to the drug, which will either disappear or cease once the course of medication has been completed.

Some adverse drug reactions may be more *permanent*. For example:

- prescription of thalidomide prescribed as a morning sickness drug for pregnant women in the 1960s is allegedly associated with deformities of 12 000 babies worldwide

- stillbestrol was allegedly linked with adenocarcinoma of the vagina in the daughters of women who took the drug.

Some adverse outcomes will *not initially be associated with consumption* of the drug. For example:

- perhexilene allegedly caused histological changes in the liver that were almost indistinguishable from those that would be caused by alcoholism

- some patients taking ACE inhibitors developed dry coughs which were not initially associated with the drugs in question.

Some adverse drug reactions will be *unexpected*, as they have not been recorded as a result of the use of other drugs in a particular therapeutic class. For example:

- benexoprofen which allegedly caused liver damage and photosensitivity in patients – outcomes that were not expected or seen as a result of the consumption of other non-steroidal anti-inflammatory drugs (NSAIDs).

The *risk of drug dependency* can be regarded as an adverse drug reaction in some classes of drugs. For example:

- it was not until after many years of use that it was established that some patients showed signs of addiction to benzodiazepines.

In clinical trials, all adverse drug reactions should be reported to the trial managers, the ethics committee that approved the trial, the trial steering committee and the trial regulators. *See* **Adverse event; Audit; Committee on the Safety of Medicines; Data-monitoring committee; Medicines Control Agency; Multicentre research ethics committee; Post-marketing surveillance; Protocol; Stopping rules; Yellow card scheme**.

○ Lagnaoui R, Moore N, Fach J *et al.* (2000) Adverse drug reactions in a department of systemic diseases-orientated internal medicine: prevalence, incidence, direct costs and avoidability. *Eur J Clin Pharmacol.* **56**: 181–6.

Adverse event

An adverse event is an undesirable clinical incident, which may or may not be related to the intervention.

Three characteristics of adverse events are that they must:

- be negative
- involve or impact on the patient
- have a line of causation.

Each of these dimensions can be used to establish accountability and, where possible, to put in place systems and procedures to reduce the likelihood of the event happening again.

Examples of adverse events include the following:

- perioperative death
- periprocedural death
- deaths from potentially remedial conditions (e.g. diabetic ketoacidosis, extradural haematoma)
- unplanned removal of an organ
- injury to a tissue or organ
- unplanned return to the operating-theatre
- unplanned readmission to hospital
- drug-dispensing errors
- development of pressure sores.

In any clinical trial there will always be the possibility of a patient experiencing an adverse event. The same, of course, is true in clinical practice. *See* **Adverse drug reaction; Critical incident techniques; Data-monitoring committee; Early stopping rule; Interim analysis.**

○ Bjerre LM and LeLorier J (2000) Expressing the magnitude of adverse effects in case–control studies: the number of patients needed to be treated for one additional patient to be harmed. *BMJ.* **320**: 503–6.

○ Laupacis A, Sackett DL and Roberts RS (1998) An assessment of clinically useful measures of the consequences of treatment. *NEJM.* **318**: 1728–33.

○ Walshe K (2000) Adverse events in health care: issues in measurement. *Qual Health Care.* **9**: 47–52.

Adverse selection

Adverse selection occurs when we inadvertently select a patient for inclusion in a trial and that patient decides not to reveal important details of the full extent of their behaviour or past history. For example, a history of heart problems may, if known, exclude a patient from a smoking cessation trial or a sexual function trial, and some patients have not revealed (or we have not picked up) their true and full history. *See* **Baseline; Entry criteria; Halo effect; Hello–goodbye effect; Transparency.**

Advisory Committee on Borderline Substances

This is a non-statutory group of experts, set up in 1971, to advise the UK government on the following:

- whether a product (e.g. food, herb, dietary supplement, toiletry) should be classified as a medicine and therefore subject to the rules regarding medicines

- whether a product should not be available on the UK publicly funded National Health Service (NHS)

- the economic use of products in the NHS.

The UK Secretary of State appoints the Chairman and seven other members. The Secretaries of State for Scotland, Wales and Northern Ireland each appoint one more person to the Committee. Although politicians select the members, party politics plays little role in the Committee's business.

Despite your first reading and initial thoughts, you may quite rightly be wondering why this particular Committee is included in this book. The reason is that the Committee is important in terms of clinical trials because if this committee deems that a particular product is a 'medicine', then that product has to satisfy the many rules and regulations that relate to medicines. These include the need to perform clinical trials on the product, the need to apply for a licence to market it, being subject to manufacturing scrutiny, and then subjecting the product to the relevant marketing and advertising rules and regulations. *See* **Committee on the Safety of Medicines; Medicines Control Agency; Medical Devices Agency; National Institute for Clinical Excellence.**

Algorithm

An algorithm should be an unambiguously defined set of rules describing how to reach a solution to a particular problem. *See* **Care path; Protocol.**

Allocation

The term allocation refers to any system of assigning patients to study groups in the trial. The system may or may not:

- be concealed (e.g. there may be lack of concealment because the doctor gets to know the system)

- be methodologically robust (e.g. there may be lack of robustness because of design flaws)

- be achieved by randomisation (e.g. non-randomising, by selecting the first two patients to go in one arm of the trial and the next two to go in another arm).

See **Bias; Blinding; Randomisation.**

Alternating allocation

This is a method of allocating patients to alternate regimens in a clinical trial.

For example, in a trial on testicular cancer, two regimens A and B were employed. If the patient you are looking at now is allocated to treatment arm A, then the next eligible patient will go to B, the third to A, the fourth to B, and so on (*see* Figure 8).

This system has been used when randomisation was not considered to be possible, practicable or ethical, and when it was not possible to wait for interim results to show which arm was providing the better results. Alternating allocation does not take into account the results of current patients in the trial when deciding where the next patient should go.

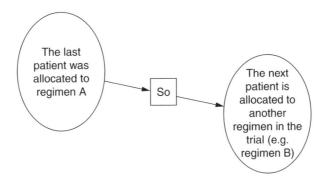

Figure 8 Alternating allocation.

See **Adaptive–adoptive trial; Play-the-winner rule; Randomisation.**

Alternative hypothesis

A statement that there is a difference or relationship between the factors under study in the clinical trial is called the alternative hypothesis. For example:

- a detoxified alcoholic taking the medicine acamprosate and abstaining from alcohol

- the hypothesis that the efficacy of sildenafil is significantly different to that of intracavernosal injection in the treatment of erectile dysfunction in terms of results with regard to the international index of erectile dysfunction.

The alternative hypothesis is usually written as

$$H_1: x \neq y$$

This means that x is not equal to y, and that there is a difference between the outcomes from regimen x or regimen y.

However, as the null hypothesis is the primary building block of the trial, after the tests and analysis we either:

• do not reject the null hypothesis *or*

• reject the null hypothesis in favour of the alternative hypothesis.

If we conclude that we 'do not reject the null hypothesis' this does not, curiously enough, mean that it is true! It only suggests that there is insufficient evidence against the null hypothesis.

If we conclude that we 'reject the null hypothesis in favour of the alternative hypothesis', this at best only suggests that the alternative hypothesis *may* be true.

It has been argued that we should never:

• reject the alternative hypothesis

• accept the alternative hypothesis.

See **Active control equivalence trial; Clinical significance; Equivalence trial; Non-inferiority trial; Null hypothesis; Statistical significance; Superiority trial.**

Analysis by administered treatment

The examination of clinical trial results based on what the patients actually received is called analysis by administered treatment. This may not be what they were assigned to receive. Whether or not it raises additional biases in a trial (e.g. if more patients went to one arm of the trial than another either through choice or because of logistics, despite being initially randomised equally to each arm) remains to be seen. For example, a trial of home care versus outpatient care may suffer if more patients prefer home care. *See* **Analysis by assigned treatment; Audit; CONSORT; Cross-over trial; Ethical issues; Intention-to-treat analysis; Last observation carried forward; Number needed to treat; Preference trial; Transparency.**

Analysis by assigned treatment

The examination of a clinical trial based on what the patients were assigned to receive is called analysis by assigned treatment.

It may not be what they actually received, and it is another more loose term for intention-to-treat analysis. *See* **Analysis by administered treatment; Care path; Intention-to-treat analysis; Last observation carried forward.**

Analytic perspective

The analytic perspective refers to the viewpoint adopted in an analysis. Examples of perspectives in clinical trials and clinical practice are shown in Figure 9.

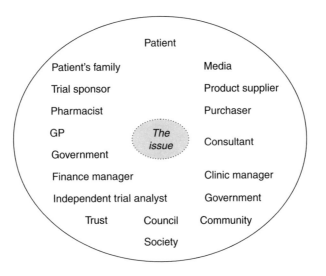

Figure 9 Analytic perspectives.

Although all of these perspectives may have some common ground (e.g. they all want better healthcare), their particular perspectives on any one issue can differ.

For example, Wellwood and colleagues found that among patients with inguinal hernias, patients preferred laparoscopic rather than open-mesh hernia repair, even though the former was more expensive. Other parties may not believe that the extra cost is justified. *See* **Accountability; Due process; Economic analysis and clinical trials; Preference trial; Research governance in the NHS.**

○ Anonymous (2000) Giving medicine a fair trial (editorial). *BMJ.* **320**: 1686.

○ Featherstone K and Donovan JL (1998) Random allocation or allocation at random? Patients' perspectives of participation in a randomised controlled trial. *BMJ.* **317**: 1177–80.

○ Grol R, Weinman J, Dale J *et al.* (1999) Patients' priorities with respect to general practice care: an international comparison. *Fam Pract.* **16**: 4–11.

○ Klein S, Tracy D, Kitchener HC and Walker LG (2000) The effects of participation of patients with cancer in teaching communication skills to medical undergraduates: a randomised study with follow-up after 2 years. *Eur J Cancer.* **36**: 273–81.

○ Wellwood J, Sculpher MJ, Stoker D *et al.* (1998) Randomised controlled trial of laparoscopic versus open-mesh repair for inguinal hernia: outcome and cost. *BMJ.* **317**: 103–10.

○ Wensing M, Mainz J, Ferreira P *et al.* (1998) General practice care and patients' priorities in Europe: an international comparison. *Health Policy.* **45**: 175–86.

Anticipated adverse effects

Anticipated adverse effects are the effects of interventions that are undesirable and known to be caused by the intervention. *See* **Adverse drug reaction; Anticipated beneficial effects; Outcome; Outcomes pyramid; Primary outcome; Unanticipated adverse effect; Unanticipated beneficial effect.**

Anticipated beneficial effects

Anticipated beneficial effects are the effects of interventions that are desirable and known to be caused by the intervention. *See* **Anticipated adverse effects; Association; Causal relationship; Outcome; Outcomes pyramid; Primary outcome; Unanticipated adverse effect; Unanticipated beneficial effect.**

Approval phase

The approval phase is the period of time between submitting an application and receiving a decision about it. Examples of approval phases include the following:

- the time period between submitting an application to start a clinical trial to the ethics committee and receiving a decision from the committee

- the time period between applying for research funding for a clinical trial and receiving a decision about the application

- the time period between applying for a market licence and receiving a decision about that application.

If all goes smoothly, the approval phase is one continuous period of time. However, it may be broken into several periods if the application is:

- incomplete

- erroneous

- opaque

- affected by the emergence of new relevant evidence

- not focussed.

See **Phases of clinical trials; Phase 1 clinical trial; Phase 2 clinical trial; Phase 3 clinical trial; Phase 4 clinical trial.**

A posteriori

A posteriori means after the event. It is sometimes also called post hoc. *See* **A priori; Data fishing.**

A priori

A priori means before the event.

For example, before the trial starts you should be able to determine from the protocol what type of clinical and statistical analysis will be performed and when. *See* **A posteriori; Data dredging; Data-monitoring committee; Interim analysis; Protocol.**

Assent

Assent is an expression of agreement. *See* **Consent**.

Assessors

Assessors are those people who are assigned the task of assessing the results of the clinical trial (they are sometimes loosely called outcome assessors). It has long been argued that assessors should not know what any patient receives in the trial. *See* **Blinding; Data dredging; Data fishing; Data-monitoring committee; Mask; Participants; Principal investigator.**

Association

An association exists when two events occur together more often than one would expect by chance. *See* **Causal relationship; Confounding factor.**

○ Hippisley-Cox J, Allen J, Pringle M *et al.* (2000) Association between teenage pregnancy rates and the age and sex of general practitioners. *BMJ.* **320**: 842–5.

Assumptions

Assumptions are the set of conditions under which an analysis or theory would give valid results. *See* **Advantages of evidence from clinical trials; Analytic perspective; Bayesian analysis; Clinical trial steering committee; Data-monitoring committee; Duhem's irrefutability theory; External validity of clinical trial results; Falsificationism; Hypothesis; Internal validity of results; Lakatosian research programme; Meta-analysis; Systematic review.**

Attrition

Attrition is the loss of patients over a period of time during the clinical trial.
    For example, attrition may occur in a trial because of the following:

* patient non-compliance with their care regimen

* protocol violation

* adverse effects

* death

* patient moving home

* poor administration (e.g. failing to remind the patient to attend a clinic for assessment).

The merits of the intervention may be misguided if attrition is not being properly taken into account. *See* **Analysis by assigned treatment; Audit; Compliance; CONSORT; Dropout; Efficacy; Intention-to-treat analysis; Lost; Missing values; Number needed to treat; Withdrawal.**

Audit

Audit is the official examination of accounts. Although common in finance, the basic principles of audit are transferable, and they can and have been applied in clinical research and clinical practice.

Recently published examples of audit include the following:

- identification of problems with data collection at a local level in NHS maternity units
- audit of antithrombolytic treatment for atrial fibrillation
- the use of an ACE inhibitor in general practice
- audit of cardiac surgery in England
- audit of death certificates
- audit of vaccine uptake among infants at risk of perinatal transmission of hepatitis B
- audit of the laterality of lower limb amputation in diabetic patients
- audit of training in bowel cancer surgery
- audit of the time it takes and the issues and changes required by regional and local research ethics committees with regard to a research application
- audit of the past year's decisions by a multicentre research ethics committee
- audit of the quality of research applications to a research ethics body
- audit of recruitment practices into a clinical trial in a primary care group
- audit of which consultants are involved in what clinical trials in the hospital.

Why bother conducting an audit? There are many reasons, some of which are listed in Table 4.

Table 4 Why conduct an audit?

1 To find out what is going on
2 To determine whether practice is satisfying rules on governance
3 To find out whether anything could be done better
4 To determine the success or failure of a programme or practice
5 To collect and share evidence of practice
6 To form the basis of quality assurance and improvement programmes
7 To satisfy other statutory regulatory requirements

Most clinical trials are subject to some type of audit, and audit is becoming a common part of clinical practice.

Like it or not, audit is going to become a much larger part of the clinical trial enterprise in the NHS. This is not only in reaction to concerns about clinical standards, and issues relating to certain research projects, but also because of the boost to audit that was given by the Department of Health's recently announced *Research Governance in the NHS*. This document indicates that NHS trusts, health authorities, general practitioners, primary care groups and primary care trusts should:

- have systems in place to review all ongoing and proposed research and development studies that they fund or intend to fund, or which involve patients in their care

- take action to ensure that good clinical practice standards for clinical trials involving NHS patients are implemented for all relevant research in which they are involved.

See **Accountability; Audit cycle; Due process; Good clinical practice; Institutional review board; Research governance in the NHS; Transparency.**

○ Earl-Slater A and Wilcox V (1997) Audit: an exploration of two models from outside the health care environment. *J Eval Clin Pract.* **3**: 265–74.

○ Johnston G, Crombie IK, Davies HTO *et al.* (2000) Reviewing audit: barriers and facilitating factors for effective clinical audit. *Qual Health Care.* **9**: 23–36.

○ Howitt A and Armstrong D (1999) Implementing evidence-based medicine in general practice: audit and qualitative study of antithrombotic treatment for atrial fibrillation. *BMJ.* **318**: 1324–7.

○ Jans MP, Schellevis FG, van Hensbergen W and van Eijk JT (2000) Improving general practice care of patients with asthma or chronic obstructive pulmonary disease: evaluation of a quality system. *Effect Clin Pract.* **3**: 16–24.

○ Steigler A, Mameghan H, Lamb D *et al.* (2000) A quality assurance audit: phase III trial of maximal androgen deprivation in prostate cancer. *Austr Radiol.* **44**: 65–71.

○ Wise P and Drury M (1996) Pharmaceutical trials in general practice: the first 100 protocols. An audit by the clinical research ethics committee of the Royal College of General Practitioners. *BMJ.* **313**: 1245–8.

Audit cycle

An audit cycle is the sequence of an audit. In terms of clinical trials and clinical practice these cycles can very quickly become very complex. Most audit cycles can be broken down into three questions as shown in Figure 10.

Thus, for example, the Department of Health gave a boost to audit of the clinical trial enterprise in their recently announced *Research Governance in the NHS* document. This document indicates that NHS trusts, health authorities, general practitioners, primary care groups and primary care trusts should:

- have systems in place to review all ongoing and proposed research and development studies that they fund or intend to fund, or which involve patients in their care

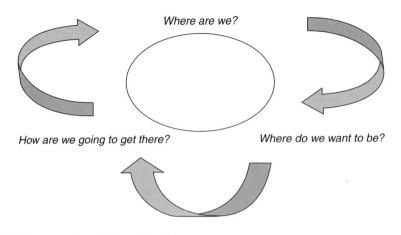

Where are we?

How are we going to get there?   *Where do we want to be?*

Figure 10 Core questions in the audit cycle.

- take action to ensure that good clinical practice standards for clinical trials involving NHS patients are implemented for all relevant research in which they are involved.

Thus according to *Research Governance in the NHS*, the NHS units have to find out where they are in terms of clinical trial enterprise, where they want to be and how they are going to get there.

You can keep the cycle going by asking the following three questions every year. Where are we? Where do we want to be? How are we going to get there? The same three questions can be asked with regard to the care of particular patient groups, to staff development, and to overseeing clinical trials or any other matter of the trust, group or board. *See* **Audit; Benchmarking; Declaration of Helsinki; Multicentre research ethics committee; Research governance in the NHS**.

- Earl-Slater A and Wilcox V (1997) Audit: an exploration of two models from outside the health care environment. *J Eval Clin Pract.* **3**: 265–74.

- Johnston G, Crombie IK, Davies HTO *et al.* (2000) Reviewing audit: barriers and facilitating factors for effective clinical audit. *Qual Health Care.* **9**: 23–36.

Autonomy

Autonomy is an individual's capacity for self-determination. When a person is in a clinical trial they remain autonomous in that they can decide whether to leave the trial at any point or to stay within it. If they are too young, too old or too infirm to decide for themselves, they will usually have a power of attorney that will make the decisions for them. *See* **Consent; Declaration of Helsinki; Ethical issues; Preference trial**.

Available case analysis

Available case analysis is the act of assessing whatever data are available.

Suppose that out of 100 patients attending a cardiovascular risk assessment clinic, you have the data shown in Table 5.

Table 5 Available cases

Data category	Number of patients for whom we have a record
Ethnicity	60
Age	95
Low-density-lipoprotein cholesterol	83
High-density-lipoprotein cholesterol	80
Systolic blood pressure	86
Diastolic blood pressure	84
Smoking status	78
Diabetes status	91
Body mass index	65

Whatever category is used (e.g. body mass index), there will be a different number of available cases.

In some clinical trials, available case analysis is performed in order to improve the power of statistical tests. It is not always made clear in the trial that available case analysis has been used. Available case analysis can affect the overall impression of how well the intervention works and lead to questions about data recording and subgroup analysis. *See* **Audit**; **Data cleaning**; **Data dredging**; **Data fishing**; **Dropout**; **External validity of clinical trial results**; **Intention-to-treat analysis**; **Missing values**; **Non-response**; **Number needed to treat**; **Protocol**; **Withdrawal**.

B

Balaam's design

Mary, a 52-year-old working mother of three, is diagnosed as having breast cancer. She is eligible for and agrees to enter a clinical trial at the local hospital, which is trying to determine whether the *order* of interventions makes any significant difference in terms of 5-year survival rates. The interventions are aggressive chemotherapy (A) and radiotherapy (B).

Suppose that clinical theory and evidence also suggest that two periods of the same treatment may be as effective as mixed doses. Thus in the trial Mary may be allocated to A and stay there, or to B and stay there, or to A then switching to B, or to B then switching to A (*see* Figure 11).

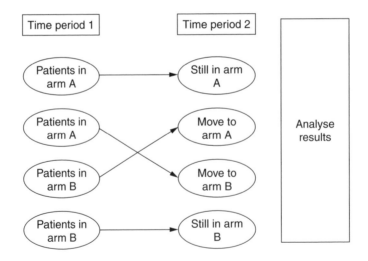

Figure 11 Balaam's design.

Therefore in a Balaam's-design clinical trial we have:

- at least two time periods
- some patients staying in the arm to which they were first allocated
- some patients crossing over to other arms in the trial.

Claimed advantages are that some patients cross over whilst other do not, yielding four groups for analysis. This system can also provide an insight into any crossover effects of patients switching regimens. One of the main disadvantages is that the number of patients may need to be large. *See* **Clinical trial; Cross-over trial; Order effects; Parallel trial; Washout period**.

Balanced design

The balanced design has been used when:

- the same numbers of patients with high and low cholesterol levels are in each arm of a cardiovascular risk reduction trial

- the same numbers of patients from rural and from urban areas are in each arm of an asthma clinical trial

- the same numbers of patients aged 45–54 years are in each arm of a type II diabetes clinical trial.

The balanced design is concerned with the number of people in each arm of the trial. It is either:

- the same number in each arm of the trial *or*

- the same proportions in each arm of the trial.

See **Adaptive–adoptive trial; Block randomisation; Clinical trial; Cross-over trial; Parallel trial; Sequential trial; Zelen's consent design**.

Barriers to clinician participation in randomised controlled trials

Table 6 provides a summary of the barriers to clinician participation in randomised controlled trials.

Table 6 Barriers to clinician participation in randomised controlled trials

1 Time constraints
2 Lack of staff training
3 Worry about impact on doctor–patient relationship
4 Concern for patients
5 Loss of professional autonomy
6 Difficulty with the consent procedure
7 Lack of rewards and recognition
8 Insufficiently interesting question

These barriers have been identified in a systematic review of the literature, and should be considered during the planning stages of clinical trials. They can also be considered in terms of planning to replicate a study, learning from others who have to some extent overcome the barriers, and as issues to think about when interpreting or trying to apply the evidence. *See* **Advantages of evidence from clinical trials; Barriers to patient participation in randomised controlled trials; Barriers to putting clinical trial evidence into practice; Causes of delay and failure to complete a clinical trial; Disadvantages of evidence from clinical trials; Evidence-based medicine; Fate of clinical research; Problems with regard to putting evidence into practice; Reasons given by the investigator for a study being abandoned or in abeyance; Reasons given by the investigator for a study never being started; Research governance in the NHS.**

Barriers to patient participation in randomised controlled trials

Table 7 provides a summary of barriers to patient participation in randomised controlled trials. Exactly which of these barriers have applied to any one trial has yet to be established. The barriers should be considered during the planning stages of clinical trials.

Table 7 Barriers to patient participation in randomised controlled trials

---

Patient concerns
1 Additional demands on the patient:
   • additional procedures and appointments
   • travel problems and cost
2 Patient preferences for a particular treatment (or no treatment)
3 Worry about uncertainty of treatment or trials
4 Patient concerns about information and consent

Clinician as a barrier to patient participation
1 Protocol causing problems with recruitment
2 Clinical concerns about information provision to patients
3 Clinician influencing patient's decision not to join

These barriers have been identified in a systematic review of the literature, and should be considered during the planning stages of clinical trials. They can also be considered in terms of replicating a study, learning from others who have to some extent overcome the barriers, and as issues to think about when interpreting or trying to apply the evidence. *See* **Advantages of evidence from clinical trials; Barriers to clinician participation in randomised controlled trials; Barriers to putting clinical trial evidence into practice; Causes of delay and failure to complete a clinical trial; Disadvantages of evidence from clinical trials; Evidence-based medicine; Fate of clinical research; Problems with regard to putting evidence into practice; Reasons given by the investigator for a study being abandoned or in abeyance; Reasons given by the investigator for a study never being started; Research governance in the NHS.**

Barriers to putting clinical trial evidence into practice

The next time you try to put evidence from a clinical trial into practice you will come across various barriers. These can be more generally and perhaps more usefully classified as problems in putting evidence into practice. *See* **Advantages of evidence from clinical trials; Disadvantages of evidence from clinical trials; Problems with regard to putting evidence into practice**.

○ Earl-Slater A (2001) Barriers to applying clinical trial evidence in practice. *J Clin Ev.* **6**: 279–82.

Baseline

The baseline refers to the patient's status at the start of the trial. Baselines can be determined in various ways, including the following:

- interview

- questionnaires

- physical examination

- observation

- laboratory tests.

It is important to find out when the baseline was actually measured. We generally said 'at the start of the trial', but more specifically we should find out exactly when the baseline was measured. For instance, it could have been when the patient enrolled for the trial, when they were allocated to an arm of the trial; or when they first received an intervention.

It is also useful to find out the following information:

- what is in the baseline

- what is not in the baseline

- what role the baseline played in subsequent allocation and analysis in the trial.

See **Adjusting for baseline; Baseline balance; Baseline characteristics; Data dredging; Data fishing**.

○ Altman DG and Dore CJ (1990) Randomisation and baseline comparisons in clinical trials. *Lancet.* **335**: 149–53.

Baseline balance

The baseline balance concerns how comparable the patients were at the start of the trial. *See* **Adjusting for baseline; Baseline; Baseline characteristics**.

○ Senn S (1994) Testing for baseline balance in clinical trials. *Stat Med.* **13**: 1715–26.

○ Roberts C and Torgerson DJ (1999) Baseline imbalance in randomised controlled trials. *BMJ.* **319**: 185.

○ Vickers AJ and Altman DG (2001) Analysing controlled trials with baseline and follow up measurements. *BMJ*. **323**: 1123–4.

Baseline characteristics

These consist of the collection of details about a patient at the start of the trial.
Key issues to consider include the following:

• what is in the baseline (and why the entries were chosen)

• what is not in the baseline

• when the baseline data were collected.

For example, the primary-care-based randomised controlled trial of Damoiseaux and colleagues of amoxicillin versus placebo for acute otitis media in children aged under 2 years reported the following baseline characteristics of 240 children:

• mean age

• gender

• whether breastfed for more than 6 months or not

• whether more than two children were in the family

• whether smoking occurred in the household

• attendance at day-care centre

• medical history – recurrent upper respiratory tract infection, recurrent acute otitis media (AOM), recurrent AOM in family, allergy

• clinical presentation (more than 3 days of complaints, earache, fever, perforation, bilateral AOM, bulging eardrum).

See **Adjusting for baseline; Audit; Baseline; Baseline balance; Case report form; Entry criteria; Protocol.**

○ Assmann SF, Pocock SJ, Enos LE and Kasten LE (2000) Subgroup analysis and other (mis)uses of baseline data in clinical trials. *Lancet*. **355**: 1064–9.

○ Damoiseaux RAMJ, van Balen FAN, Hoes AW *et al.* (2000) Primary-care-based randomised, double-blind trial of amoxicillin versus placebo for acute otitis media in children aged under 2 years. *BMJ*. **320**: 350–4.

○ Vickers AJ and Altman DG (2001) Analysing controlled trials with baseline and follow up measurements. *BMJ*. **323**: 1123–4.

Baskerville trial

In a Baskerville trial, patients determine how long they will stay in any arm of the trial.

The Baskerville trial works as follows.

- Those who are happy to continue with their current regimen in the trial generally do so.

- Those who are not happy to continue with the regimen that they are receiving in the trial and who want to try something else are allocated to another regimen (exactly how they are reallocated depends on the specifics of the trial).

- Those who want to withdraw from the clinical trial, for whatever reason, leave it.

Figure 12 illustrates this.

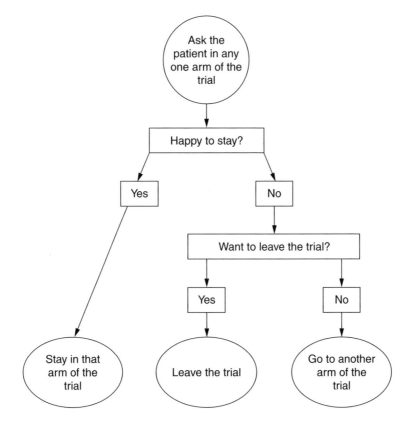

Figure 12 A Baskerville trial.

According to both the ethical principle of autonomy and the Declaration of Helsinki, in reality all patients can determine whether they wish to continue in any arm of a trial.

The distinguishing features of the Baskerville trial are as follows.

- Patients are asked if they wish to continue.
- Those who wish to switch arms of the trial are allowed to do so.

This method has been used in a phase 4 study to detect patient preferences in care regimes. Baskerville trials may quite reasonably reflect clinical practice. *See* **Analysis by administered treatment; Analysis by assigned treatment; Autonomy; Belmont Report; Bernoulli trial; Consent; Declaration of Helsinki; Ethical issues; Follow-up; Generalisability of trial results; Preference trial; Zelen's consent design**.

Bayesian analysis

A Bayesian analysis involves updating the probability of events in the light of new evidence, experience or understanding. Lilford and Braunholtz suggest that Bayesian techniques allow all of our current knowledge to be explicitly represented and synthesised with new data. They indicate that health issues are now much more complex and that the amount of disparate evidence which impacts on belief has increased.

Spiegelhalter and colleagues defined a Bayesian approach to health technology assessment as 'the explicit quantitative use of external evidence in the design, monitoring, analysis, interpretation and reporting of a health technology assessment study'.

For example, before you send a patient to be examined by a consultant, you may have a prior probability of her having Alzheimer's dementia. Your prior probability will be based on prior objective evidence, experience and opinion. You then receive the test results, and once you have reflected on these results you transform what you thought before the test to what you now believe. You then have what is called a *posterior probability distribution* of her likelihood of having Alzheimer's dementia.

Figure 13 illustrates this.

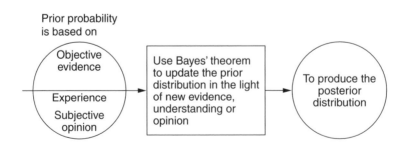

Figure 13 A Bayesian scheme.

The approach has been considered to be controversial as it relies on one's experience and subjective opinion, and these vary both between practitioners and over time. *See* **Bayes' theorem; Meta-analysis; Systematic review.**

○ Berry DA and Stangl DK (1996) *Bayesian biostatistics.* Dekker, New York.

○ Freedman L (1996) Bayesian statistical methods: a natural way to assess clinical evidence. *BMJ.* **313**: 569–70.

○ Lilford RJ and Braunholtz D (1996) The statistical basis of public policy: a paradigm shift is overdue. *BMJ.* **313**: 603–7.

○ Spiegelhalter DJ, Myles JP, Jones DR and Abrams KR (1999) An introduction to Bayesian methods in health technology assessment. *BMJ.* **319**: 508–12.

○ Stevens A, Abrams K, Brazier J, Fitzpatrick R and Lilford R (eds) (2001) *The Advanced Handbook of Methods in Evidence-Based Healthcare.* Sage Publishing, London.

Bayes' theorem

This is a theory, named after the eighteenth-century English vicar, Thomas Bayes, that describes the procedures for updating the probability of an event in the light of new evidence. *See* **Bayesian analysis.**

Before-and-after analysis

Before-and-after analysis is an evaluation of factors before and after a particular event (*see* Figure 14).

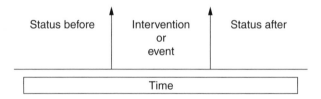

Figure 14 Before-and-after analysis.

For example, Hawton and colleagues used a before-and-after study to report on the effects of legislation restricting the pack size of paracetamol and salicylate on self-poisoning in the UK. There is a series of letters in response to this in the *British Medical Journal* of May and June 2001 which should be read in conjunction with the original paper. *See* **Association; Audit; Case–control study; Causal relationship; Primary question; Research questions and research methods; Types of study.**

○ Hawton K, Townsend E, Deeks J *et al.* (2001) Effects of legislation restricting pack size of paracetamol and salicylate on self-poisoning in the United Kingdom: before and after study. *BMJ.* **322**: 1203.

Belmont Report

The Belmont Report is a report from the US National Commission for the Protection of Human Subjects of Biomedical and Behavioral Research on the ethical principles and guidelines for the protection of human subjects of research. Produced in April 1979, the report describes three basic ethical principles:

- *respect for persons*: individuals should be treated as autonomous agents, and persons with diminished autonomy are entitled to protection

- *beneficence*: acts of kindness and charity that go beyond strict obligation with rules such as 'do not harm', 'maximise possible benefits' and 'minimise possible harm'

- *justice*: in the sense of fairness of distribution or what is deserved. These terms can be formulated in various contrasting ways (e.g. equal shares to each person, to each person according to individual need, to each person according to individual merit, to each person according to societal contribution, or to each person according to merit).

The Belmont Report is currently being considered for revision. *See* **Declaration of Helsinki; Ethical considerations in a randomised clinical trial; Ethical issues**.

○ US National Commission for the Protection of Human Subjects of Biomedical and Behavioral Research (1979) *The Belmont Report: Ethical Principles and Guidelines for the Protection of Human Subjects of Research*, 18 April 1979. The full report is available at http://www.fda.gov/.

Benchmarking

Every day you will be making comparisons between x and y, whatever x and y may be. Benchmarking is simply another term for comparison.

- In clinical trials you will often see a comparison between a new product and a placebo.

- You can compare the results from different clinical trials.

- You can make comparisons between what happens in a clinical trial and what happens in practice.

- You can compare the results obtained from different clinical settings.

See **Audit; Critical incident techniques; Equivalence trial; Gold standard; Non-inferiority trial; Randomised controlled trial; Superiority trial; Transparency**.

○ Donovan MI, Evers K, Jacobs P and Mandleblatt S (1999) When there is no benchmark: designing a primary-care-based chronic pain management program from the scientific basis up. *J Pain Symptom Manage*. **18**: 38–48.

○ Rippon TJ (2000) Aggression and violence in healthcare professions. *J Adv Nurs*. **32**: 452–60.

○ Weissman NW, Alison JJ, Kiefe CI *et al.* (1999) Achievable benchmarks of care: the ABCs of benchmarking. *J Eval Clin Pract.* **5**: 269–81.

Beneficence

The moral principle of doing good. It is one of four standard principles in healthcare ethics. *See* **Belmont Report**; **Ethical issues**; **Morality**.

Bernoulli trial

A Bernoulli trial is one in which only two outcomes are considered.
Examples of Bernoulli trials include the following:

- whether or not the patient died after surgery

- whether or not the patient had another stroke after receiving a new medication

- whether or not the patient continued to experience incontinence after treatment

- whether or not varicose veins became clinically worse after using four-layer compression bandages in a trial

- whether or not patients with Parkinson's disease suffered a relapse during a 6-month period in a trial.

Although there may be more than two outcomes of any possible intervention, the focus of the Bernoulli clinical trial is to look at only two of the possible outcomes.
If you only see two outcomes reported in a clinical trial (e.g. survived/did not survive, had a stroke/did not have a stroke, relapsed/did not relapse), ask the following questions.

- Was the trial initially conceived as being Bernoulli?

- What were the reasons for that choice?

- What other outcomes could be important but were not recorded or not reported in the trial?

See **Baskerville trial**; **Clinical trial**; **Composite endpoint**; **Outcomes pyramid**; **Primary outcome**.

Bias

Bias is any systematic deviation from the truth, or any process that leads to a systematic deviation from the truth.
Bias can occur in various areas of clinical trials and clinical practice (*see* Table 8).

Table 8 Types of bias and meaning

Type of bias	Meaning
Allocation bias	A systematic distortion of the data resulting from the way in which the patients are allocated to the arms of the trial
Selection bias	Occurs because those who enter a trial are not a random sample of the wider population from which they are drawn. It can be argued that it may not matter much if the selection is similar to that which would occur in clinical practice (i.e. reality)
Ascertainment bias	Occurs when results are systematically distorted by knowledge of which intervention was received
Inappropriate handling of dropouts, withdrawals, protocol violations bias	Occurs when those who fail to continue in the trial are not properly accounted for in the analysis of the results
Publication bias	Occurs when you look at the available publications and not at all of the relevant documents pertaining to the clinical trial
Language bias	Occurs in two ways – when you rate a clinical trial lower if it is in a foreign language (i.e. not in your mother tongue) or higher if it has been published, for example, in English
Source and country of trial bias	Occurs when you rate a trial lower if it did not occur in the authors' country or higher if it did
Potential breakthrough bias	Occurs when you are too optimistic about the importance of a particular set of results
Financial support bias	Occurs either when you place more importance on the trial results because of the body that sponsored the trial, or when you come up with the easy criticism 'They would say that, wouldn't they?'
Vested interest bias	A mixed bag of bias including, for example, the claim that 'They would say that, wouldn't they?' or the claim that negative results are not publicised
Clinical practice bias	Occurs when the trial results threaten your current clinical practice or those of your favoured colleagues
Change bias	Occurs when you either inflate the results if they favour your ideas for change, or deflate the results if they do not favour your ideas for change
Professional esteem and progress bias	Occurs when the trial results show the importance of a particular group of professionals, and these professionals over-rate the idea
Professional threat bias	Occurs when the trial results threaten a particular group of professionals. Some of these professionals will consciously misinterpret the results or find unimportant limitations in the evidence

continued opposite

Table 8 continued

Type of bias	Meaning
Journal bias	Occurs when you rate the trial results according to the journal in which they appeared. The more prestigious the journal, the more important the results (supposedly)
Empiricism–narcissism bias	Occurs when you deflate the results because they are just 'numbers' and are claimed not to reflect the wider reality of practice
Famous person or institution bias	Occurs when you inflate the trial results because they come from a famous person or institution
Unknown person or unknown institution bias	Occurs when you deflate the trial results because they come from a relatively unknown person or institution
Rivalry bias	Occurs when you understate the strength of the trial and amplify its weaknesses, because it was conducted by a rival (professional, author, organisation or sponsor)
'I owe him/her one' bias	Occurs in various ways – for example, when you promote the results or papers because the author/institution/ sponsor did the same for one of your pieces of work, or when you deflate the results or papers because the author/institution/sponsor deflated one of yours
Regret–rejoice bias	More general than the above, but occurs when you say that you regret putting out a negative review or judgement of a paper or presentation (e.g. at a conference), but you in fact rejoice and relish in the fact that you have the chance (strangely to show your bias!). This occurs particularly in cases when someone (and there is always going to be someone) says that they could have done better than you at whatever it was you did
Ageism bias	Occurs when certain age groups (e.g. children, the elderly) are not included in a trial, even though there is no robust reason for that exclusion
Ethnic bias	Occurs when certain ethnic groups are not included in a trial, even though there is no robust reason for that exclusion
Moral bias	Occurs when the study affects your morals, whatever they may be (e.g. clinical trials on patients with multiple sclerosis and cannabis use, trials on methods used for abortion, trials on teenage sex education, trials using animal organ transplantation in humans)
Do something bias	Sometimes linked to the above, but often driven by a political imperative (let's do something even if there is no real evidence that it works!)
Do nothing bias	Occurs when you under-rate a study that suggests something should be done or, less likely, over-rate a study which states that nothing can be done

continued overleaf

Table 8 continued

Type of bias	Meaning
Method-up bias (favoured design bias)	Occurs when you over-rate a study or its results because it used a method that you favour (e.g. a double-blind randomised placebo-controlled multicentre trial with a 6-month follow-up)
Method-down bias (disfavoured design bias)	Occurs when you under-rate a study or its results because it used a method that you do not favour
Multicentre trial bias	Occurs when you either prefer such trials and over-rate their results or do not prefer such trials and under-rate their results
International trials bias	Occurs when you either favour these trials and over-rate their results or do not favour them and under-rate their importance
Large trial bias	Occurs when you distort the truth because the trial is large, so that if you like large trials you increase the importance of the results, and if you dislike large trials you belittle the importance of the results
Small trial bias	Occurs when you distort the truth because the trial is small, so that if you like small trials you increase the importance of the results, and if you dislike small trials you belittle the importance of the results
Favoured resource allocation bias	Occurs when you over-rate the implications of the trial if it suggests that more resources should be put into the areas of healthcare which you prefer
Disfavoured resource allocation bias	The opposite of favoured resource allocation bias
Prominent author bias	Occurs when you over-rate the results of the trial because it has a famous name somewhere in the list of authors
Unknown author bias	Occurs when you think of weaknesses in the paper just because you have not heard of the author(s)
Sexy title bias	Occurs either when you favour papers or presentations that have a sexy title, or when you do not favour papers or presentations because of their title (e.g. because you think it is unscientific, common, vulgar, cheap, journalese, populist, etc.)
Flashy title bias	As above, but relates to flashy titles (not all of which are sexy)
Substituted question bias	Occurs when you change focus from the question that the paper addressed to the one that you think should have been addressed
He/she is/was my student bias	Occurs when you over-rate a paper because it comes from one of your current or previous students

continued opposite

Table 8 continued

Type of bias	Meaning
He/she is/was my mentor bias	Occurs when you over-rate a trial because it comes from someone who is or was one of your mentors
Not my scene bias	Often occurs when you belittle the importance of a trial because it does not relate to your particular interests or work environment
Belligerence bias	Involves fighting and being difficult 'just for the hell of it'
I want a job bias	Occurs when you over-rate the importance of a trial because you want a job at the institution, or you want to work with the authors or the sponsors
Money-bags bias	Occurs generally when you over-rate the importance of the results of a paper just because it comes from a wealthy source, was written by a wealthy author, was sponsored by a wealthy organisation, could help to make you wealthy, or because you want to nestle up to apparently wealthy people

Get a group of colleagues together and look at the evidence from one particular product. From the literature and your own experiences, identify which biases could exist, which ones you think do exist, how important they may be, and what can be done about them. Many but not all of the entries and further discussion can be found in Alejandro Jadad's excellent book. *See* **Accountability; Advantages of evidence from clinical trials; Clinical trial; Due process; Error; Hierarchies of the evidence; Meta-analysis; Peer review; Pooled analysis; Randomisation; Research governance in the NHS; Systematic review; Transparency; William's agreement measure.**

○ Jadad A (1998) *Randomised Controlled Trials.* BMJ Books, London.

○ McCormack J and Greenhalgh T (2000) Seeing what you want to see in randomised controlled trials. Versions and perversions of UKPDS data. *BMJ.* **320**: 1720–3.

Biased coin method

If you toss a standard coin, heads will come up half the time and tails will come up half the time. A biased coin is one for which the probability of heads is not the same as the probability of tails. In terms of clinical trials, the biased coin method means that the likelihood of going into any arm of the trial is not equal. The reasons for choosing a biased coin method should be made clear in the trial protocol, the application for ethical approval and the writing up. *See* **Adaptive–adoptive trial; Alternating allocation; Balanced design; Bias; Equipoise; Play-the-winner rule; Random; Randomisation; Two-armed bandit allocation.**

Blind

Blind means not being able to see. *See* **Bias; Blinding**.

Blinding

Blinding refers to procedures of concealment or masking. It aims to keep certain individuals in the trial ignorant as to what regimen a patient received.

These individuals could be:

- the patients

- the clinicians

- the outcome assessors

- the statisticians.

For example, one may wish to:

- conceal how patients are allocated to regimens in the trial

- conceal what intervention any one patient is receiving

- conceal from the caregiver what a particular patient received in the trial

- conceal from the analysts what a particular patient received in the trial.

Blinding is used to reduce bias. It is frequently employed in clinical trials, but not in clinical practice.

Some care has to be taken when using the term, for the following reasons.

- A single-blind trial usually refers to the blinding of the patients, but sometimes we have seen single-blind trials where it is the clinician who is blinded, or where it is the statisticians who were blinded.

- A double-blind trial usually refers to the blinding of the patients and the clinicians or caregivers, but the term has also been used when the clinicians and statisticians were blinded.

- A triple-blind trial usually refers to the blinding of the patients, clinicians and statisticians.

If blinding is involved in a trial, you need to ask the following questions.

- Who was blinded?

- How were they actually blinded?

- Why were they blinded?

See **Blind; Double-blind trial; Efficacy; Meta-analysis; Quadruple-blind trial; Single-blind trial; Systematic review; Triple-blind trial; Unblinded clinical trial.**

○ Colditz GA, Miller JN and Mosteller F (1989) How study design affects outcomes in comparisons of therapy. *Stat Med.* **8**: 441–54.

○ Jadad AR, Moore RA, Carroll D *et al.* (1996) Assessing the quality of reports on randomised controlled trials: is blinding really necessary? *Control Clin Trials.* **12**: 195–208.

Block

A block is a homogenous group of subjects. *See* **Block randomisation; Homogenous product.**

Block randomisation

Block randomisation is a procedure that tries to ensure that similar numbers of patients are in each arm of the trial at any one time.

For example, suppose that you set patients into groups (or blocks) of four. Suppose that there are two arms in the trial, A and B. Then for any group of four patients, two individuals will be assigned to each arm of the trial, A or B. According to this design, the numbers in the arms of the trial will not differ by more than two subjects.

Block randomisation is useful when you do not want the numbers in the blocks to be inordinately different in magnitude. It is sometimes also called random permuted blocks or restricted randomisation. *See* **Bias; Blocking; Cluster randomisation; Group randomisation; Randomisation; Stratified randomisation.**

○ Altman DG and Bland JM (1999) How to randomise. *BMJ.* **319**: 703–4.

Blocking

Blocking techniques aim to increase the statistical power of the results of a clinical trial. They do this by eliminating from analysis those factors that have an effect but which are of no interest to the particular trial. Blocking has more accurately been termed *stripping out*, because the techniques strip out factors that are not of interest to the study.

Blocking can be achieved by omitting from the data set those variables that are of no interest to the particular study. Statistical advice should be obtained if possible before blocking or stripping out. *See* **Association; Causal relationship; Data dredging; Data fishing; Equivalence trial; Factor analysis; Non-inferiority trial; Parsimony principle; Primary question; Statistical tests: ten ways to cheat with statistical tests; Superiority trial.**

Boundary approach

In any clinical trial there will be limits which determine whether or not the trial should continue in its current form. The boundary approach is a system whereby a trial is stopped if the results cross a certain boundary. That boundary should be specified before the trial commences.

For example:

- you may allow up to a 10% difference in outcomes between arms A and B of the trial, but if at any time the analysis shows a difference greater than 10% the trial is then stopped

- a trial might be stopped if more than 2% of the patients who were allocated to any arm of the clinical trial died within 28 days of starting the trial.

Suppose that the trial protocol stated that if the difference in primary results between arms A and B exceeded 10%, the trial would be stopped. This situation is illustrated in Figure 15.

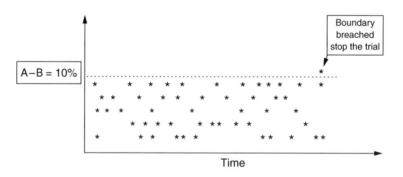

Figure 15 A simple boundary approach example: one breach and it is stopped.

The asterisks denote the difference in results between treatment arms A and B measured over time. Other boundary approaches exist, some of which are based on complicated statistical formulae and sophisticated clinical criteria.

In some circumstances you may allow more than one breach (e.g. to help to reduce the possibility that a breach occurred purely by chance). The key issues are to determine what boundary approach is in the protocol, how the results from the trial are going to be measured, what statistical tests will be performed, and how many breaches will be allowed before the trial is stopped (in Figure 15 you used one breach to stop the trial). *See* **Data-monitoring committee; Early stopping rule; Interim analysis; Primary outcome; Stopping rules; Truncated data**.

Caldicott Guardians

Caldicott Guardians made their appearance throughout the National Health Service from April 1999. Their duty is essentially to safeguard and protect the handling of confidential patient information as it passes between and outwith NHS organisations.

The Caldicott Committee was set up in response to a threatened British Medical Association boycott of the NHS Net because of the vulnerability of patient data flowing from clinical to administrative settings. Led by Dame Fiona Caldicott, principal of Somerville College, Oxford, and past president of the Royal College of Psychiatrists, the Caldicott Committee Report appeared in 1997.

The introduction of 'local guardians of patient confidentiality' was a key recommendation of the Caldicott Report, and an NHS Executive circular ordered NHS units to have them appointed by 1 April 1999. The individuals in what has become a network of Caldicott Guardians were appointed by each health authority, NHS trust, and primary care group. The NHS circular said that, ideally, the guardians should be board members and senior health professionals, with some responsibility for clinical governance within the organisation. According to the NHS Executive circular their work should not be delegated:

'It is intended that Caldicott Guardians will be central to the development of a new framework for handling patient information in the NHS.'

In support of the guardians, NHS boards developed protocols for:

- the disclosure of patient information to other organisations

- access

- reviewing the uses of patient data

- improving database design, staff training and compliance.

The Caldicott Report offered six principles of good practice for the health service when handling patient identifiable information (*see* Table 9).

Table 9 Caldicott Principles of Good Practice

Principle 1	*Justify the purpose(s)* Every proposed use or transfer of patient-identifiable information within or from an organisation should be clearly defined and scrutinised, with continuing uses regularly reviewed by an appropriate guardian.
Principle 2	*Don't use patient-identifiable information unless it is absolutely necessary* Patient-identifiable information items should not be used unless there is no alternative.
Principle 3	*Use the minimum necessary patient-identifiable information* Where use of patient-identifiable information is considered to be essential, each individual item of information should be justified with the aim of reducing identifiability.
Principle 4	*Access to patient-identifiable information should be on a strict need to know basis* Only those individuals who need access to patient-identifiable information should have access to it, and they should only have access to the information items that they need to see.
Principle 5	*Everyone should be aware of their responsibilities* Action should be taken to ensure that those handling patient-identifiable information – both clinical and non-clinical staff – are aware of their responsibilities and obligations to respect patient confidentiality.
Principle 6	*Understand and comply with the law* Every use of patient-identifiable information must be lawful. Someone in each organisation should be responsible for ensuring that the organisation complies with legal requirements.

Caldicott Guardians should have the authority to exercise the necessary influence on local policy and strategic planning in the NHS. Candidates might include directors of public health and clinical or nursing directors of trusts. Each primary care group and trust should have its Caldicott Guardian, and each practice should nominate a liaison point for confidentiality issues. Preserving patient confidentiality is considered a cornerstone of the NHS information strategy. The then Junior Health Minister Baroness Hayman said that the Caldicott Guardians would have a vital role to play as the NHS learns to harness the enormous potential of information technology. Dr Ian Bogle, as chairman of council of the BMA, welcomed the initiative. In 1999, Ian is reported to have said that the process had a long way to go but that the setting up of a system of guardians was a vital first step. Dr Sandy Macara, then chairman of the British Medical Association council, reportedly said 'there is still much to be done, but we can all now see where the start line is'. However, Dr Fleur Fisher of the Campaign for Medical Privacy is reported as saying 'we still have databases built in an unacceptable and unethical way'.

It is clear that the six principles in Table 9 could be used in any research study whether or not NHS patients are involved.

The health service circular on Caldicott Guardians is available from the Department of Health: http://www.open.gov.uk/doh/coinh.htm.

See **Accountability; Analytic perspective; Consent: eight key questions on law and consent; Due process; European Union Directive on clinical trials of medicinal products for humans; Patient information sheet and consent forms; Patient preferences; Research governance in the NHS; Transparency**.

○ Anderson R (2001) Undermining data privacy in health information. *BMJ*. **322**: 442–3.

○ Caldicott Committee (1997) *Report on the Review of Patient Identifiable Information*. Department of Health, London.

○ Carnall D (1997) Report urges widespread reform of handling NHS data. *BMJ*. **315**: 1559.

○ NHS Executive (1999) *Protecting and Using Patient Information: a manual for Caldicott Guardians*. NHS Executive, London.

○ Strobl J, Cave E and Walley T (2000) Data protection legislation: interpretation and barriers to research. *BMJ*. **321**: 890–2.

○ Warden J (1999) Guardians to protect patient data. *BMJ*. **318**: 284.

Capture–recapture sampling

On many occasions it would be impossible or prohibitively expensive to obtain a complete record of every person, and to work out who has what characteristics. Therefore techniques have been developed to estimate the number of cases with a particular characteristic of interest (e.g. alcohol dependence) in an area. Capture–recapture sampling is one of these techniques.

Try to answer the following questions.

- How many crack-cocaine abusers live in your town?

- How many people working in your nearest factory are dependent on alcohol?

- How many children at your nearest school regularly smoke cigarettes?

- How many people in your primary care group over 50 years of age suffer from walking-mobility problems?

- How many female patients in your primary care group are clinically obese?

- How many people in your nearest health action zone programme have dementia?

- How many elderly people in the local council's homes for the elderly have grip-strength problems?

How many questions were you able to answer? How did you actually find the answers?

Capture–recapture sampling works as follows. An initial sample is obtained from the population, (tested) marked and replaced in the population. A second sample is obtained from the population, and one then establishes how many of the marked individuals are in this second sample.

A simple capture–recapture study is the Peterson system. The calculation proceeds as follows.

- Let A be the number of individuals captured in the first foray, tested, marked and released.

- Let B be the number of individuals captured in the second foray.

- Let C be the number of marked individuals found inside B who are marked.

- Then the capture–recapture estimate of the population with the attribute is:

$$P = \frac{A}{C} \times B$$

Suppose that from 5000 patients we randomly pick 100 individuals. Then we have A = 100, and suppose we go on to find B = 20, C = 5. Therefore the estimated number of people with the attribute of interest is:

$$P = \frac{100}{5} \times 20 = 400$$

This suggests that approximately 400 of the 5000 individuals have the condition of interest (e.g. drug addiction, clinical obesity, walking-mobility problems).

There are various models of this (e.g. those by Seber or Bailey). It is important to check to see what version is being used, as they have different methodologies and therefore different implications for unbiased estimation.

More traditionally, capture–recapture sampling has been used to estimate wildlife populations and changes over time. Quite recently capture–recapture techniques have been adjusted and used to test the coverage of different literature databases. *See* **Sampling strategies; Sampling with replacement; Sampling without replacement; Two-stage sampling**.

○ EURODIAD ACE Study Group (2000) Variation and trends in incidence of childhood diabetes in Europe. *Lancet*. **355**: 873–6.

○ Jarvis SN, Lowe PJ, Avery A *et al*. (2000) Children are not goldfish: mark–recapture techniques and their application to injury data. *Injury Prevent*. **6**: 46–50.

○ La Porte R (1994) Assessing the human condition: capture–recapture techniques. *BMJ*. **308**: 5–6.

○ Maxwell JC (2000) Methods for estimating the number of 'hardcore' drug users. *Subst Use Misuse*. **35**: 399–420.

○ Spoor P, Airey M, Bennett C, Greensill J and Williams R (1996) Use of capture–recapture technique to evaluate the completeness of systematic literature searches. *BMJ*. **313**: 342–3.

Care path

The care path is the route that a patient follows while receiving care. In a clinical trial, well-defined care paths are normally set out in advance of the trial starting.

Care path records can be used to help to identify who received what care, where, when and why, with what results and at what cost.

Holzbeierlein and Smith have described the development, implementation and evaluation of a collaborative care pathway for radical retropubic prostatectomy, and the reader is referred to their paper for more detail.

In some cases there will be a difference between the planned care path and the actual care path that the patient followed in the clinical trial. *See* **Analysis by administered treatment; Analysis by assigned treatment; Audit; Baseline; Clinical pathway; Intention-to-treat analysis; Protocol.**

○ Holzbeierlein JM and Smith JA (2000) Radical prostatectomy and collaborative care pathways. *Semin Urol Oncol.* **18**: 60–5.

Carry-over effects

Suppose that for the last 6 weeks you have been taking a course of medication and today, for whatever reason, you suddenly stop taking it. In general, the effects of the medicine will not immediately stop at that point. Any effects that the medicine continues to have once you have stopped taking it are called carry-over effects.

In clinical trials, carry-over effects are important for the following reasons:

- patients may have to come off their existing medication before they start in a trial

- the effects of their previous medication may affect recordings in the trial

- when patients switch treatments in the trial (e.g. from A to B), the effects of one treatment can carry over into their new regimen.

More generally, therefore, carry-over effects occur when the effects of an intervention continue after the intervention has stopped. *See* **Baseline; Confounding factor; Cross-over trial; Follow-up; Run-in period; Washout period.**

Case–control study

A case–control study is an observational study in which the cases have the issue of interest but the controls do not. The 'issue' could be anything (e.g. a specific disease, a specific clinical reading, exposure to a particular risk, or a specific genetic profile).

For example:

- Agerbo and colleagues reported a nested case–control study of the risk of suicide in relation to income level in people admitted to hospital with mental illness

- Fioretti and colleagues reported on a case–control study of menopause and the risk of non-fatal acute myocardial infarction

- Fleming and colleagues reported on a population-based case–control study of the UK's accelerated immunisation programme and sudden unexpected death in infancy

- Fraser and colleagues reported on a hospital-based case–control study of deprivation and late presentation of glaucoma

- Nuesh and colleagues reported on a prospective case–control study of the relationship between insufficient response to antihypertensive treatment and poor compliance with treatment

- Pierfitte and colleagues reported on a case–control study of benzodiazepines and hip fractures in elderly people.

The advantages of a case–control study are as follows.

- They can shed light on unexpected clinical events.

- They are usually easier to conduct than a clinical trial.

The disadvantages of case–control studies are as follows.

- They cannot prove causation.

- They cannot generally discover new events.

- Cases and controls need to be carefully determined in order to dilute bias.

In reality, case–control studies can be retrospective (i.e. looking back in time) or prospective (i.e. looking forward in time). There is some debate about this, and some people think that case–control studies can only be retrospective. You can simply ask whether the study looks forward or backward. *See* **Baseline; Clinical trial; Cohort study; Prospective study; Randomised controlled trial; Research questions and research methods; Retrospective studies; Types of research questions**.

○ Agerbo E, Mortensen PB, Eriksson T *et al*. (2001) Risk of suicide in relation to income level in people admitted to hospital with mental illness: nested case–control study. *BMJ*. **322**: 334–5.

○ Bjerre LM and LeLorier J (2000) Expressing the magnitude of adverse effects in case–control studies: the number of patients needed to be treated for one additional patient to be harmed. *BMJ*. **320**: 503–6.

○ Fioretti F, Tavani A, Gallus S *et al*. (2000) Menopause and risk of non-fatal acute myocardial infarction: an Italian case–control study and a review of the literature. *Hum Reprod*. **15**: 599–603.

○ Fleming PJ, Blair PS, Platt MW *et al*. (2001) The UK accelerated immunisation programme and sudden unexpected death in infancy: case–control study. *BMJ*. **322**: 822.

○ Fraser S, Bunce C, Wormald R and Brunner E (2001) Deprivation and late presentation of glaucoma: case–control study. *BMJ*. **322**: 639–43.

○ Nuesh R, Schroeder K, Dieterle T *et al*. (2001) Relation between insufficient response to antihypertensive treatment and poor compliance with treatment: a prospective case–control study. *BMJ*. **323**: 142–6.

○ Pierfitte C, Macouillard G, Thicoipe M *et al*. (2001) Benzodiazepines and hip fractures in elderly people: case–control study. *BMJ*. **322**: 704–8.

Case finding

Case finding is any procedure that leads to the detection of a case of interest – for example, looking through patients' notes to see which ones may meet the clinical trial entry criteria. *See* **Audit; Feasibility trial**.

Case report

A case report is a description of a particular patient or event – for example, a case report of managing an elderly patient with a fractured neck of femur. Other case reports have described unusual aspects of a patient's disease or condition, or an adverse event. Some case reports have been used to build up a wider, clearer picture with regard to evidence-based medicine in their practice. On many occasions case reports will be used for teaching purposes.

Case reports can feed into considerations of the following:

- an audit

- the design of a clinical trial

- the primary question for a clinical trial

- the outcomes to consider for a clinical trial

- the design of systems and procedures that are used to implement evidence from a clinical trial.

The advantages of case reports are as follows.

- They can convey a great deal of evidence that could be missed in a clinical trial.

- They can be completed quite quickly.

- They are relatively easy to complete.

- They are usually cheaper to undertake than other types of research.

The disadvantages of case reports are as follows.

- They have no control group.

- They may not be generalisable.

Sometimes a case report is called a case study. *See* **Audit; Case report form; Generalisability of trial results; Primary question; Protocol; Research questions and research methods**.

○ Fowkes FGR and Fulton PM (1991) Critical appraisal of published research: introductory guidelines. *BMJ*. **302**: 1136–40.

Case report form

A case report form is a document (paper or electronic) that is used to record information about each patient in the clinical trial. *See* **Audit**; **Baseline**; **Case report**; **Missing values**.

Case series

A case series is a description of more than one case.

Examples include the following:

- a review of the results of screening tests
- a review of medical practice on a ward
- a review of Caesareans in a particular hospital
- community pharmacy advice to elderly patients with dementia
- whether patients gave written consent to enter a trial
- whether a group of patients followed the protocol in a particular trial.

See **Case report**; **Case report form**.

- ○ Fowkes FGR and Fulton PM (1991) Critical appraisal of published research: introductory guidelines. *BMJ*. **302**: 1136–40.

Case study

See **Case report**.

Causal hypothesis

A causal hypothesis is a statement that a particular event is caused by a particular named factor. An example would be the link between cigarette smoking and certain cancers. *See* **Association**; **Bayesian analysis**; **Causal relationship**; **Duhem's irrefutability theory**; **Factor analysis**; **Falsificationism**; **Hypothesis**; **Hypothesis testing**.

Causal relationship

When a patient receives a particular intervention and it has an effect on him or her, then it can be *suggested* that there is a causal relationship between the intervention and the outcomes.

For example, taking aspirin after myocardial infarction increases life expectancy. Although the relationship is not yet fully understood, it does indeed exist. Burns and Spangler looked at the relationship between psychotherapy homework compliance and changes in depression. *See* **Association; Causal hypothesis; Confounding factor; Statistical tests: ten ways to cheat with statistical tests**.

○ Burns DD and Spangler DL (2000) Does psychotherapy homework lead to improvements in depression in cognitive–behaviour therapy or does improvement lead to increased homework compliance? *J Consult Clin Psychol*. **68**: 46–56.

○ Heitjan DF (1999) Causal inference in a clinical trial: a comparative example. *Control Clin Trials*. **20**: 309–18.

Causes of delay and failure to complete a clinical trial

Good edited a book in 1976 which included a table listing some of the causes of delay and reasons for failing to complete a clinical trial. The table is reproduced here, as many of us still experience these delays (*see* Table 10).

Table 10 Causes of delay and failure to complete a clinical trial

Area	Aspect	Example
Plan	Protocol	Asking wrong question Incorrect trial design
Planners	Statistician Consultant Medical adviser	Not consulted Consulted late in the trial Inexperienced
Powers	Ethical committee Consultant Registrar	Delay Loses interest Over-committed
Pilots	Medical adviser Clinical trial team Nurse observer	Inadequate follow-up Badly managed Poorly motivated
Passenger (product)	Therapeutic substance	Badly formulated Appearance of toxicity Inadequate clinical trials stock
Patients		Bad selection Inadequate recruitment Unco-operative Not attending for assessment
Patients' records		Badly designed Incompletely filled in Not properly identified
Pharmacists	Company Hospital	Faults in supply of clinical material Faults in dispensing of clinical trial materials
Publishing		Lack of impetus to write up trial and submit to journal Incomplete results Poor writing up Lack of journal space

Table 10 is not a complete list of all causes of delay or failure to complete a trial, nor does it give an indication of how prevalent the problems are, how they are resolved and why some of them are not resolved.

The issues listed in Table 10 should be considered before starting or getting involved in a trial, and also when writing up or interpreting a trial. *See* **Fate of clinical research; Local research ethics committee; Multicentre research ethics committee; Reasons given by the investigator for a study being abandoned or in abeyance; Reasons given by the investigator for a study never being started; Research governance in the NHS.**

○ Altman DG (1994) The scandal of poor medical research. *BMJ.* **308**: 283–4.

○ Good CS (ed.) (1976) *The Principles and Practice of Clinical Trials.* Churchill Livingston, London.

Censoring

Censoring is the act of deleting data from analysis in a clinical trial.

For example, when you look at survival rates in breast cancer, some patients will be alive for quite some time after the trial. You do not know how long they will live, nor can you wait for them all to die before you study the results. Some trials with advanced breast cancer patients have reported 5-year survival rates. The data have been censored to the 5-year survival point. This may mask differences in survival before or after that particular point (e.g. 1-year and 10-year survival rates). *See* **Data dredging; Data fishing; Missing values; Statistical test diagram; Statistical tests: ten ways to cheat with statistical tests; Surrogate endpoint.**

○ Leung KM, Elashoff RM and Afifi AA (1997) Censoring issues in survival analysis. *Ann Rev Pub Health.* **18**: 83–104.

Chronic

A chronic condition is generally a slow or gradual onset of a condition. *See* **Acute; Clinical trial; Cross-over trial; Long term; Parallel trial.**

Clinical governance

According to the UK Government, 'clinical governance can be defined as a framework through which NHS organisations are accountable for continuously improving the quality of their services and safeguarding high standards of care by creating an environment in which excellence in clinical care will flourish'. The exact systems of accountability, and the meaning of the terms 'quality' and 'excellence', have yet to be clarified. The impact of clinical governance on research, and vice versa, is really only just emerging. *See* **Accountability; Audit; Due process; Research governance in the NHS; Transparency.**

○ Donaldson L (1998) *A First-Class Service: Quality in the New NHS.* HMSO, London.

○ Lugon M and Seker-Walker J (eds) (2001) *Advancing Clinical Governance.* Royal Society of Medicine Press, London.

Clinical pathway

A clinical pathway is a course of clinical care that a patient follows in a clinical trial. It relates only to the clinical issues and not to the complete care path. Sometimes the terms are loosely amalgamated and called the care path, but not all care involves clinical aspects. *See* **Analysis by administered treatment**; **Analysis by allocated treatment**; **Audit**; **Care path**; **Clinical practice guidelines**; **Protocol**.

Clinical practice guidelines

These are a set of guidelines which can aid clinical practice. They are an aid to – not an escape from – clinical decision making. Some clinical practice guidelines are an amalgamation of what is considered to be best practice, expert opinion and the results of clinical trials. At best, clinical practice guidelines are systematically developed statements designed to assist practitioner and patient decisions about appropriate healthcare for specified clinical circumstances. *See* **Guidelines, clinical trials and change**; **Hierarchies of the evidence**; **National Institute for Clinical Excellence**; **Protocol**; **Research governance in the NHS**; **Transparency**.

○ Hurwitz B (1999) Legal and political considerations of clinical practice guidelines. *BMJ*. **318**: 661–4.

○ Sackett D and Oxman A (1999) Guidelines and killer Bs. *Evidence-Based Med*. **4**: 100–1.

○ Scottish Intercollegiate Guidelines Network (SIGN) (1999) *Guidelines: an Introduction to SIGN Methodology for the Development of Evidence-Based Clinical Guidelines*. SIGN, Edinburgh.

○ Shaneyfelt TM, Mayo-Smith MF and Rothwangl J (1999) Are guidelines following guidelines? The methodological quality of clinical practice guidelines in the peer-reviewed medical literature. *JAMA*. **281**: 1900–5.

○ Woolf SH, Grol A, Hutchinson A *et al. (*1999) Potential benefits, limitations and harms of clinical guidelines. *BMJ*. **318**: 527–30.

Clinical protocols

Clinical protocols are precise and explicit rules for a clinical study or clinical practice. They have to be followed. Clinical protocols should always have escape routes so that in some instances they need not be followed to the letter. *See* **Clinical practice guidelines**; **Protocol**; **Research governance in the NHS**; **Transparency**.

Clinical significance

A result is said to be clinically significant if it is generally considered on clinical grounds to be important. A key question is who deems it to be clinically important. Is it the clinician, the patient, someone else, or a committee?

Reducing the weight of an obese person by 10 kg reduces their risk of having a stroke by 20%. This 20% reduction in risk is considered by a group of clinicians to be clinically significant.

A clinically significant result may or may not be statistically significant. Conversely, a statistically significant result may not be considered to be clinically significant. *See* **Analytic perspective; Barriers to putting clinical trial evidence into practice; Clinical versus statistical significance; Significance; Statistical significance; Statistical tests: ten ways to cheat with statistical tests.**

Clinical trial

A clinical trial is a prospective experiment that is used to identify and assess the nature and results of intervention(s).

Basically patients are allocated to an arm of the trial and followed up over a period of time. In its simplest form, some patients (called cases) will be allocated to the new intervention of interest, while others (called controls) will be allocated to another arm of the trial. The controls may be allocated to receive a placebo, nothing at all, the current care option in practice, or another regimen of interest to the study. In due course the cases may differ from the controls in terms of both compliance and outcomes. The task then is to identify the causes of the differences, where these exist.

The purpose of a clinical trial can be to:

- improve diagnostic procedures

- improve therapeutic procedures

- improve prophylactic procedures

- aid the understanding of the aetiology and pathogenesis of disease

- improve knowledge and understanding of patient risk profiles

- improve care

- improve the use of services, technology and personnel.

If you cannot find out the primary purpose of a clinical trial, be very careful about getting involved in or interpreting the results of such a study.

Clinical trials in healthcare are undertaken on the following:

- humans

- animals

- tissues

- cultures

- plants

- genetically modified organisms

- systems of care arrangements (e.g. midwife-led clinic versus standard care).

See **Clinical trial steering committee; Control group; Cross-over trial; Ethical considerations in a randomised clinical trial; Evidence-based medicine; Experimental study; Fate of clinical research; Hierarchies of the evidence; Meta-analysis; Observational study; Parallel trial; Phases of clinical trials; Placebo; QUOROM; Randomised controlled trial; Reasons given by the investigator for a study being abandoned or in abeyance; Reasons given by the investigator for a study never being started; Research question; Research questions and research methods; Systematic review; Types of research questions**.

○ Chow SC and Liu JP (1998) *Design and Analysis of Clinical Trials*. John Wiley & Sons, Chichester.

○ Jadad A (1998) *Randomised Controlled Trials*. BMJ Books, London.

○ Mathews J (2000) *Introduction to Randomised Controlled Clinical Trials*. Edward Arnold, London.

○ Meinert CL (1996) *Clinical Trials Dictionary: terminology and usage recommendations*. Johns Hopkins University Press, Baltimore, MD.

○ Peto R and Baigent C (1998) Trials: the next 50 years. *BMJ*. **317**: 1170–1.

○ Raven A (1993) *Clinical Trials: an introduction*. Radcliffe Medical Press, Oxford. Out of print.

Clinical trial ethical approval committee: primary purpose

In general, the primary purpose of clinical trial ethical committees varies over time and across settings. Their primary aim has been to protect subjects and to promote high-quality studies. Other purposes can include the following:

- to protect investigators

- to give advice on ethical problems

- to maintain research standards

- to support high-quality research

- to make that which is emotionally unacceptable to some people seem more respectable and acceptable

- to maintain public support for clinical research

- to assess the ethical and scientific nature of research proposals.

Before applying for ethical approval, it is always worth speaking to the secretary or chairperson of the committee to make sure that you know what their primary purpose is. Also, if you are getting involved in a clinical trial as a trial recruiter or as a patient, then it may be helpful for you to establish with certainty the primary purpose of the ethical committee. *See* **Clinical trial steering committee; Ethical issues; Institutional review board; Local research ethics committee; Multicentre research ethics committee; Research governance in the NHS**.

Clinical trial steering committee

A clinical trial steering committee is a group of people who are responsible for directing the clinical trial. It has been argued that each member of the committee should:

- be experienced in clinical trials
- be expert in project management
- have accomplished interpersonal skills
- be authoritative
- be financially independent from the trial sponsors.

Before a trial starts, the clinical trial steering committee should have:

- a well-defined set of rights and responsibilities, open and available for all to see
- a democratically elected chairman
- a written declaration of any interests that they or their family have in the trial or with the trial sponsors.

Clinical trial steering committees are sometimes called clinical trial executive committees. *See* **Accountability; Data-monitoring committee; Institutional review board; Principal investigator; Sponsor; Transparency.**

Clinical versus statistical significance

In an early publication of a trial of donepezil for patients with mild to moderate Alzheimer's disease, a statistically significant difference in cognitive function was found between patients who were prescribed donepezil compared with those who were prescribed placebo. Some healthcare professionals argued that the results were of little or no clinical significance, and would not be seen or valued in everyday clinical practice. Since then, more robust results have emerged from additional donepezil trials.

The early results from the donepezil trials once again raised an important issue, namely the possibility that there can be a difference between clinically significant results and statistically significant results. Figure 16 illustrates this point.

Figure 16 shows that:

- some results in a clinical trial may be clinically significant
- some results may be statistically significant
- some results may be both clinically and statistically significant.

See **Clinical significance; Significance; Statistical significance; Statistical test diagram; Statistical tests: ten ways to cheat with statistical tests.**

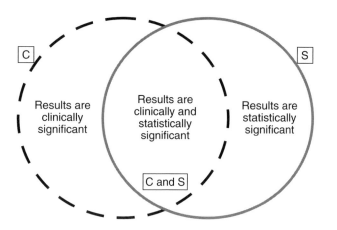

Figure 16 Clinical versus statistical significance.

Closed question

A closed question in a clinical trial is one that has a pre-set list of answers.
For example:

- (to the patient) 'Would you say that your health is excellent, good, average, not so good or poor?'

- (to the doctor) 'Do you understand the Declaration of Helsinki, yes or no?'

- (from the trial sponsor to the potential trial manager) 'Have you read the UK's *Research Governance in the NHS* document, yes or no?'

- (from an interested doctor to the trial sponsor) 'Does this trial have ethical approval, yes or no?'

- (from the patient to the doctor) 'If I did not enter this trial that you are advocating, would it affect our relationship, yes or no?'

The advantages of closed questions are as follows.

- They need to be of good design.

- They may help to categorise answers.

- They may provide better motivation to answer.

- The answers are relatively easy to analyse.

- They enable rapid analysis.

- They are relatively cheap to undertake.

- The answers can lead to a series of further, more detailed questions.

The disadvantages of closed questions are as follows.

- They can create false options.
- They can create bias if sufficient options are not available.
- They may create a loss of spontaneity in answering the questions.

See **Primary question; Types of research questions**.

Closed sequential trial
When there is a limit to the number of patients recruited into a sequential trial, then it is called a closed sequential trial. *See* **Clinical trial; Open sequential trial; Sequential trial**.

Cluster
A cluster is a group of cases with something in common. *See* **Cluster analysis; Cluster randomisation; Cluster randomised trial; Group randomisation**.

Cluster analysis
Cluster analysis involves the classification of data into meaningful groups, and the subsequent analysis of these groups.

Examples of cluster groups include the following:

- patient's age
- gender
- socio-economic status
- ethnicity
- geographical location
- intervention
- treatment history
- disease history
- clinic attending
- clinical outcome
- health status.

See **Cluster; Cluster randomisation; Cluster randomised trial; Ethical issues; Group randomisation**.

○ Donner A and Klar N (2000) *Design and Analysis of Cluster Randomization Trials in Health Research.* Edward Arnold, London.

Cluster randomisation

Patients are classified into one of the group 'clusters', and that cluster is randomly allocated to an arm of the trial.

This approach has been used when it is not possible to obtain a complete list of members of a population one wishes to study, but one can obtain a list of the groups (e.g. clinics) that one wishes to include in the trial. The clinics are then randomly allocated to an arm of the trial.

Cluster randomisation has also been used in tests of the safety and bacteriology of certain foodstuffs from shops across the country, and pesticides used on farms in England.

Cluster randomisation is sometimes called group randomisation. *See* **Cluster; Cluster analysis; Cluster randomised trial; Ethical issues; Group randomisation**.

○ Donner A and Klar NS (2000) Cluster randomization trials. *Stat Methods Med Res.* **9**: 79–80.

○ Donner A and Klar NS (2000) *Design and Analysis of Cluster Randomization Trials in Health Research.* Edward Arnold, London.

○ Reading R, Harvey I and Mclean M (2000) Cluster randomised trials in maternal and child health: implications for power and sample size. *Arch Dis Child.* **82**: 79–83.

○ Torgerson DJ (2001) Contamination in trials: is cluster randomisation the answer? *BMJ.* **322**: 355–7.

Cluster randomised trial

This is a clinical trial in which clusters and not individuals are randomised to the arms of the trial.

According to Edwards and colleagues, the two main reasons for using cluster randomised trials in healthcare are as follows:

- the regimen itself may be administered to and affect entire groups (e.g. fluoridation)

- although an intervention may be given to individuals, it affects groups.

For example, Montgomery and colleagues reported on a cluster randomised unblinded controlled trial with 1-year follow-up of an evaluation of a computer-based clinical decision support system and risk chart management of hypertension in primary care. General practices were randomly allocated to one of the following:

- a computer-based clinical decision support system plus a risk chart (10 practices, 229 patients), *or*

- a risk chart only (10 practices, 228 patients), *or*

- usual care (7 practices, 157 patients).

Morrison and colleagues reported on a pragmatic cluster randomised controlled trial to evaluate guidelines for the management of infertility across the primary care–secondary care interface. However, in a response to their paper, Professor Nick Freemantle argued strongly, among other fundamental concerns (e.g. with regard to primary endpoints, statistical methods and the impact of 'evidence'), that an analysis at the wrong level in a cluster study is never appropriate. He cited a recent meeting organised by the UK's Medical Research Council at which cluster randomised trials were discussed, and it was acknowledged that it is always incorrect to use the patient as the unit of analysis from trials in which the doctor or healthcare provider forms the natural subject.

Other recently published examples of cluster randomised trials include the following:

- an intervention to improve the management of asthma (the Greenwich asthma study)

- a trial of expert systems based on the transtheoretical (stages of change) model for smoking prevention and cessation in schools

- prevention of injuries in children

- vitamin and beta-carotene supplementation and mortality related to pregnancy in a city.

See **Clinical trial; Cluster; Cluster analysis; Cluster randomisation; Ethical issues; Group randomisation; Multilevel modelling.**

○ Campbell MJ (2000) Cluster randomized trials in general (family) practice research. *Stat Methods Med Res.* **9**: 81–94.

○ Donner A (1998) Some aspects of the design of cluster randomized trials. *Appl Stat.* **47**: 95–113.

○ Donner A and Klar NS (2000) Cluster randomization trials. *Stat Methods Med Res.* **9**: 79–80.

○ Donner A and Klar NS (2000) *Design and Analysis of Cluster Randomization Trials in Health Research.* Edward Arnold, London.

○ Edwards SJL, Braunholtz DA, Lilford RJ and Steven AJ (1999) Ethical issues in the design and conduct of cluster randomised controlled trials. *BMJ.* **318**: 1407–9.

○ Freemantle N (2001) Methodological weakness and poor reporting undermine author's conclusions. *BMJ.* **323**: 808.

○ Freemantle N, Wood J, Campbell MK *et al.* (1999) Cluster randomised trials. *BMJ.* **318**: 1286.

○ Murray DM (1998) *The Design and Analysis of Group Randomised Trials.* Oxford University Press, Oxford.

○ Montgomery AA, Fahey T, Peters TJ *et al.* (2000) Evaluation of computer-based clinical decision support system and risk chart for management of hypertension in primary care: randomised controlled trial. *BMJ.* **320**: 686–90.

○ Morrison J, Carroll L, Twaddle S *et al.* (2001) Pragmatic randomised controlled trial to evaluate guidelines for the management of infertility across the primary care–secondary care interface. *BMJ.* **322**: 1282–4.

○ Reading R, Harvey I and Mclean M (2000) Cluster randomised trials in maternal and child health: implications for power and sample size. *Arch Dis Child.* **82**: 79–83.

○ Ukoumunne OC, Gulliford MC, Chinn S *et al.* (1998) Evaluations of health care interventions at area and organisation level. In: N Black, JK Brazier, R Fitzpatrick and B Reeves (eds) *Health Services Research Methods: a guide to best practice.* BMJ Books, London.

Cochrane Collaboration

The Cochrane Collaboration is an international network of organisations and individuals who are committed to preparing, maintaining and disseminating reviews of health service research.

The Cochrane Collaboration aims to:

* work in collaboration

* build on people's enthusiasm and interests

* minimise duplication of effort

* avoid bias

* remain up to date

* ensure reasonable access to its reports (www.update-software.com).

See **Cochrane Controlled Trials Register; Cochrane Database of Reviews; National Research Register**.

Cochrane Controlled Trials Register

The Cochrane Controlled Trials Register is an electronic database of references to controlled trials in healthcare. More details can be found on the Cochrane website (www.update-software.com or www.cochrane.org) *See* **Cochrane Collaboration; Cochrane Database of Reviews; National Research Register**.

Cochrane Database of Reviews

The Cochrane Database of Reviews is an electronic database of all currently available Cochrane reviews. Tables 11 and 12 illustrate just some of the new and updated Cochrane reviews available in summer 2001. The full text of these reviews and others, including the protocols, is available from the Cochrane Library.

The Cochrane Library is prepared and published by Update Software Ltd. *See* www.update-software.com or contact Update Software, info@update.co.uk, for information on subscribing to the Cochrane Library in your area. Update Software Ltd, Summertown Pavilion, Middle Way, Oxford OX2 7LG, UK. Tel: +44 1865 513902. Fax: +44 1865 516918. *See* **Cochrane Collaboration; Cochrane Controlled Trials Register; Systematic review**.

Table 11 Some new Cochrane reviews

1. Active chest compression–decompression for cardiopulmonary resuscitation
2. Bronchodilators for the prevention and treatment of chronic lung disease in preterm infants
3. Condom effectiveness in reducing heterosexual HIV transmission
4. Day-hospital versus outpatient care for psychiatric disorders
5. Early versus late anti-epileptic drug withdrawal for patients with epilepsy in remission
6. Formula milk versus preterm human milk for feeding preterm or low-birth-weight infants
7. Herbal and dietary therapies for primary and secondary dysmenorrhoea
8. Information provision for stroke patients and their caregivers
9. Multifocal versus monofocal intra-ocular lenses after cataract extraction
10. Nasal intermittent positive pressure ventilation (NIPPV) versus nasal continuous positive airway pressure (NCPAP) for preterm neonates after extubation
11. Occupational therapy for patients with Parkinson's disease
12. Physiotherapy for patients with Parkinson's disease
13. Routine intracranial pressure monitoring in patients with acute coma
14. Stapled versus handsewn methods for colorectal anastomosis surgery
15. Transcutaneous electrical nerve stimulation (TENS) for chronic pain
16. Valproic acid, valproate and divalproex in the maintenance treatment of bipolar disorder
17. What is the role of stimulant laxatives in the management of childhood constipation and soiling?

Table 12 Some updated Cochrane reviews

1. Antipsychotic medication for challenging behaviour in people with learning disability
2. Biopsy versus resection for malignant glioma
3. Caregiver support for postpartum depression
4. Depot pipothiazine palmitate and undecylenate for schizophrenia
5. Elective high-frequency oscillatory ventilation versus conventional ventilation for acute pulmonary dysfunction in preterm infants
6. Furosemide for symptomatic patent ductus arteriosus in indomethacin-treated infants
7. Hospital at home versus in-patient hospital care
8. Interventions for preventing obesity in children
9. Lamotrigine add-on for drug-resistant partial epilepsy
10. Lithium for maintenance treatment of mood disorders
11. Methylxanthine treatment for apnoea in preterm infants
12. Screening of newborns for cystic fibrosis
13. Osteotomy, compression and reaming techniques for internal fixation of extracapsular hip fractures
14. Palliative radiotherapy regimens for non-small-cell lung cancer
15. Reduced or modified dietary fat intake for preventing cardiovascular disease
16. Suburethral sling operations for urinary incontinence in women
17. Thioridazine for dementia
18. Vaginal misoprostol for cervical ripening and induction of labour
19. Zuclopenthixol acetate in the treatment of acute schizophrenia and similar serious mental illnesses

Cohort

A cohort is a particular group of people.
  For example, it might include:

- those in your primary care group who have been recorded as having hypertension

- those attending your monthly type II diabetes clinic

- those attending the fast-track chest clinic at the general hospital

- a group of people who have been exposed to a risk factor.

See **Cohort study; Research questions and research methods.**

Cohort study

A cohort study is an observational study of a particular group over a period of time.

- A retrospective cohort study looks back over time (e.g. at all those who had antithrombotic treatment for atrial fibrillation, or all those who had paediatric cardiac surgery).

- Ely and colleagues sought to determine whether there was any evidence that greater medical knowledge was associated with increased malpractice claims. They used a cohort study linking data from medical directories and family practice certification examination scores with medical malpractice insurance claims.

- In a 5-year retrospective cohort study of 138 acute care hospitals, Glasgow and colleagues sought to determine whether higher hospital volume was associated with lower operative mortality and shorter length of stay after hepatic resection.

- Reid and colleagues reported on a retrospective cohort study of medically unexplained symptoms in frequent attenders for secondary healthcare services.

- A prospective cohort study looks forward over time (e.g. to determine how many people with a specified risk factor go on to develop the disease of interest). For example, Doll and colleagues used a prospective study of 34 439 male doctors in the UK to assess the possible association between smoking and dementia.

- Evans and colleagues used a cohort study to identify and examine depression in pregnant women during pregnancy and after childbirth.

The advantages of cohort studies include the following.

- They are relatively cheaper to perform than a clinical trial.

- They may be completed more quickly than a clinical trial.

- They can be used to examine cause and effect.

- They follow patients over a period of time.

Some of the disadvantages of cohort studies include the following.

- They do not involve a control group.

- They can be more prone to loss of subjects over time.

- They may not be generalisable.

See **Before-and-after analysis; Care path; Case–control study; Clinical trial; Cohort; Comparing research methods; Dropout; Generalisability of trial results; Lost; Lost in follow-up; Missing values; Research questions and research methods.**

○ Bull C, Yates R, Sarkar D, Deanfield J and de Leval M (2000) Scientific, ethical and logistical considerations in introducing a new operation: retrospective cohort study from paediatric cardiac surgery. *BMJ.* **320**: 1168–73.

○ Doll R, Peto R, Boreham J and Sutherland I (2000) Smoking and dementia in male British doctors: a prospective study. *BMJ.* **320**: 1097–102.

○ Edmond SL and Felson DT (2000) Prevalence of back symptoms in elders. *J Rheumatol.* **27**: 220–5.

○ Ely JW, Dawson JD, Young PR *et al.* (1999) Malpractice claims against family physicians: are the best doctors sued more? *J Fam Pract.* **48**: 23–30.

○ Evans J, Heron J, Francomb H *et al.* (2001) Cohort study of depressed mood during pregnancy and after childbirth. *BMJ.* **323**: 257–60.

○ Fowkes FGR and Fulton PM (1991) Critical appraisal of published research: introductory guidelines. *BMJ.* **302**: 1136–40.

○ Glasgow RE, Showstack J, Katz PP *et al.* (1999) The relationship between hospital volume and outcomes of hepatic resection for hepatocellular carcinoma. *Arch Surg.* **134**: 30–5.

○ Reid S, Wessely S, Crayford T and Hotopf M (2001) Medically unexplained symptoms in frequent attenders of secondary health care: retrospective cohort study. *BMJ.* **322:** 767.

Co-intervention

A co-intervention simply means more than one intervention. *See* **Adjunctive therapy; Combination trial; Confounding factor.**

Combination trial

A combination trial is a clinical trial in which patients receive combinations of interventions.

Recently published examples include the following:

- in the thrombolysis in myocardial infarction (TIMI) 14 trial, patients received abciximab plus reduced-dose tissue plasminogen activator (tPA), and this was compared with tPA alone

- a comparison was made of dacarbazine, alkylating agent 1,3-bis(2-chloroethyl)-1-nitrosourea, cisplatin and tamoxifen with dacarbazine and interferon in the treatment of advanced melanoma

- ziprasidone and the pharmacokinetics of a combined oral contraceptive

- the efficacy of inhaled budesonide plus oral prednisone in reducing relapses in patients with acute asthma

- the efficacy of beta-agonists plus ipratropium bromide in the emergency treatment of adults with acute asthma

- the efficacy of loperamide and simethicone versus loperamide alone, simethicone alone or placebo in reducing the duration of acute diarrhoea and relieving gas-related abdominal discomfort

- comparison of two doses of misopristone in combination with misoprostol for early medical abortion

- transmyocardial laser revascularisation combined with coronary artery bypass grafting.

Some issues to consider with regard to combination trials include the following.

- The order of combinations may matter, but it is not always fully addressed.

- The effect of any single intervention may not be clear.

- The way in which the combinations were provided, when and by whom may matter more than is normally suggested.

See **Additive effect; Adjunctive therapy; Clinical trial; Multiplicative effect.**

○ Allen KB, Dowling RD, DelRossi AJ *et al.* (2000) Transmyocardial laser revascularization combined with coronary artery bypass grafting: a multicentre, blinded, prospective, randomised controlled trial. *J Thorac Cardiovasc Surg.* **119**: 540–9.

○ Comella P, Frasci G, Panza N *et al.* (2000) Randomized trial comparing cisplatin, gemcitabine and vinorelbine with either cisplatin and gemcitabine or cisplatin and vinorelbine in advanced non-small-cell lung cancer: interim analysis. *J Clin Oncol.* **18**: 1451–7.

○ de Lemos JA, Antman EM, Gibson CM *et al.* (2000) Abciximab improves both epicardial flow and myocardial reperfusion in ST-elevation myocardial infarction. Observations from the TIMI 14 Trial. *Circulation.* **101**: 239–43.

○ Middleton MR, Lorigan P, Owen J *et al.* (2000) A randomized phase III study comparing dacarbazine, BCNU, cisplatin and tamoxifen with dacarbazine and interferon in advanced melanoma. *Br J Cancer.* **82**: 1158–62.

○ Muirhead GJ, Harness J, Holt PR, Oliver S and Anziano RJ (2000) Ziprasidone and the pharmacokinetics of a combined oral contraceptive. *Br J Clin Pharmacol.* **49(Supplement 1)**: 49–56S.

○ WHO Task Force on Post-Ovulatory Methods of Fertility Regulation (2000) Comparison of two doses of misopristone in combination with misoprostol for early medical abortion. *Br J Obstet Gynaecol.* **107**: 524–30.

Committee on the Safety of Medicines

The Committee on the Safety of Medicines is a UK committee composed of around 34 independent experts, with secretariat support, that meets every fortnight with the responsibility of assessing an application for a product licence and making recommendations to the UK ministers of health (politicians) as to whether, and on what terms, the product should be licensed for use in the UK.

Why, you may ask, is this committee included in this book? The answer is because quite crucially and critically it assesses the evidence put forward in support of a product licence and most of the evidence pertains to clinical trials. *See* **Medicines Control Agency; Yellow card scheme**.

Common areas of non-compliance in clinical studies

Where there are sets of standards to be complied with in clinical research it would be interesting and useful to know to what extent these are in fact being complied with. The present UK government, the Medicines Control Agency and the UK National Health Service are neither able nor legally required to provide information to the public on common areas of non-compliance in clinical studies.

Nevertheless, there is some evidence from the USA so we shall use that. The US Food and Drug Administration (FDA) has initiated a number of enforcement actions, including warning letters to investigators and review boards about non-compliance in clinical studies. Whilst every action, warning and enforcement letter to non-compliers is specific, Table 13 provides an insight into the FDA's citations against non-compliant clinical study investigators.

Table 13 Common areas of non-compliance in clinical studies

Area of concern	Percentage of official actions since 1994 in which these violations were cited
Adherence to the investigational plan and study protocols	82%
Control over the test article	44%
Documentation	85%
Reporting	74%
Subject protection	67%

It would be interesting to see whether that information now becomes available in the new research-based NHS in the UK and via moves at a European level to harmonise clinical trials. It would also be interesting to see whether public reports become available from the major non-profit-making trial sponsors in the UK (e.g. Medical Research Council, Wellcome Trust, British Heart Foundation). What do they do about detecting and dealing with non-compliance, and can they share their lessons with a wider audience in order to reduce the problems in the future? *See*

Audit; Fate of clinical research; Institutional review board; Local research ethics committee; Medicines Control Agency; Medical Research Council Guidelines for Good Practice in Clinical Trials; Multicentre research ethics committee; Questions to ask before getting involved in a clinical trial; Research governance in the NHS.

○ Food and Drug Administration (2000) *Oversight of Clinical Investigators.* HHS Office of the Inspector General, FDA, Bethesda, MD.

Community trial

A community trial is a trial involving a group of people from a specified community. The community may be defined by the following:

- geographical location (e.g. your town)
- administrative region (e.g. your health authority area)
- ethnicity
- schooling
- where people work (e.g. in a retail park, office or factory)
- where people live.

Recently reported community-based trials have included the following:

- Fleming and colleagues, who used a community-based trial to study brief physician advice in older patients with potentially excessive drinking problems
- Scott and colleagues, who conducted a trial to compare the safety and efficacy of two products for treating acute seizures in children and adolescents with refractory epilepsy at a residential centre in Surrey
- Steinberg and colleagues, who looked at the prevention of falls and near falls of the elderly in a community dwelling.

See **Clinical trial; Multicentre trial; Multilevel modelling; Trial site.**

○ Fleming MF, Manwell LB and Barry KL (1999) Brief physician advice for alcohol problems in older adults. A randomized community based trial. *J Fam Pract.* **48**: 378–84.

○ Scott RC, Besag FM and Neville BG (1999) Buccal midazolam and rectal diazepam for treatment of prolonged seizures in childhood and adolescence: a randomised trial. *Lancet.* **353**: 623–6.

○ Steinberg M, Cartwright C, Peel N and Williams G (2000) A sustainable programme to prevent falls and near falls in community-dwelling older people: results from a randomised trial. *J Epidemiol Commun Health.* **54**: 227–32.

Comparative bioavailability trial

A trial using different formulations of a product to assess their *in-vivo* performance. *See* **Dose comparison trial; Equivalence trial**.

Comparing research methods

Although this book is essentially about clinical trials, there are other methods of analysis that can be used in clinical research. Table 14 provides a summary of four different research methods.

Table 14 gives a general overview, a set of general issues if you like, of the differences between the research methods along different dimensions (e.g. cost, requirement for ethical approval). In reality you will encounter some exceptions to the entries in Table 14. If you do so, try to find out why the exception exists. In general there is no robust evidence to support the statements in the table. It is indicative, intuitive, suggestive and based on experience rather than on a systematic review of the evidence.

You should be considering the dimensions in Table 14 when:

- setting up a study

- getting involved in someone else's study

- sponsoring a study

- recommending a study

- analysing a study

- trying to put the research results into everyday clinical practice.

The actual research method that you use will depend on the primary question you want to address, the resources available, and the ability to have the relevant study samples in place for analysis. Whatever method is chosen, all research would benefit from a clear primary question, good-quality research protocols, appropriate data collection, robust data-recording systems, pertinent analysis and publication (at least on the Internet). *See* **Bias; Case–control study; Clinical trial; Cohort study; Meta-analysis; Observational study; Primary question; Randomised controlled trial; Research question; Systematic review; Triangulation**.

○ Crombie IK and Davies HTO (1998) *Research in Healthcare*. John Wiley & Sons, Chichester.

○ Elwood M (1998) *Critical Appraisal of Epidemiological Studies and Clinical Trials* (2e). Oxford Medical Press, Oxford.

○ Jenkinson C (ed.) (1997) *Assessment and Evaluation of Health and Medical Care*. Open University Press, Buckingham.

○ Stevens A, Abrams K, Brazier J, Fitzpatrick R and Lilford R (eds) (2001) *The Advanced Handbook of Methods in Evidence-Based Healthcare*. Sage Publishing, London.

Table 14 Some dimensions of different research methods

Dimension	Method			
	Observational	Cohort	Case–control	Randomised control trial
Typical question addressed (roughly – yet to be refined and made more specific)	How widespread is this condition?	What are the effects on patients of exposure to a particular risk?	What caused this particular problem?	What are the merits of care regimen A compared with regimen B?
Cost	Can be relatively low	Moderate	Moderate	Higher
Time to perform study	Relatively short	Can be short	Moderate	Moderate to long
Is it retrospective or prospective?	Either, but often prospective	Can be either	Can be either	Prospective
Is a research protocol required?	Desirable	Desirable	Desirable	Generally required
Is ethical approval required?	Desirable	Desirable	Desirable	Required
Must patient sign informed consent forms?	No	No	Not usually	Usually
Must doctor say that they do not know what is the best course of action (treatment), and must the patient understand and accept this position?	Not required	Not required	Not usually required	Required
Ability to establish what is going on?	Quite often	Quite often	Quite often	Usually
Ability to determine association?	Sometimes	Not often	Quite often	Quite often
Ability to determine why certain things are happening (causation)?	Not often	Not often	Quite often	Quite often
Ability to generalise to a wider patient group?	Sometimes	Sometimes	Sometimes	Sometimes
Ability to be repeated?	Not often (each observation is time and 'situation' dependent)	Quite often	Quite often	Often (but rarely happens)

Competing cause

A competing cause occurs when an effect may have been caused by a rival factor. For example, myocardial infarction can be caused by many possible underlying factors, such as poor diet, lack of exercise, smoking, stress or obesity. *See* **Confounding factor**.

Completed treatment

This refers to a patient who completes the course of treatment under the clinical trial conditions (sometimes called a 'completer'). *See* **Analysis by administered treatment; Analysis by assigned treatment; Care path; Completer; Compliance; CONSORT; Dropout; Intention-to-treat analysis; Protocol**.

Completer

A completer is a patient who completes a trial. *See* **Audit; Available case analysis; Completer analysis; CONSORT; Dropout; Intention-to-treat analysis; Missing values; Number needed to treat; Withdrawal**.

Completer analysis

Completer analysis is the analysis of data only from those patients who complete the trial. Trials should report how many individuals started the study and how many completed it. *See* **Attrition; Available case analysis; Completer; Intention-to-treat analysis; Last observation carried forward; Lost; Lost in follow-up; Missing values; Withdrawal**.

Compliance

Compliance is the extent to which patients adhere to the advice given.

- One trial showed that most clinically obese patients complied with their medication, stayed on a mildly hypocaloric diet with 30% of calories as fat, and took multivitamin supplements.

- Studies of clinical practice show that 30–50% of patients do not comply with their treatment regimen.

- Non-compliance is not necessarily always detrimental to the patient.

Sometimes compliance has been loosely called concordance, although the two phenomena are not the same. *See* **Concordance; Efficacy**.

○ Cuzick J, Edwards R and Segnan N (1997) Adjusting for non-compliance and contamination in randomized clinical trials. *Stat Med.* **16**: 1017–29.

○ Foulkes MA (1999) Drug regimen compliance: issues in clinical trials and patient management. *Control Clin Trials.* **20**: 473–5.

○ Heitjan DF (1999) Causal inference in a clinical trial. A comparative example. *Control Clinl Trials.* **20**: 309–18.

○ Hartigan C, Rainville J, Sobel JB and Hipona M (2000) Long-term exercise adherence after intensive rehabilitation for chronic low back pain. *Med Sci Sports Exerc.* **32**: 551–7.

○ Johnson BF, Hamilton G, Fink J, Lucey G, Bennet N and Lew R (2000) A design for testing interventions to improve adherence within a hypertension clinical trial. *Control Clin Trials.* **21**: 62–72.

○ Tulsky JP, Pilote L, Hahn JA, Burke M, Chesney M and Moss AR (2000) Adherence to ioniazide prophylaxis in the homeless: a randomized controlled trial. *Arch Intern Med.* **160**: 697–702.

Composite endpoint

A composite endpoint is a combination of more than one endpoint or outcome. Some examples are listed below.

- Brown and colleagues reported on a randomised trial of long-acting calcium-channel-blocker or diuretic in a hypertension treatment study. A composite endpoint of cardiovascular events, cerebrovascular death, non-fatal myocardial infarction, stroke and heart failure was the primary outcome measure.

- Hansson and colleagues reported on a randomised trial of the effects of calcium antagonists compared with diuretics and beta-blockers on cardiovascular morbidity and mortality in patients with hypertension, using as their main outcome measures diastolic blood pressure, and a composite endpoint including fatal and non-fatal stroke, fatal and non-fatal myocardial infarction and other cardiovascular death.

- Rubins and colleagues used the composite endpoint of the combined incidence of non-fatal myocardial infarction or death from coronary artery disease.

The components may not be of equal importance (e.g. death and myocardial infarction), so you need to ask the following questions.

- Why was a composite endpoint used?
- What is in the composite?
- What really is the most important outcome?
- Did the trial report on single endpoints as well (and if not, why not)?

See **Additive effect; Composite hypothesis; Multiple endpoints; Outcomes pyramid; Primary outcome; Primary question.**

○ Brown MJ, Palmer CR, Castaigne A *et al.* (2000) Morbidity and mortality in patients randomised to double-blind treatment with a long-acting calcium-channel blocker or diuretic in the International

Nifedipine GITS Study: Intervention as a Goal in Hypertension Treatment (INSIGHT). *Lancet.* **356**: 366–72.

○ European Agency for the Evaluation of Medicinal Products (1999) *Concept paper on the development of a Committee for Proprietary Medical Products (CPMP). Points to consider on biostatistical/methodological issues arising from recent CPMP discussions on licensing applications: adjustment for multiplicity and related topics.* EMEA, London.

○ Hansson L, Hedner T, Lund-Johanson P et al. for the NORDIL study group (2000) Randomised trial of effects of calcium antagonists with diuretics and beta-blockers on cardiovascular morbidity and mortality in hypertension: the Nordic Diltiazem (NORDIL) study. *Lancet.* **356**: 359–65.

○ Rubins HB, Robins SJ, Collins D et al. (1999) Gemfibrozil for the secondary prevention of coronary heart disease in men with low levels of high-density-lipoprotein cholesterol. *NEJM.* **341**: 410–18.

Composite hypothesis

In general a composite hypothesis either:

- does not fully specify the distribution of one or more random variables, e.g. H_0: $z > 2$, or

- it sets up a combination of hypothesis, e.g. H_0: A = B and C = D.

The former definition is most often used in medical statistics but the latter one is also becoming vogue in certain circles, even if some statistician aficionados would quibble on its definition and it is more accurately a 'combination hypothesis' (it combines two statements A = B, C = D).

Suppose you think a new drug reduces cholesterol levels in particular patients. You may not wish to say exactly how much of a reduction in a new trial but may think of a minimum number. So for example you can set up a composite hypothesis as:

$$H_0: x > 1.5 \text{ mmol/l}$$

Using the first definition this can be taken as a composite hypothesis because if the results are that $x = 1.6, 1.7, 1.8$ or $1.9\ldots$ then they are all regarded as $x > 1.5$.

Another example comes from the European clinical trial guidelines on Alzheimer's dementia. The guidelines suggested that one appropriate test for the products in question is that the drug should reduce the Alzheimer's Disease Assessment Scale-cognitive subscore (ADAS-cog) by at least 4 units. So a composite hypothesis could be:

$$H_0: \text{ADAS-cog} > 4$$

That is, this new intervention reduces the ADAS-cog by more than 4 units.

If you have more than one adjustable parameter in the hypothesis then this is considered by some to be a composite hypothesis. For example:

$$H_0: A = B \text{ and } C = D$$

A recent composite hypothesis has been where the null hypothesis is that counselling regimen A has the same effects as regimen B for helping to keep detoxified alcoholics off the alcohol, and patient satisfaction measured by method C is the same result as measured by method D.

Remember that we set up the null hypothesis and hope to prove it false. The trial would hope to prove A is not equal to B and C is not equal to D. Various problems arise. Suppose only half the hypothesis holds: suppose you found that A is equal to B but C is not equal to D, what do you do with the evidence? Another problem arises in composite hypothesis where the data are censored or truncated as would occur in the ADAS-cog or cholesterol scores.

Exactly what the composite hypothesis is, helps determine the appropriate statistical tests. If you see a composite hypothesis, ask why it was not set out in two distinct tests. Equally, if you see a simple, standard hypothesis, ask if clinical practice would be more enlightened if a composite hypothesis was used.

See **Additive effect**; **Composite endpoint**; **Hypothesis**; **Multiplicative effect**; **Outcomes pyramid**; **Primary outcome**; **Statistical test diagram**; **Statistical tests: ten ways to cheat with statistical tests**.

Comprehensive cohort design

The comprehensive cohort design is a special type of clinical trial involving patient preferences.

The design works as follows.

- Eligible patients are asked whether they consent to be randomised.

- If they do not consent, they get the intervention that they prefer.

- If they do consent, they are randomly allocated to one of the arms of the trial.

- All eligible patients are followed throughout the period of the trial.

Figure 17 shows an example.

This method has been used to test for any differences in compliance and outcomes between those who accept randomisation and those who do not. It is also used to examine preferences. However, one problem is the possibility of having an unbalanced trial (e.g. if a large number of people end up in one arm of the trial). See **Preference trial**; **Wennberg's design**; **Zelen consent design**.

○ Schmoor C, Olschewski M and Schumacher M (1996) Randomised and non-randomised patients in clinical trials: experiences with comprehensive cohort studies. *Stat Med*. **15**: 236–71.

○ Olschewski M and Scheurlen H (1985) Comprehensive cohort study: an alternative to randomised consent design in breast preservation trial. *Methods Inf Med*. **24**: 131–4.

○ Torgerson DJ, Klaber-Moffett J and Russell IT (1996) Patient preferences in randomised trials: threat or opportunity? *J Health Serv Res Policy*. **1**: 194–7.

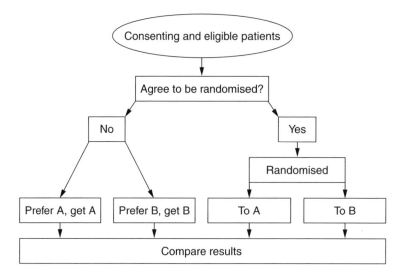

Figure 17 Comprehensive cohort design.

Concealment

To conceal means to disguise or hide. *See* **Blinding; Concealment of method of allocation; Mask.**

Concealment of method of allocation

Concealment of method of allocation occurs when we do not allow the doctor or patient to see how patients are allocated to regimens in the trial. It is used to prevent, as far as is possible, any foreknowledge of assignment. *See* **Bias; Blinding; Concealment.**

Concomitant therapy

Concomitant therapy occurs when a patient receives more than one intervention at the same time in the trial. *See* **Adjunctive therapy; Co-intervention; Combination trial; Efficacy; Generalisability of trial results.**

○ Vockes EE, Kies MS, Haraf DJ *et al.* (2000) Concomitant chemoradiotherapy as primary therapy for locoregionally advanced head and neck cancer. *J Clin Oncol.* **18:** 1652–61.

Concordance

Concordance means agreement after discussion between, say, the patient and the doctor or the pharmacist. It involves a discussion between the parties involved and then an agreement. *See* **Compliance.**

Confidence interval

The confidence interval is that range of numbers within which we are confident that the true value lies. It quantifies the degree of uncertainty in measurement. The width of the confidence interval gives us some idea of how uncertain we are about the unknown parameter. A wide confidence interval may suggest that more data should be collected before anything definite can be concluded about the parameter.

The rationale for using the confidence interval is the uncertainty which is always associated with the use of sampling.

One published clinical trial has shown that alendronate reduced new fractures in postmenopausal women who had low bone mineral density and existing vertebral fractures. In the subgroup of patients under 75 years of age, the trial showed that 15 patients would need to be treated in order to avoid one vertebral fracture. In a 95% confidence interval the number needed to treat in order to avoid one vertebral fracture was found to be 11 to 27 patients. Thus one can conclude that according to this evidence there is 95% confidence that the number of patients needed to treat in order to avoid one vertebral fracture is between 11 and 27.

We could have any other level of confidence (e.g. 90%, 93%, 99%). The standard is usually 95%. Wide confidence intervals are more conservative and suggest greater uncertainty. Narrow confidence intervals are less conservative and suggest less uncertainty. *See* **Acceptance area; Confidence limits; P-value; Statistical significance; Statistical tests: ten ways to cheat with statistical tests**.

○ Ensrud KE, Black DM, Palermo L *et al.* for the Fracture Intervention Trial Research Group (1997) Treatment with alendronate prevents fractures in women at highest risk. Results from the Fracture Intervention Trial. *Arch Intern Med.* **157**: 2617–24.

○ Petrie A and Sabin C (2000) *Medical Statistics at a Glance.* Blackwell Science, Oxford.

Confidence limits

Confidence limits are the lower and upper values of a confidence interval. In the example given above we had a lower limit of 11 and an upper limit of 27 for the 95% confidence interval. *See* **Confidence interval**.

Conflict of interest

This is the notion that there may be a conflict of interest between some parties related to the clinical trial. The parties may, for example, be:

• those hosting the trial

• those paying for the trial

• those conducting the trial

• those overseeing the trial

- those writing up the trial

- those peer reviewing the trial

- the publishers of the trial or summary reports thereof

- those promoting or otherwise publicising the trial (positively or negatively).

In some places full disclosure of any possible conflict of interest is required to be made transparent, while in other places only certain facts have to be disclosed (e.g. shares in the company, consultancy agreements, contingent staff support). In some places only certain interests above a threshold (e.g. trips involving fees above $500) need to be declared.

Many journals require authors to state whether they have any conflict of interest, but it is certainly not clear to many people how that system is actually policed by the journal or an independent person, if indeed it is policed at all. The policies at scientific conferences with regard to conflicts of interest remain unclear.

What is to be declared, by whom, when and to whom remains a matter of serious debate, as there is no one consensus on best practice. See **Accountability; Bias; Clinical trial steering committee; Ethical issues; European Union Directive on clinical trials of medicinal products for humans; Institutional review board; Local research ethics committee; Medical Research Council Guidelines for Good Practice in Clinical Trials; Multicentre research ethics committee; Peer review; Problems with regard to putting evidence into practice; Research governance in the NHS; Transparency.**

○ Bernard L, Wolfe LE and Berkeley A (2000) Conflict of interest policies for investigators in clinical trials. *NEJM.* **343**: 1616–20.

○ Drazen JM and Koski G (2000) To protect those who serve. *NEJM.* **343**: 1643–5.

○ Marco CA (2001) Guidelines for research co-operation with biomedical industry organisations. *Acad Emerg Med.* **8**: 756–7.

○ Topol EJ, Nurok M, Ratain MJ *et al.* (2001) Conflict on interest policies. *NEJM.* **344**: 1017–18.

Confounding factor

When it is impossible to distinguish clearly what factor caused a result, confounding factors are present. For example, we may look for a relationship between A and B but fail to account for another factor, say C, which affects the results. See **Adjunctive therapy; Causal relationship.**

Consent

To consent means to agree.

Consent may be given orally or in writing. For example, in 1999 the Association of Anaesthetists of Great Britain and Ireland stated that express consent should be obtained for any procedure which carries a material risk. According to this Association, the consent could be obtained orally or in writing.

Guidelines on securing consent vary across the professions, as may the interpretation of guidelines within the professions. Consent is an issue not just for clinical trials but also for clinical practice.

The issues of consent, or the lack of it, have received much publicity in the wake of problem cases (e.g. in the NHS in the UK involving trials on babies, heart surgery and organ donation).

There are issues relating to consent by proxy, situations when consent is not required, and what truly constitutes consent.

A record of the consent should always be kept in the form of an official written letter stating the following:

- what the patient was told

- who told them

- when they were told

- confirmation that they said that they understood what they were told

- confirmation that they knew their rights.

The letter should be signed and dated by the patient and a representative of the trial team. If the patient has a power of attorney, then they may sign the letter on behalf of the patient. *See* **Assent; Consent: eight key questions on law and consent; Declaration of Helsinki; Deferred consent; Informed consent; Patient information sheet and consent forms.**

○ Aitkinhead A (1999) Anaesthetists need consent, but not written consent. *BMJ*. **319**: 1135.

○ Smith R (2000) Babies and consent. *BMJ*. **320**: 1285–6.

○ Smith R (1997) Informed consent: the intricacies. *BMJ*. **314**: 1059–60.

○ Tobias J and Doyal L (2000) *Informed Consent: respecting patients in research and practice.* BMJ Books, London.

○ Wolf AM and Schorling JB (2000) Does informed consent alter elderly patients' preferences for colorectal cancer screening? Results of a randomized trial. *J Gen Intern Med*. **15**: 24–30.

Consent: eight key questions on law and consent

Whilst the laws on consent vary across countries and over time, the following information is a summary of the Department of Health's answers to eight questions. The answers are based on the Department of Health's understanding of the current laws in England (as of March 2001). The answers given relate in general to interventions in living people.

Q1 When do health professionals need consent from patients?
Before you examine, treat or care for competent adult patients you must obtain their consent.

Adults are always assumed to be competent unless demonstrated otherwise. If you have doubts about their competence, the question to ask is: 'can this patient understand and weigh up the information needed to make this decision?' Unexpected decisions do not prove the patient is incompetent, but may indicate a need for further information or explanation.

Patients may be competent to make some healthcare decisions, even if they are not competent to make others.

Giving and obtaining consent is usually a process, not a one-off event. Patients can change their minds and withdraw consent at any time. If there is any doubt, you should always check that the patient still consents to your caring for or treating them.

Q2 Can children consent for themselves?
Before examining, treating or caring for a child, you must also seek consent. Young people aged 16 and 17 are presumed to have the competence to give consent for themselves. Younger children who understand fully what is involved in the proposed procedure can also give consent (although their parents will ideally be involved). In other cases, someone with parental responsibility must give consent on the child's behalf, unless they cannot be reached in an emergency. If a competent child consents to treatment, a parent cannot override that consent. Legally, a parent can consent if a competent child refuses, but it is likely that taking such a serious step will be rare.

Q3 Who is the right person to seek consent?
It is always best for the person actually treating the patient to seek the patient's consent. However, you may seek consent on behalf of colleagues if you are capable of performing the procedure in question, or if you have been specially trained to seek consent for that procedure.

Q4 What information should be provided?
Patients need sufficient information before they can decide whether to give their consent: for example, information about the benefits and risks of the proposed treatment, and alternative treatments. If the patient is not offered as much information as they reasonably need to make their decision, and in a form they can understand, their consent may not be valid.

Q5 Is the patient's consent voluntary?
Consent must be given voluntarily: not under any form of duress or undue influence from health professionals, family or friends.

Q6 Does it matter how the patient gives consent?
Consent can be written, oral or non-verbal. A signature on a consent form does not itself prove the consent is valid – the point of the form is to record the patient's decision, and also, increasingly, the discussions that have taken place. Your trust or organisation may have a policy setting out when you need to obtain written consent.

Q7 What about refusals of treatment?
Competent adult patients are entitled to refuse treatment, even where it would clearly benefit their health. The only exception to this rule is where the treatment is for a mental disorder and the patient is detained under the Mental Health Act 1983. A competent pregnant woman may refuse any treatment, even if this would be detrimental to the foetus.

Q8 What about adults who are not competent to give consent?
No-one can give consent on behalf of an incompetent adult. However, you may still treat such a patient if the treatment would be in their best interests. 'Best interests' go wider than best medical interests, to include factors such as the wishes and beliefs of the patient when competent, their current wishes, their general well-being and their spiritual and religious welfare. People close to the patient may be able to give you information on some of these factors. Where the patient has never been competent, relatives, carers and friends may be best placed to advise on the patient's needs and preferences.

If an incompetent patient has clearly indicated in the past, while competent, that they would refuse treatment in certain circumstances (an 'advance refusal'), and those circumstances arise, you must abide by that refusal.

Naturally, the eight questions and the summary answers from the Department of Health cannot cover all situations. Ethical, legal and professional advice should be sought if there is any doubt about the proposed intervention.

See **Assent; Caldicott Guardians; Consent; Declaration of Helsinki; Deferred consent; Informed consent; Patient information sheet and consent forms; Patient preferences; Patient preferences in clinical trials; Research governance in the NHS.**

○ Ashcroft RE (2001) Ethics of clinical trials: social, cultural and economic factors (Chapter 2). In: A Stevens *et al.* (eds) *The Advanced Handbook of Methods in Evidence Based Healthcare*. Sage Publishing, London.

○ Department of Health's *Reference Guide to Consent for Examination or Treatment* available at http://www.doh.gov.uk.

○ Gostin LO (1995) Informed consent, cultural sensitivity and respect for persons. *JAMA*. **274**: 844–5.

CONSORT

CONSORT is an acronym for Consolidated Standard of Reporting Trials. In 1996, the Standards Of Reporting Trials (SORT) Group and the Asilomar Working Group on Recommendations for Reporting of Clinical Trials in the Biomedical Literature met and published the first CONsolidated Standard Of Reporting Trials. Various experts were involved in developing CONSORT, including clinical trialists, methodologists, epidemiologists, statisticians and journal editors. In May 1999, 13 members of the CONSORT group met with the objective of revising and refreshing the original CONSORT system. After various deliberations, the revised CONSORT system was produced. These deliberations concerned the merits of each item in the light of current evidence. The revisions to the checklist were circulated to the CONSORT group for comment and feedback. CONSORT participants met in May 2000 to discuss the new system, and the revised CONSORT was completed shortly afterwards. The revised CONSORT system was published simultaneously in journals such as the *Lancet*, *Annals of Internal Medicine* and the *Journal of the American Medical Association* in early 2001.

As with the old CONSORT system, the new CONSORT system has two parts, namely a flow chart (*see* Figure 18) and a Table (*see* Table 15). The third part of the CONSORT system is its website (http://www.consort-statement.org) where there are options to click through words in the table and to move into quite helpful explanatory documents.

In the flow chart you can determine how many people were assessed for eligibility (*n* = …), obtain the number of individuals who were excluded (and reasons for this), obtain the numbers allocated to each arm of the trial, record how many were lost and why (e.g. dropouts), and then enter the number of patients who were and were not analysed (*see* Figure 18).

The second part of the revised CONSORT system is a table consisting of a checklist of items to report on (*see* Table 15).

Although Table 15 is already quite long and taxing, it is not comprehensive.

Of course, when some of us see tables like this there is a temptation to skip through the table and carry on reading (or skipping through!) the rest of the text. Yet if you want to understand and critique more effectively the evidence from certain clinical trials and other people's reports of them, or if you want to submit an application for research funding, or to summarise a trial along the lines of an international standard template, you can start by using the new CONSORT system. From experience, probably the best way to begin to get to grips with the new CONSORT system is for you and some colleagues to find a recently published paper on a clinical trial, read through it, and on the basis of what you have read to complete, as best you can, Figure 18 and Table 15. Then share your findings and thoughts with your colleagues and reflect on what else you would need to know for the evidence from that trial to have an influence on your clinical practice.

Who uses the CONSORT system? Various journals adopted the old CONSORT system, including the *British Medical Journal*, the *Lancet*, the *Journal of the American Medical Association* and *Annals of Internal Medicine*. Professor Doug Altman and

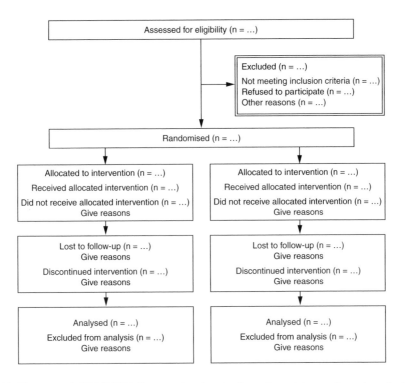

Figure 18 The revised CONSORT diagram showing the flow of participants through each stage of a randomised trial.

colleagues suggested that 'about 80 journals from around the world have adopted (old) CONSORT or are seriously thinking of doing so'. It is expected that those who have adopted the old version will subsequently adopt the revised version, and those who have not adopted the CONSORT system will now be encouraged to do so.

The CONSORT system can be used both as a guide for authors to frame their papers, and as templates for reviewers of submitted papers. Interestingly, relatively few papers that appear in journals actually report the trial in terms of the old CONSORT figure and the CONSORT table.

In addition, the CONSORT system can be used by clinical trialists to help to frame their reports. It can also be used even earlier as a template to help to consider the design, recording and management of a clinical trial. Writing in the *British Medical Journal*, Liam O'Toole, trials manager at the Medical Research Council (MRC) in London, indicated that the MRC required all investigators who sought MRC funds for clinical trials to present their applications in a structured format with headings similar to those of CONSORT. The benefits of doing so, according to O'Toole, were that the use of a structured format would make the peer-review process more cost-effective for applicants and reviewers, and that it would increase awareness of the requirements for a good trial at an early stage in its development.

The main strengths of the CONSORT system are outlined in Table 16.

Table 15 The CONSORT table (items that should be included in reports of randomised trials)

Paper section and topic	Item description	Reported on page …
Title and abstract	1 How participants were allocated to interventions (e.g. 'random allocation', 'randomised' or 'randomly assigned')	
Introduction		
Background	2 Scientific background and explanation of rationale	
Methods		
Participants	3 Eligibility criteria for participants and the settings and locations where the data were collected	
Interventions	4 Precise details of the interventions intended for each group, and how and when they were actually administered	
Objectives	5 Specific objectives and hypothesis	
Outcomes	6 Clearly defined primary and secondary outcome measures and, when applicable, any methods used to enhance the quality of measurements (e.g. multiple observations, training of assessors)	
Sample size	7 How sample size was determined and, when applicable, explanation of any interim analysis and stopping rules	
Randomisation sequence generation	8 Method used to implement the random allocation sequence, including details of any restrictions (e.g. blocking, stratification)	
Randomisation allocation concealment	9 Method used to generate the random allocation sequence (e.g. numbered containers or central telephone), clarifying whether the sequence was concealed until interventions were assigned	
Randomisation implementation	10 Who generated the allocation sequence, who enrolled participants, and who assigned participants to their groups	
Blinding (masking)	11 Whether or not participants, those administering the interventions and those assessing the outcomes were blinded to group assignment. When relevant, how the success of blinding was evaluated	
Statistical methods	12 Statistical methods used to compare groups for primary outcome(s); methods for additional analysis, such as subgroup analysis and adjusted analysis	

continued opposite

Table 15 continued

Paper section and topic	Item description	Reported on page ...
Results		
Participant flow	13 Flow of participants through each stage (a diagram is strongly recommended). Specifically, for each group report the numbers of participants randomly assigned, receiving the intended treatment, completing the study protocol, and analysed for the primary outcome. Describe the protocol deviations from the study as planned, together with reasons	
Recruitment	14 Dates defining the periods of recruitment and follow-up	
Baseline data	15 Baseline demographic and clinical characteristics of each group	
Numbers analysed	16 Number of participants (denominator) in each group included in each analysis, and whether the analysis was by 'intention to treat'. State the results in absolute numbers when feasible (e.g. 10/50, not 50%)	
Outcomes and estimation	17 For each of the primary and secondary outcomes, a summary of the results for each group, and the estimated effect (e.g. 95% confidence interval)	
Ancillary analysis	18 Address multiplicity by reporting any other analyses performed, including subgroup analyses and adjusted analyses, indicating those that were pre-specified and those that were exploratory	
Adverse events	19 All important adverse events or side-effects in each intervention group	
Discussion		
Interpretation	20 Interpretation of the results, taking into account the study hypothesis, sources of potential bias or imprecision, and the dangers associated with multiplicity of analysis and outcomes	
Generalisability	21 Generalisability (external validity) of the trial findings	
Overall evidence	22 General interpretation of the results in the context of current evidence	

To obtain a more complete and accurate understanding of the trial, one would need to have answers to the following questions (which address some weaknesses of the CONSORT system (*see* Table 17).

If you use the CONSORT system with the series of points outlined in Tables 15 and 16, including other questions and issues that are important to you, of course, you will begin to obtain a more accurate, complete and helpful insight into certain types of clinical trials and their relevance to your clinical practice. In fact, you will also be putting yourself in an enviable position to begin to appraise critically certain types of clinical trial as well as the work of anyone else who uses the CONSORT system as it currently stands.

Table 16 Strengths of the CONSORT system

1 It can be used to aid the orderly design of certain clinical trials.
2 It can be used as part of a wider template for submitting bids for funding for a clinical trial.
3 It offers a structured framework for reporting some aspects of certain types of clinical trials.
4 It offers a standard against which to compare – with care – certain different trials.
5 It is available in other languages, thus facilitating comparison of trials reported in different languages.
6 It can be used to show the completion and attrition rates of patients through a clinical trial.
7 It can be used to outline some aspects of the methodology and results of the trial.
8 It can focus debate about the gaps between what is known and what we want to know or need to know about a clinical trial.
9 It can be used to focus debates about the application of evidence to clinical practice.

Table 17 Weaknesses of the CONSORT system

1 Can the system cope in practice with more than two arms in a trial?
2 The system cannot readily cover cluster trials, in which clusters of people and not individuals are randomised to treatment interventions. Are these trials to be excluded?
3 Is placebo really an intervention? If not, then are placebo-controlled trials excluded?
4 Is an option of 'watchful waiting' an intervention? It is certainly something that happens in clinical practice. If 'watchful waiting' or even 'doing nothing for a period of time' is not an intervention, then are all of these trials to be excluded?
5 The CONSORT system pays little attention to the major and fundamental issues of consent and informed consent.
6 The CONSORT system asks nothing about who funded the study, why, and what links the trialists and trial report authors have with the sponsors.
7 Nothing is said about ethical approval. Who approved it and who, if anyone, did not approve it?
8 There is no proper trace made of the demographic and clinical characteristics of patients going through each stage of the trial, and not enough on compliance support systems used.
9 Insufficient attention is paid to the time-scales of the trial.
10 No information is sought as to whether the interim analysis and stopping rules were generated in the design stage of the trial (i.e. in advance).
11 Nothing is said about the systems of data quality assurance in the trial.
12 The CONSORT system could and should develop closer links with non-researching healthcare practitioners, managers, implementers of the evidence, patient groups and patients.

However, if you want to use that information in your practice, knowing about the trials is only part of the story. In trying to apply clinical trial evidence to practice, one needs to know about practice and other research evidence. It is poor practice to advocate change in the light of evidence from clinical trials or via CONSORT reports if one is not aware of what is going on in clinical reality.

More generally, then, you should note the following points.

• The CONSORT flow chart is not a full audit of patient flows, but just at best a descriptor of some progress.

- The CONSORT set of descriptors in Table 15 is not comprehensive.

- The individual descriptors in Table 15 are not of equal value.

- Other systems for reporting other types of research exist and continue to be developed, but there is a risk of too many templates, so common questions should be developed and then supplemented by tailor-made questions for each method (e.g. covering quality of reporting meta-analysis (QUOROM), quality of reporting systematic reviews (QSR), meta-analysis of observation studies in epidemiology (MOOSE), standardised health economics reporting (SHER), standardised reporting of qualitative analysis (SROQA), and so on).

- As Moher and colleagues suggest, CONSORT is usually used to assess certain clinical trials as stated in published reports not to assess certain clinical trials *per se*. What are the gaps between the trial and the published report, and how important are they?

- Finally, what are the gaps between research evidence and research practice?

For further details of the CONSORT system, you could visit the CONSORT system website. *See* **Advantages of evidence from clinical trials; Questions to ask before getting involved in a clinical trial**.

○ Altman DG (1996) Better reporting of randomised controlled trials: the CONSORT statement. *BMJ*. **313**: 570–1.

○ Begg C, Cho M, Eastwood S *et al*. (1996) Improving the quality of reporting of randomised controlled trials – The CONSORT Statement. *JAMA*. **276**: 7–9.

○ Earl-Slater A (2001) The new CONSORT system. *J Clin Govern*. **6**: 211–18.

○ Egger M, Juni P and Bartlet C for the CONSORT group (2001) Value of flow diagrams in reports of randomized controlled trials. *JAMA*. **285**: 1996–9.

○ Elbourne DR and Campbel MK (2001) Extending the CONSORT statement to cluster randomized trials: for discussion. *Stat Med*. **20**: 489–96.

○ Moher D (1998) CONSORT: an evolving tool to help improve the quality of reports of randomised controlled trials. *JAMA*. **279**: 1489–91.

○ Moher D, Jadad AR, Nichol G *et al*. (1995) Assessing the quality of randomised controlled trials: an annotated bibliography of scales and checklists. *Control Clin Trials*. **124**: 485–9.

○ Moher D, Jones A and Lapage L (2001) Use of CONSORT statement and quality reports of randomized trials: comparative before-and-after evaluation. *JAMA* **285**: 1992–5.

○ Moher D, Shultz KF and Altman DG for the CONSORT Group (2001) The CONSORT statement: revised recommendations for improving the quality of reports of parallel-group randomised trials. *Lancet*. **357**: 1191–4.

○ Rennie D (2001) CONSORT revised – improving reporting of randomized trials. *JAMA*. **285**: 2006–7.

Context

The context relates to the particular conditions, time, circumstances and setting of the clinical trial or clinical practice.

There is usually a difference between the context of the trial and the context of your practice. The key issue is to determine whether the differences are important in terms of putting trial evidence into practice. *See* **Advantages of evidence from clinical trials; Analytic perspective; Disadvantages of evidence from clinical trials; Generalisability of trial results; Problems with regard to putting evidence into practice; Qualitative analysis.**

Contingency fees

Contingency fees are those fees that are paid if a particular event occurs.
   For example:

* some large pharmaceutical companies pay smaller companies fees if the clinical trial that the smaller company is running makes specific progress

* doctors and consultants usually receive fees if they recruit a certain number of patients into a clinical trial.

See **Questions to ask before getting involved in a clinical trial; Research governance in the NHS; Transparency.**

Continuous variable

A continuous variable is one that can differ by an infinitesimally small amount.
   Examples include the following:

* blood pressure

* high-density-lipoprotein cholesterol

* body mass

* temperature.

See **Data types; Outcome; Outcomes pyramid.**

Control

A control is a patient who does not receive the experimental intervention of interest. The control usually receives standard care, watchful waiting, a placebo or nothing at all. In some types of trials (e.g. active control equivalence trials) the control group receives another regimen (e.g. another medication).
   See **Active control equivalence trial; Case-control study; Clinical trial; Control group; Controlled trial; Randomised controlled trial.**

Control group

A control group is a group of patients in a study who do not receive the experimental intervention of interest. The aim of using controls in a clinical trial is to give a benchmark against which the experimental intervention can be compared. The baseline characteristics of the control group should be as similar as possible to those of the other groups in the trial.

The control group is usually given standard care, 'watchful waiting' or a placebo. For example:

- in a trial of cystic fibrosis patients, the control group took their 'usual physical activity'

- in a multicentre trial to determine whether clinics run by nurses in primary care improved secondary prevention in patients with coronary heart disease, the control group was allocated to 'standard care'

- in a trial of patients with persistent otitis media with effusion at a children's hospital, the control group was allocated to the 'watchful-waiting' programme, whereas the experimental group received early surgery.

It is always worth finding out exactly what the control group received.

If you find out that the controls were allocated to receive:

- 'standard care', find out more precisely what was meant by 'standard care', as this usually differs over time and between practices, and it may not be your standard

- 'placebo control', remember that the control patients will otherwise be receiving exactly the same care management as the experimental group

- 'watchful waiting', find out if it was true, and ask yourself if it would be an option in clinical practice that you could or currently do adopt.

See **Baseline; Benchmarking; Clinical trial; Control; Controlled trial; Generalisability of trial results; Placebo; Placebo-controlled trial; Problems with regard to putting evidence into practice; Treatment group: experimental.**

○ Campbell NC, Ritchie LD, Thain J *et al.* (1998) Secondary prevention in coronary heart disease: a randomised trial of nurse-led clinics in primary care. *Heart.* **80**: 447–52.

○ Chambers I (1997) Assessing comparison groups to assess the effects of healthcare. *J R Soc Med.* **90**: 379–86.

○ Maw R, Wilks J, Harvey I *et al.* (1999) Early surgery compared with watchful waiting for glue ear and effect on language development in preschool children: a randomised trial. *Lancet.* **353**: 960–3.

○ Schneiderman-Walker J, Pollock SL, Corey M *et al.* (2000) A randomised controlled trial of a 3-year home exercise program in cystic fibrosis. *J Pediatrics.* **136**: 304–10.

Controlled trial

A controlled trial is an experimental study which compares one or more interventions in one or more groups of patients.

The 'controlled' aspect of the trial is that the experimental group is compared with another group – the control group.

Sometimes the control group receives what is termed 'usual care', standard care, a placebo, watchful waiting or nothing at all. However, what is classified as 'usual care' may not be that common or even match your usual practice. The same argument applies to standard care, as it may not be your standard.

For example, one controlled trial looked at recovery from depression in elderly patients receiving home care. One group of patients (the experimental group) received an individualised management plan formulated by the psychogeriatric team. The plan included physical and psychological interventions. The other group of patients (the control group) received their usual care from their general practitioner. The trial found that among frail elderly patients who were receiving home care, those who received the psychogeriatric management plan were more likely to recover from depression than those receiving usual care from their doctor.

Remember that not all controlled trials are randomised, whereas all randomised trials are controlled. *See* **Baseline**; **Clinical trial**; **Control**; **Control group**; **Randomised controlled trial**.

○ Banerjee S, Shamash K, Macdonald AJ and Mann AH (1996) Randomised controlled trial of effect of intervention by psychogeriatric team on depression in frail elderly people at home. *BMJ*. **313**: 1058–61.

○ Stevens A, Abrams K, Brazier J, Fitzpatrick R and Lilford R (eds) (2001) *The Advanced Handbook of Methods in Evidence-Based Healthcare*. Sage Publishing, London.

Correlation

Correlation is a measure of the *association* between factors of interest in the clinical trial. It is *not* a measure of *cause and effect*.

Correlation may be:

- positive (i.e. values rise and fall together) *or*

- negative (i.e. values go in opposite directions, so that as one increases the other decreases).

See **Causal relationship**; **Confounding factor**; **Statistical test diagram**; **Statistical tests: ten ways to cheat with statistical tests**.

Correlation coefficient

The correlation coefficient is a numerical number ranging from –1 through 0, to +1, which represents the measure of the association between the variables under study. For example, if the formula of X and Y is linear, say $X = a + bY$, then the correlation coefficient is represented by b. If $b = -1$, this denotes a negative association (e.g. Y goes up and X goes down). If $b = 0$, this denotes a lack of association. If $b = 1$, this denotes a positive association (e.g. Y goes up and X goes up). *See* **Association**; **Causal relationship**; **Statistical test diagram**; **Statistical tests: ten ways to cheat with statistical tests**.

Critical appraisal

Critical appraisal techniques are methods that are used to analyse evidence systematically, consciously and explicitly.

Although there are many templates that can be used to appraise any piece of evidence critically, there is no consensus as to which template is to be preferred in any particular situation.

Probably the most important general questions to ask when you are faced with any piece of evidence are as follows.

1 Is the research question clearly stated?

2 Is that question important to you?

3 What is already known about the issue under study?

4 What methods are used to answer the research question?

5 What are the patient, intervention and study setting characteristics?

6 What are the results?

7 Do the results actually seem to be plausible?

8 Where were the results published?

9 Who sponsored the study and why?

10 What can you now do with the evidence in clinical practice?

See **Advantages of evidence from clinical trials; Bias; Cochrane Database of Reviews; Data-display formats; Disadvantages of evidence from clinical trials; Local research ethics committee; Meta-analysis; Multicentre research ethics committee; Outcome measures; Problems with regard to putting evidence into practice; Questions to ask before getting involved in a clinical trial; Systematic review; Ways of presenting results.**

○ Earl-Slater A (1999) Advantages and disadvantages of evidence from clinical trials. *Evidence-Based Healthcare*. **3**: 53–4.

○ Earl-Slater A (2001) Critical appraisal of clinical trials: barriers to putting trial evidence into clinical practice. *J Clin Govern*. **6**: 279–82.

○ Stevens A, Abrams K, Brazier J, Fitzpatrick R and Lilford R (eds) (2001) *The Advanced Handbook of Methods in Evidence-Based Healthcare*. Sage Publishing, London.

○ Rosser WM (1999) Application of evidence from randomised controlled trials to general practice. *Lancet*. **353**: 661–4.

Critical incident techniques

Critical incident techniques are methods of analysing critical incidents. Figure 19 shows the key issues to be addressed.

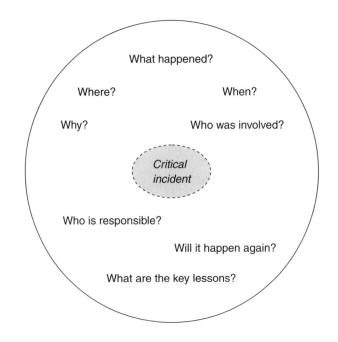

Figure 19 Critical incident techniques: key questions to ask.

As Figure 19 shows, critical incident techniques usually look at where, when and why the event took place, who was involved and what the outcomes were. They would also look at the implications and possibly give recommendations on how to avoid a repetition of the event. The UK Department of Health recently announced the idea of setting up an early warning system to aid the collection, audit, analysis and management of critical incidents.

Figure 19 offers a useful framework for analysing critical incidents in clinical trials or clinical practice. *See* **Adverse drug reaction; Audit; Multicentre research ethics committee; Research governance in the NHS; Yellow card scheme**.

Critical region
A critical region is a range of data which leads us to reject a statement. *See* **Acceptance area; Critical value; Equivalence trial; Non-inferiority trial; Null hypothesis; Superiority trial**.

Critical value
A critical value is a particular number in a clinical trial that marks the turning point between accepting something and rejecting it, or between continuing and not continuing. *See* **Acceptance area; Critical region; Early stopping rule; Interim analysis; Null hypothesis**.

Cross-over

A cross-over occurs when a patient moves from one regimen in the clinical trial to another regimen. *See* **Cross-over rate; Cross-over trial; Preference trial; Washout period**.

Cross-over rate

The cross-over rate is the proportion of patients who switch from one arm of the trial to another. For example, if 40 patients start in regimen 1 and 35 of them move to regimen 2, then the cross-over rate is 87.5% (i.e. 35/40).

Cross-over rates may be planned at the outset of the trial or occur in the course of running the trial. Whenever they arise, you must ask questions about why they occurred and their likely effects on outcomes. *See* **Carry-over effects; Cross-over; Cross-over trial; Protocol; Washout period**.

Cross-over trial

A cross-over trial is a clinical trial in which patients switch, by design, between the different arms of the trial.

A *forced* cross-over trial is one in which patients cross over at a particular point in time. An *open* cross-over trial is one in which the patients themselves decide when to cross to another arm of the trial.

Recent examples include the following.

- Allan and colleagues reported on a randomised cross-over trial of transdermal fentanyl and sustained-release oral morphine for treating chronic non-cancer pain.

- Cromheecke and colleagues reported on a randomised cross-over trial of oral anticoagulation self-management compared with management by a specialist anticoagulation clinic.

- Engleman and colleagues used a cross-over design to study continuous positive air-way pressure (CPAP) in patients with mild sleep apnoea/hypopnoea syndrome. Patients were assigned to CPAP therapy or placebo for 4 weeks and then, with no washout period, crossing over for a subsequent 4 weeks.

- Richter and colleagues reported on a randomised controlled trial of the effects of on-demand beta-2-agonist inhalation in patients with moderate to severe asthma.

- Schrader and colleagues reported on a randomised placebo-controlled cross-over trial of prophylactic treatment of migraine with angiotensin-converting-enzyme inhibitor (lisinopril).

- Zhu and colleagues used a cross-over trial with a 23-day washout period to compare the bioequivalence of two sertraline tablet formulations in healthy male volunteers.

The advantages of cross-over trials include the following.

- Each patient acts as his or her own control.
- A smaller number of patients need to be recruited.
- They require baseline data recording.
- They require data monitoring and recording at the cross-over points.

The disadvantages of cross-over trials include the following.

- There is a possibility of treatment effects carrying over from one period to the other.
- There is a possibility of requiring a washout period between the crossover points.
- They could take a long time to conduct.
- Some types of interventions cannot be studied using this method.

In general, therefore, if you are studying care regimens involving drugs A or B, then one group of patients would receive A then B, and the other group would receive B then A. Figure 20 illustrates this.

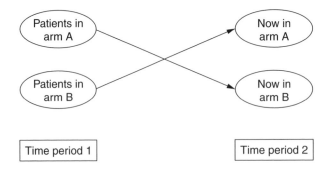

Figure 20 Cross-over trial (simplified).

One of the main issues with cross-over trials is that the effects of one intervention may carry over into the next period in the trial. This makes it difficult to tease out the precise cause of certain effects. Other issues include the length of the washout period, and why a certain length was chosen. *See* **Carry-over effects; Clinical trial; Confounding factor; Cross-over rate; Parallel trial; Preference trial; Run-in period; Sequential trial; Washout period.**

○ Allan L, Hays H, Jensen N-H *et al.* (2001) Randomised cross-over trial of transdermal fentanyl and sustained-release oral morphine for treating chronic non-cancer pain. *BMJ.* **322**: 1154–8.

○ Cromheecke ME, Levi M, Colly LP *et al.* (2000) Oral anticoagulation self-management and management by a specialist anticoagulation clinic: a randomized cross-over comparison. *Lancet.* **356**: 97–102.

○ Engleman HM, Kingshott RN, Wraith PK *et al.* (1999) Randomised placebo-controlled cross-over trial of continuous positive airway pressure for mild sleep apnea/hypopnea syndrome. *Am J Resp Crit Care Med.* **159**: 461–7.

○ Matthews JNS (2000) *An Introduction to Randomized Controlled Clinical Trials.* Edward Arnold, London.

○ Richter B, Bender R and Berger M (2000) Effects of on-demand beta-2-agonist inhalation in moderate to severe asthma. A randomized controlled trial. *J Intern Med.* **247**: 657–66.

○ Senn S (1993) *Cross-over trials in clinical research.* John Wiley & Sons, Chichester.

○ Schrader H, Stovner LJ, Helde G *et al.* (2001) Prophylactic treatment of migraine with angiotensin-converting-enzyme inhibitor (lisinopril): randomised, placebo-controlled crossover study. *BMJ.* **322**: 19–22.

○ Zhu CJ, Wu JF, Qu ZW *et al.* (1999) Bioequivalence evaluation of two sertraline tablet formulations in healthy male volunteers after a single-dose administration. *Int J Pharmacol Ther.* **37**: 120–4.

Cross-sectional study

A cross-sectional study is an analysis of a defined group of subjects at a particular point in time.

The advantages of cross-sectional studies are as follows.

• They can generally be conducted faster and more cheaply than clinical trials.

• They can generate new hypotheses.

The disadvantages of cross-sectional studies are as follows.

• The data that are collected relate to a particular moment in time.

• They do not follow patients through time.

• They cannot be easily used to test a hypothesis.

• There is a lack of generalisabilty.

Recently published examples of cross-sectional studies include the following:

• reporting of epileptic seizures to general practitioners

• error, stress and teamwork in medicine and aviation

• quality of general practitioner consultations

• lifetime prevalence, characteristics and associated problems of non-consensual sex in men

• profiling disability in elderly non-institutionalised people

• breastfeeding and obesity

- role of vaccinations as risk factors for ill health in veterans of a war

- a cross-sectional study of primary care groups in London looking to calculate socio-economic and health status measures and examine the association between these measures and hospital admission rates

- a community-based cross-sectional study in Bristol of the effect of *Helicobacter pylori* infection on blood pressure

- a cross-sectional study evaluating a range of diagnostic tests for risk assessment of left ventricular systolic dysfunction in primary care.

See **Case–control study; Clinical trial; Cohort; Comparing research methods; Fate of clinical research; Prospective study; Research questions and research methods**.

○ de Jonge J, Bosma H, Peter R and Siegrist J (2000) Job strain, effort–reward imbalance and employee well-being: a large-scale cross-sectional study. *Soc Sci Med*. **50**: 1317–27.

○ Majeed A, Bardsley M, Morgan D *et al*. (2000) Cross-sectional study of primary care groups in London: association of measures of socio-economic and health status with hospital admission rates. *BMJ*. **321**: 1057–60.

Cross-validation

Cross-validation is a method of testing the validity of relationships in a clinical trial.

Cross-validation in a clinical trial works as follows.

- The results from the trial are divided into subsets.

- One subset is used to estimate relationships.

- Another subset is used to validate (or not) the estimated relationship.

Figure 21 illustrates this.

Another way to look at cross-validation is as follows. Suppose that you have results from 1000 participants in a clinical trial. You can randomly select 500 records and analyse them, then randomly select another 500 records and analyse those. After this you can compare the results. You do not have to use all of the data – you could have randomly chosen sets of 100 records each. *See* **Data dredging; Hypothesis testing; Split-half method of analysis; Statistical test diagram; Statistical tests: ten ways to cheat with statistical tests**.

Cumulative meta-analysis

Suppose that you have five clinical trials bearing on a particular topic, and it is possible to summarise their results. You consider performing a cumulative meta-analysis. Table 18 shows an example of cumulative meta-analysis.

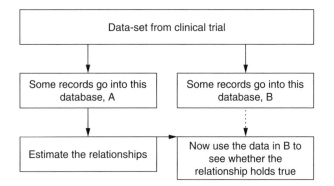

Figure 21 Cross-validation of clinical trial data.

Table 18 Cumulative meta-analysis

Paper	Meta-analysis of:
1	Paper 1
2	Papers 1 and 2
3	Papers 1, 2 and 3
4	Papers 1, 2, 3 and 4
5	Papers 1, 2, 3, 4 and 5

An advantage is that cumulative meta-analysis can show how the conclusions change in the light of new evidence. A disadvantage is that it is not clear how the papers should be ordered, even if we can overcome the inherent problems of adding data together.

The way in which the papers are ordered should be made clear. For example, the order could be determined by the date when the trial results first appeared in a peer-reviewed medical journal, the date when the trials stopped, or the date when the trials started.

One important point to establish is whether the cumulative meta-analysis comes from the original data in the trials or from the data as reported in the published papers. The former usually provide a stronger database from which to work, but may not always be accessible even if they are compatible. *See* **Cochrane Collaboration; Meta-analysis; Sensitivity analysis.**

○ Lau J, Schmid CH and Chalmers TC (1995) Cumulative meta-analysis of clinical trials: builds evidence for exemplary medical care. *J Clin Epidemiol.* **48**: 45–57.

○ Whiting GW, Lau J, Kupelnick B and Chalmers TC (1995) Trends in inflammatory bowel disease therapy: a meta-analytic approach. *Can J Gastroenterol.* **9**: 405–11.

D

Data cleaning

Data cleaning involves the checking of data from clinical trials or clinical practice in terms of inconsistent or erroneous codes and entries. For example, data cleaning can be used to identify negative ages, numbers well away from those expected, or double entries in the database. *See* **Data-monitoring committee; Dirty data**.

Data-display formats

When presenting the results of a clinical trial, there is always a choice of which format to use to present the data.

Elting and colleagues examined the influence of different data-display formats on clinical trialists' decisions as to whether to continue a hypothetical trial or stop for an unplanned statistical analysis. The authors found that more correct decisions were made with icon displays than with tables, pie charts or bar graphs (correct decisions were 82% versus 68%, 56% and 43%, respectively). They also found that more correct decisions were made when the data were framed negatively rather than positively (93% versus 47%).

A data-display format is simply a particular way of displaying data.

Examples of data-display formats include the following:

- tables

- pie charts

- bar graphs

- line graphs

- icon displays.

The term 'data-display format' is of interest in clinical trials for the following reasons.

- The way in which data are presented can affect the way in which they are interpreted, examined and understood.

- Clinical trialists' decisions may be affected by factors that are unrelated to the trial results.

- Decisions in clinical practice may be affected by factors that are unrelated to the actual results.

See **Bias; Clinical trial; Due process; Problems with regard to putting evidence into practice; Research governance in the NHS; Transparency; Ways of presenting results**.

○ Elting LS, Martin CG, Cantor SB and Rubenstein EB (1999) Influence of data-display formats on physician investigators' decisions to stop clinical trials: prospective trial with repeated measures. *BMJ*. **318**: 1527–31.

Data dredging

Data dredging occurs when a database is subject to analysis that was not part of the original clinical trial protocol. Although data dredging sounds somewhat improper and unprofessional, you must remember that the patients underwent the clinical trial in good faith. Data dredging therefore allows greater use of existing data – indeed it may be considered unethical not to do any data dredging. Why is this?

There are several reasons.

- The data exist.

- Much effort goes into collecting the data.

- Collecting trial data is expensive.

- Cleaning that data takes time.

- As much information and analysis as possible should be gleaned from whatever data currently exist.

Key problems include the lack of prior ethical approval, and the possibility that the dredging will turn into data fishing.

Data dredging has been used to analyse international databases on adverse drug reactions, run by the World Health Organisation.

Data dredging is sometimes also called exploratory data analysis or data mining. *See* **Data fishing; Data-monitoring committee; Exploratory data analysis; Protocol; Subgroup analysis**.

○ Coulter DM, Bate A, Meyboom RHB *et al.* (2001) Antipsychotic drugs and heart muscle disorder in international pharmacovigilance: data-mining study. *BMJ*. **322**: 1207–9.

Data fishing

Data fishing is action that seeks to 'get a result' if the analysts try long and hard enough.

With the availability of computerised databases and more sophisticated statistical software packages, data fishing is very easy to do, and is becoming more difficult to detect. *See* **Data dredging; Data-monitoring committee; Multicentre research ethics committee; Protocol; Research governance in the NHS; Statistical test diagram; Statistical tests: ten ways to cheat with statistical tests**.

Data-monitoring committee

A data-monitoring committee is a group of people who have access to the complete data for the clinical trial. The committee can, if necessary, identify which patient received which intervention.

The primary role of this committee is to make recommendations as to whether or not the trial should be continued in its current form. They make their recommendations to the trial steering committee and the principal or lead investigator.

According to the UK's Medical Research Council, membership of data-monitoring and ethics committees should be completely independent of the principal investigators, the trial steering committee and the host institution. What is meant by 'completely independent' and what investigations are undertaken to check 'independence' remain the subject of debate.

Not all clinical trials in the NHS have data-monitoring committees, and some people in the UK and continental Europe are against the existence of such independent data-monitoring committees. One eminent professor has even recently claimed, without supporting evidence, that 'the money spent on data-monitoring committees would be better used to provide more care for patients'.

Remember that more and more people are looking at the evidence from clinical trials. For various reasons, people will want to find a weakness in a particular clinical trial. If they can discount your trial and raise a concern among others because of an issue regarding data monitoring, all of the time and expense involved in performing that trial and all of the goodwill you have established with the patients and the host institution could be completely wasted if it has been compromised in any way. *See* **Accountability; Clinical trial steering committee; Data dredging; Due process; Early stopping rule; Ethics committee; Guidance on good practice in clinical research; Institutional review board; Interim analysis; National Research Register; Research governance in the NHS; Transparency.**

○ deMets DL (2000) Relationships between data-monitoring committees. *Control Clin Trials.* **21**: 54–5.

○ Freidlin B, Korn EL and George SL (1999) Data-monitoring committees and interim monitoring guidelines. *Control Clin Trials.* **20**: 395–407.

○ CL Meinert (1998) Clinical trials and treatment effects monitoring. *Control Clin Trials.* **19**: 515–22.

Data types

One of the key issues when analysing data from clinical trials is to determine what type of data one is dealing with.

The type of data will help to:

- determine what statistical tests can or should be performed on the data

- reveal how the trialists identified, categorised and possibly captured the data.

Data can be either categorical or quantitative. If they are categorical, they may or may not be ordered. If they are quantitative, they may be discrete or continuous. Table 19 shows a simple way to remember the types of data, and also provides examples.

Table 19 Different types of data

Categorical	
Ordinal (ordered)	*Nominal (unordered)*
For example, grade of breast cancer, grade of dementia, agree/indifferent/disagree, better/same/worse	For example, alive or dead, male or female, blood group

Quantitative	
Continuous	*Discrete*
For example, age, body mass, cholesterol level, blood pressure, height, tumour size, weight	For example, the number of offspring, number of asthma attacks in a week, number of epileptic fits in a month

See **Data format; Data-monitoring committee; Scales of measurement; Statistical test diagram; Statistical tests**.

Decision tree

A decision tree is a framework representing choices available, outcomes and probabilities of achieving those outcomes.

Referring to Figure 22, suppose in a clinical trial that the patient could be allocated to one of two alternative courses of action, namely treatment regimen A or treatment regimen B. If they are allocated to regimen A, then they may secure outcome 'O1' with a probability of X, or outcome 'O2' with a probability of $1 - X$ in the clinical trial. However, if they are allocated to regimen B, then they may secure outcome 'O3' with a probability of Y, or outcome 'O4' with a probability of $1 - Y$.

To find out what is the best option, we compare the results of the following:

- $O1 \times X$
- $O2 \times (1 - X)$
- $O3 \times Y$
- $O4 \times (1 - Y)$.

The best option is whichever result is highest.

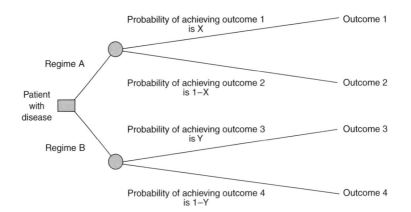

Figure 22 Decision tree.

Decision trees can be used for the following purposes:

- to share knowledge

- to represent issues

- to clarify points

- to encourage debate

- to show what data are required to make a decision

- to open discussion about the difficulties of obtaining those data

- to indicate the treatment paths that patients follow

- to indicate the treatment paths to which patients are allocated

- to improve decision making

- to deceive rather than enlighten (e.g. missing options, incorrect data).

See **Accountability; Clinical practice guidelines; Due process; Evidence-based medicine; Transparency.**

○ Berry DA, Wolff MC and Slack D (1994) Decision making during a phase-III randomised controlled trial. *Control Clin Trials.* **15**: 360–78.

○ Detsky AS, Naglie G, Krahn MD, Redelmeier DA and Naimark D (1997) Primer on medical decision analysis: Part 2. Building a tree. *Med Decis Making.* **17**: 126–35.

○ Enthoven VA, Sowden A and Watt I (1998) Evaluating interventions to promote patient involvement in decision making: by what criteria should effectiveness be judged? *J Health Serv Res Policy.* **3**: 100–7.

○ Lilford RJ, Pauker SG, Braunholtz DA and Chard J (1998) Getting research findings into practice: decision analysis and implementation of research findings. *BMJ.* **317**: 405–9.

○ O'Conner AM, Fiset V, Tetroe JM *et al.* (2000) Decision aids for people facing health treatment or screening. *Cochrane Library.* Update Software, Oxford.

Declaration of Helsinki

The Declaration of Helsinki is a set of recommendations for guiding physicians in biomedical research involving human subjects.

For those who are interested in the development of the Declaration, it was first adopted by the 18th World Medical Association in Helsinki, Finland, in June 1964, and subsequently amended at various times (29th WMA General Assembly in Tokyo, Japan, in October 1975; 35th WMA General Assembly in Venice, Italy, in October 1983; 41st WMA General Assembly in Hong Kong in September 1989; 48th WMA General Assembly in Somerset West, Republic of South Africa, in October 1996; and 52nd WMA General Assembly in Edinburgh, Scotland, in October 2000).

Due to the inexorable rise in interest in clinical trials worldwide, the revised version of the Declaration of Helsinki (Edinburgh edition) is reproduced in its entirety below.

Introduction

1 The World Medical Association has developed the Declaration of Helsinki as a statement of ethical principles to provide guidance to physicians and other participants in medical research involving human subjects. Medical research involving human subjects includes research on identifiable human material or identifiable data.

2 It is the duty of the physician to promote and safeguard the health of the people. The physician's knowledge and conscience are dedicated to the fulfilment of this duty.

3 The Declaration of Geneva of the World Medical Association binds the physician with the words, 'The health of my patient will be my first consideration', and the International Code of Medical Ethics declares that 'A physician shall act only in the patient's interest when providing medical care which might have the effect of weakening the physical and mental condition of the patient'.

4 Medical progress is based on research which ultimately must rest in part on experimentation involving human subjects.

5 In medical research on human subjects, considerations related to the well-being of the human subject should take precedence over the interests of science and society.

6 The primary purpose of medical research involving human subjects is to improve prophylactic, diagnostic and therapeutic procedures and the understanding of the aetiology and pathogenesis of disease. Even the best proven prophylactic, diagnostic and therapeutic methods must continually be challenged through research for their effectiveness, efficiency, accessibility and quality.

7 In current medical practice and in medical research, most prophylactic, diagnostic and therapeutic procedures involve risks and burdens.

continued overleaf

8 Medical research is subject to ethical standards that promote respect for all human beings and protect their health and rights. Some research populations are vulnerable and need special protection. The particular needs of the economically and medically disadvantaged must be recognised. Special attention is also required for those who cannot give or refuse consent for themselves, for those who may be subject to giving consent under duress, for those who will not benefit personally from the research and for those for whom the research is combined with care.

9 Research investigators should be aware of the ethical, legal and regulatory requirements for research on human subjects in their own countries as well as applicable international requirements. No national ethical, legal or regulatory requirement should be allowed to reduce or eliminate any of the protections for human subjects set forth in this Declaration.

Basic principles for all medical research

10 It is the duty of the physician in medical research to protect the life, health, privacy and dignity of the human subject.

11 Medical research involving human subjects must conform to generally accepted scientific principles, be based on a thorough knowledge of the scientific literature, other relevant sources of information and on adequate laboratory and, where appropriate, animal experimentation.

12 Appropriate caution must be exercised in the conduct of research which may affect the environment, and the welfare of animals used for research must be respected.

13 The design and performance of each experimental procedure involving human subjects should be clearly formulated in an experimental protocol. This protocol should be submitted for consideration, comment, guidance and, where appropriate, approval to a specially appointed ethical review committee, which must be independent of the investigator, the sponsor or any other kind of undue influence. This independent committee should be in conformity with the laws and regulations of the country in which the research experiment is performed. The committee has the right to monitor ongoing trials. The researcher has the obligation to provide monitoring information to the committee, especially any serious adverse events. The researcher should also submit to the committee, for review, information regarding funding, sponsors, institutional affiliations, other potential conflicts of interest and incentives for subjects.

14 The research protocol should always contain a statement of the ethical considerations involved, and should indicate that there is compliance with the principles enunciated in this Declaration.

15 Medical research involving human subjects should be conducted only by scientifically qualified persons and under the supervision of a clinically competent medical person. The responsibility for the human subject must always rest with a medically qualified person and never rest on the subject of the research, even though the subject has given consent.

continued opposite

16 Every medical research project involving human subjects should be preceded by careful assessment of predictable risks and burdens in comparison with foreseeable benefits to the subject or to others. This does not preclude the participation of healthy volunteers in medical research. The design of all studies should be publicly available.

17 Physicians should abstain from engaging in research projects involving human subjects unless they are confident that the risks involved have been adequately assessed and can be satisfactorily managed. Physicians should cease any investigation if the risks are found to outweigh the potential benefits or if there is conclusive proof of positive and beneficial results.

18 Medical research involving human subjects should only be conducted if the importance of the objective outweighs the inherent risks and burdens to the subject. This is especially important when the human subjects are healthy volunteers.

19 Medical research is only justified if there is a reasonable likelihood that the populations in which the research is carried out stand to benefit from the results of the research.

20 The subjects must be volunteers and informed participants in the research project.

21 The right of research subjects to safeguard their integrity must always be respected. Every precaution should be taken to respect the privacy of the subject and the confidentiality of the patient's information, and to minimise the impact of the study on the subject's physical and mental integrity and on the personality of the subject.

22 In any research on human beings, each potential subject must be adequately informed of the aims, methods, sources of funding, any possible conflicts of interest, the institutional affiliations of the researcher, the anticipated benefits and potential risks of the study and the discomfort it may entail. The subject should be informed of the right to abstain from participation in the study or to withdraw consent to participate at any time without reprisal. After ensuring that the subject has understood the information, the physician should then obtain the subject's freely given informed consent, preferably in writing. If the consent cannot be obtained in writing, the non-written consent must be formally documented and witnessed.

23 When obtaining informed consent for the research project the physician should be particularly cautious if the subject is in a dependent relationship with the physician or may consent under duress. In that case the informed consent should be obtained by a well-informed physician who is not engaged in the investigation and who is completely independent of this relationship.

24 For a research subject who is legally incompetent, physically or mentally incapable of giving consent or is a legally incompetent minor, the investigator must obtain informed consent from the legally authorised representative in accordance with applicable law. These groups should not be included in research unless the research is necessary to promote the health of the population represented and this research cannot instead be performed on legally competent persons.

continued overleaf

25 When a subject who is deemed legally incompetent, such as a minor child, is able to give assent to decisions about participation in research, the investigator must obtain that assent in addition to the consent of the legally authorised representative.

26 Research on individuals from whom it is not possible to obtain consent, including proxy or advance consent, should be done only if the physical/mental condition that prevents obtaining informed consent is a necessary characteristic of the research population. The specific reasons for involving research subjects with a condition that renders them unable to give informed consent should be stated in the experimental protocol for consideration and approval of the review committee. The protocol should state that consent to remain in the research should be obtained as soon as possible from the individual or a legally authorised surrogate.

27 Both authors and publishers have ethical obligations. In publication of the results of research, the investigators are obliged to preserve the accuracy of the results. Negative as well as positive results should be published or otherwise publicly available. Sources of funding, institutional affiliations and any possible conflicts of interest should be declared in the publication. Reports of experimentation not in accordance with the principles laid down in this Declaration should not be accepted for publication.

Additional principles for medical research combined with medical care

28 The physician may combine medical research with medical care only to the extent that the research is justified by its potential prophylactic, diagnostic or therapeutic value. When medical research is combined with medical care, additional standards apply to protect the patients who are research subjects.

29 The benefits, risks, burdens and effectiveness of a new method should be tested against those of the best current prophylactic, diagnostic and therapeutic methods. This does not exclude the use of placebo, or no treatment, in studies where no proven prophylactic, diagnostic or therapeutic method exists.

30 At the conclusion of the study, every patient entered into the study should be assured of access to the best-proven prophylactic, diagnostic and therapeutic methods identified by the study.

31 The physician should fully inform the patient which aspects of the care are related to the research. The refusal of a patient to participate in a study must never interfere with the patient–physician relationship.

32 In the treatment of a patient, where proven prophylactic, diagnostic and therapeutic methods do not exist or have been ineffective, the physician, with informed consent from the patient, must be free to use unproven or new prophylactic, diagnostic and therapeutic measures, if in the physician's judgement these offer hope of saving life, re-establishing health or alleviating suffering. Where possible, these measures should be made the object of research designed to evaluate their safety and efficacy. In all cases, new information should be recorded and, where appropriate, published. The other relevant guidelines of this Declaration should be followed.

Further details are available at the World Medical Association website (www.wma.net).

From previous experience, you may have been tempted to skip some of the content in the above Declaration. If you have, you are not doing yourself or your profession any favours. Read through it again and write down at the side of the page one example for each issue raised in the Declaration.

It is only by doing this at least once that you will gain a pretty clear understanding of the seriousness with which medical research should be undertaken. It may be worth asking some of your colleagues to share their examples with you. *See* **Assent; Belmont Report; Consent; Equipoise; Ethical issues; Institutional review board; Local research ethics committee; Medical Research Council Guidelines for Good Practice in Clinical Trials; Multicentre research ethics committee; Preference trial; Research governance in the NHS**.

○ Altman DG (1994) The scandal of poor medical research. *BMJ*. **308**: 283–4.

○ Anon. (1999) Declaration of Helsinki – nothing to declare? *Lancet*. **353**: 1285.

○ Christie B (2000) Doctors revise Declaration of Helsinki. *BMJ*. **321**: 913.

○ Ferriman A (2001) WMA agree to refine changes to Declaration of Helsinki. *BMJ*. **322**: 1142.

Deferred consent

Deferred consent is consent that is sought and given after the patient has been allocated to a particular regimen of the trial or after the regimen has started.

Deferred consent is generally best avoided in clinical trials, as it raises a tangle of clinical, moral, ethical, professional and, increasingly, legal concerns.

There is also the issue of patient entrapment. The patient's decision may be affected by their current state (e.g. already allocated or in an arm of the trial). In practice, it may be difficult to free the patient from their position. The patient may be more likely to consent if they are already somewhere in the trial. Their position affects their judgement. Your local clinical trial ethics review board should be contacted for guidance on what to do. However, if it was the same board that gave the go-ahead for the trial without patient consent, consider also going to another review board for a second opinion. Do not worry about offending the local review board's feelings – they themselves will be delighted to have a second opinion on what to do. *See* **Consent; Equipoise; Ethical issues; Local research ethics committee; Multicentre research ethics committee; Questions to ask before getting involved in a clinical trial**.

Definitive clinical trial

A definitive clinical trial is a trial that is intended to answer an important question, significantly changing practice or understanding. Some argue that this term is best avoided, even though many leading researchers who are running a clinical trial, or looking for funding for a trial, claim (and continue to do so) that their trial is definitive. The questions then are how definitive it is, and to whom it is really definitive. *See* **Clinical trial; Comparing research methods; Duhem's irrefutability** theory; Falsificationism; Lakatosian research programme; Mega-trial; Primary question; Problems with regard to putting evidence into practice; Research questions and research methods.

Delphi technique

This involves methods of reaching a consensus on a particular question by using a group of people who review the evidence, issues and arguments in an iterative manner until a consensus is reached. Thus they operate in stages or rounds in an effort to achieve convergence of opinion on a particular issue. *See* **Advantages of evidence from clinical trials; Focus group; Qualitative research; Research questions and research methods.**

○ Barbour RS (2001) Checklists for improving rigour in qualitative research: a case of the tail wagging the dog? *BMJ.* **322**: 1115–17.

○ Giacomini MK (2001) The rocky road: qualitative research as evidence. *Evidence-Based Med.* **6**: 406.

○ Goodare H and Smith R (1995) The rights of patients in research. *BMJ.* **310**: 1277–8.

○ Greenhalgh T and Taylor R (1997) Papers that go beyond numbers (qualitative research). *BMJ.* **315**: 740–3.

○ Kitzinger J (1995) Introducing focus groups. *BMJ.* **311**: 299–302.

○ Pope C and Mays N (eds) (2000) *Qualitative Research in Health Care.* BMJ Books, London.

○ Singer PA (2000) Recent advances: medical ethics. *BMJ.* **321**: 282–5.

Demographic profile

A demographic profile is a list of attributes of a population. Age, gender, fertility, birth rates, mortality, health status, and incidence and prevalence of diseases are standard elements of demographic profiles. Some of these attributes are identified and used in clinical trials. *See* **Baseline; Entry criteria; Multilevel modelling.**

Demonstrative trial

Another term for a feasibility trial or pilot trial. *See* **Feasibility trial.**

Derogation

Derogation occurs when a person or organisation legitimately exercises an option not to comply with certain rules and regulations that would otherwise affect them. *See* **Care path; Declaration of Helsinki; Discretion; Duration; Protocol; Research governance in the NHS.**

Dirty data

Dirty data is a collection of data that has not been cleaned, checked or edited, and may therefore contain errors and omissions. *See* **Data cleaning.**

Disadvantages of evidence from clinical trials

For various reasons, more and more attention is being focused on clinical trials as a source of evidence.

Today, when you make a decision, someone is more likely than ever to ask you where the evidence is to support that decision. Even if you have that evidence, you may be cross-examined on it. Therefore it will be useful to understand the main limitations of evidence derived from clinical trials.

Table 20 provides an indication of the key disadvantages of evidence derived from clinical trials.

Table 20 Ten disadvantages of securing and using evidence from clinical trials

1	Trial patients are not representative of general patients.
2	Trial centres and physicians are not representative of all centres or physicians.
3	Trials have strong entry and exclusion criteria.
4	Patient monitoring in trials is not the same as monitoring in practice.
5	Health professionals may not act as they would in practice.
6	Information systems and data gathering differ from those in practice.
7	Placebos do not reflect a realistic or practical option in practice.
8	Outcomes may not be the same as those found in practice.
9	Statistically significant results do not mean that the results are clinically important.
10	Trial periods are relatively short.

Therefore you must think about the limitations of the evidence if you are receiving summaries of evidence from the following:

- colleagues in a committee

- others in practice

- conferences, symposia, workshops or educational meetings

- sales executives

- agents of the government advising on practice

- professional bodies

- consultancies.

Get two of your colleagues together for a working lunch one day next week. Your joint task is to look at one recently published clinical trial and reflect on your own experiences. Then at the working lunch use Table 20 above to identify whether or not each limitation applies to the evidence.

In everyday practice you should not expect other people to determine the disadvantages or limitations of evidence from any clinical trial. It is important to find out for yourself.

Remember to keep a sense of balance because, just as there is a set of disadvantages of evidence derived from clinical trials, so there is also a set of advantages. *See* **Advantages of evidence from clinical trials; Clinical trial; External validity of clinical trial results; Meta-analysis; Multicentre research ethics committee; Problems with regard to putting evidence into practice; Protocol; Questions to ask before getting involved in a clinical trial; Research governance in the NHS; Systematic review; Transparency.**

○ Earl-Slater A (2001) Critical appraisal of clinical trials: advantages and disadvantages of evidence from clinical trials. *J Clin Govern.* **6**: 136–9.

Discretion

Discretion is a decision made outside the strict bounds of the rules of a decision-making framework. *See* **Accountability; Derogation; Due process; European Union Directive on clinical trials of medicinal products for humans; Institutional review board; Local research ethics committee; Multicentre research ethics committee; Research governance in the NHS; Transparency.**

Documentary analysis

Documentary analysis is the study of documents in terms of the following:

- source

- date

- targeted audience

- content

- logic

- strengths and weaknesses.

Sources of documents include, for example, government, regulatory, company, individual or academic bodies, proceedings of conferences or symposia, professional bodies, patient advocacy groups and charitable bodies.

The documents may or may not be in the public domain.

The advantages of documentary research and analysis include the following:

- their non-reactivity with the investigator

- the permanence of the records

- their accessibility (in general).

The disadvantages of documentary analysis include the following:

- questions about their authenticity and accuracy

- questions of interpretation

- questions of completeness

- the fact that no document provides a complete and accurate representation of the phenomenon of interest

- few documents indicate their process of construction

- they are time dependent and often become out of date.

See **Pooled analysis; Qualitative analysis; Systematic review; Transparency.**

Dose comparison trial

This is a trial that compares different doses of a medicine.

In the general type of dose comparison trial, different groups of patients are given different doses of the drug at the same time (see the example by Black and colleagues referred to below).

Sometimes the term is more loosely used when the same group of people are given different doses of the drug at different times in the clinical trial (more accurately this is called a titration trial).

Recent examples of dose comparisons include the following:

- the study reported by Black and colleagues, on a multicentre placebo-controlled dose comparison trial of oral iloprost in patients with Raynaud's phenomenon secondary to systemic sclerosis

- the study by Packer and colleagues of high-dose lisinopril compared with low-dose lisinopril for reducing combined mortality and cardiovascular events in patients with congestive heart failure

- Annand and Yusuf's meta-analysis of randomised trials of high-dose and moderate-dose oral anticoagulants in patients with coronary artery disease.

Dose comparison trials (also often called dose-ranging trials) are used to establish the optimum doses of the drug for particular patients. For example, Stevenson and colleagues used a dose-ranging randomised trial to study the efficacy and safety of cyclosporin A ophthalmic emulsion in the treatment of moderate to severe dry eye disease. *See* **Dose escalation; Dose response; Subgroup analysis; Titration.**

○ Anand SS and Yusuf S (1999) Oral anticoagulation therapy in patients with coronary artery disease: a meta-analysis. *JAMA.* **282**: 2058–67.

○ Black CM, Halkier-Sorensen L, Belch JJ *et al.* (1998) Oral iloprost in Raynaud's phenomenon secondary to systemic sclerosis: a multicentre placebo-controlled dose comparison study. *Br J Rheumatol.* **37**: 952–60.

○ Packer M, Poole-Wilson PA, Armstrong PW *et al.* on behalf of the ATLAS Study Group (1999) Comparative effects of low and high doses of the angiotensin-converting-enzyme inhibitor lisinopril on morbidity and mortality in chronic heart failure. *Circulation.* **100**: 2312–18.

○ Stevenson D, Tauber J and Reis BL (2000) Efficacy and safety of cyclosporin A ophthalmic emulsion in the treatment of moderate to severe dry eye disease: a dose-ranging randomized trial. The Cyclosporin A Phase 2 Study Group. *Ophthalmology.* **107**: 967–74.

Dose escalation

Dose escalation occurs when the dose given in a clinical trial is increased. For example, you may wish to find out how toxicity and safety change as the dose of a particular drug is increased.

This is particularly important when you are assessing an appropriate dosage for the medication during, say, a phase 1 trial. *See* **Dose comparison trial; Dose response; Phase 1 clinical trial; Titration**.

Dose response

The dose response is the change in measured outcome that results from a change in the dose administered.

For some drugs the response does not continue after a particular dose. Usually there is a ceiling above which an increase in the dose does not produce any corresponding change in outcome.

For example, Johnson and colleagues sought to establish whether a dose–response relationship existed for aspirin in patients with a history of previous transient ischaemic attack or stroke. *See* **Dose escalation; Dose comparison trial; J-shaped distribution**.

○ Johnson ES, Lanes SF, Wentworth CE *et al.* (1999) A metaregression analysis of the dose–response effect of aspirin on stroke. *Arch Intern Med.* **159**: 1248–53.

Double-blind trial

A double-blind trial is generally one in which two parties to the trial are blind as to what certain patients are receiving or have received. Usually the two blinded parties are the patients themselves and the doctors, but sometimes the two blinded parties are the patient and the data analyst.

One reason for blinding the patient is to dilute performance bias. For example, if they find out that they are on the new experimental regimen, they may believe that 'new' is better and this may have an effect on the results of the trial.

One reason for blinding the doctor is to dilute allocation bias (i.e. they may otherwise allocate certain patients to certain regimens which they think will be best for the patients).

Double-blind trials do need close attention because the 'blindness' implies a large degree of ignorance of the specific intervention involved. *See* **Bias; Blind; Blinding; Quadruple-blind trial; Single-blind trial; Triple-blind trial.**

Dropout

A dropout is a patient who, for whatever reason(s), fails to continue in a study and leaves without permission. The patient may for instance:

- become dissatisfied with the trial

- leave the area

- experience changes in home and family circumstances.

Trial managers cannot force anyone to stay in a trial and the reason(s) for dropping out should wherever possible be established. Sometimes the term 'dropout' is used as an impolite way of saying 'withdrawal' but it may be better to say that 'withdrawals' leave with permission, whereas dropouts don't. *See* **Analysis by assigned treatment; Audit; CONSORT; Intention-to-treat analysis; Lost; Withdrawal.**

Due process

Due process occurs when a decision maker explicitly states the following:

- what their decision is

- how they reached it

- what the benefits will be

- what the cost will be

- what resources (e.g. staff and equipment) will be required.

See **Accountability; Clinical trial steering committee; Data-monitoring committee; Evidence-based medicine; Systematic review; Transparency.**

Duhem's irrefutability theory

Duhem's irrefutability theory is that no hypothesis can be comprehensively falsified or refuted, as any particular hypothesis always has a series of auxiliary conditions or underlying hypotheses, in that no one can ever be sure of the exact location of any refutation. Thus refutation is not definite. Figure 23 gives an example of this.

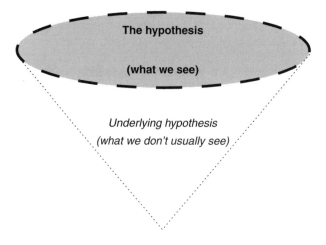

Figure 23 Duhem's irrefutability theory.

If the results of a randomised clinical trial comparing a new drug with current best practice suggest that the new drug is more cost-effective than current best practice, then according to Duhem's irrefutability theory one cannot conclude without reservation that the new drug is more cost-effective than current best practice. *See* **Bayesian analysis; Hypothesis testing; Lakatosian's hard-core, protective belt**.

E

Early stopping rule

An early stopping rule is a predefined rule in a clinical trial that sets out the conditions under which the trial would be prematurely stopped.

There are very few, if any, occasions when a clinical trial should be stopped on the basis of statistical results alone.

Examples of the early stopping rule include the following.

- The HOPE trial was stopped early after planned interim analysis showed the merits of one intervention over another in high-risk patients.

- Kearon and colleagues addressed the question of whether or not extended prophylaxis with warfarin reduced the rate of recurrence of venous thrombo-embolism, deep venous thrombosis and pulmonary embolism in patients who had had a first episode of idiopathic venous thromboembolism. The trial was stopped early when a highly favourable effect was shown at a planned interim analysis.

- The trial reported by Hjalmarson and colleagues was designed to determine whether in patients with symptomatic chronic heart failure, controlled- and extended-release metoprolol succinate reduced mortality, symptoms and hospital admission. This trial was stopped early because interim analysis showed a 34% reduction in mortality.

See **Data-monitoring committee; Interim analysis; Multiple endpoints; Statistical test diagram; Statistical tests: ten ways to cheat with statistical tests; Stopping rules**.

○ Heart Outcomes Prevention Evaluation Study Investigators (HOPE) (2000) Effects of an angiotensin-converting-enzyme inhibitor, ramipril, on death from cardiovascular causes, myocardial infarction and stroke in high-risk patients. *NEJM*. **342**: 145–53.

○ Hjalmarson A, Goldstein S, Fagerberger B *et al*. for the MERIT-HF Study Group (2000) Effects of controlled-release metoprolol on total mortality, hospitalizations and well-being in patients with heart failure: the Metoprolol CR/XL Randomized Intervention Trial in Congestive Heart Failure (MERIT-HF). *JAMA*. **283**: 1295–302.

○ Kearon C, Gent M, Hirsh J *et al*. (1999) A comparison of three months of anticoagulation with extended anticoagulations for a first episode of idiopathic venous thromboembolism. *NEJM*. **340**: 901–7.

○ Meinert CL (1998) Clinical trials and treatment effects monitoring. *Control Clin Trials*. **19**: 515–22.

○ O'Neill R (1994) Early stopping rules workshop: conclusion. *Stat Med*. 13: 1493–9.

Economic analysis and clinical trials

Every clinical trial has economic implications, but relatively few clinical trials involve formal economic analysis.

In a 1994 report from the Department of Health, Professor Michael Peckham, then Director of Research and Development, stated that 'the requirement of the NHS for sound information on cost-effectiveness is such that trials which do not include an economic component should not be conducted by or in the NHS without a valid reason'. As yet neither the reformed ethics committees in the NHS nor the trial sponsors have put in place a mandatory requirement for economic analysis to be in any way part of a clinical trial. In fact, there is no mention of any such economic requirement or move towards it in the recently announced overarching European Union's Directive on clinical trials in human subjects, or in the international guidelines on clinical trials. So is economic analysis in clinical trials a barren field? The answer is not quite.

From another quarter there is a growing emphasis on the economic implications of products and services. For example, in the UK this comes from the National Institute for Clinical Excellence, which is looking at the clinical and economic implications of products, services and health technologies. Across the world, health-care purchasers are in various ways increasingly demanding economic evidence as well as clinical evidence to help to formulate their decisions.

Table 21 provides an overview of some of the key issues that you need to tackle if you want to integrate economic analysis into a clinical trial, or to run economic analysis parallel to the clinical trial or (less useful but more common) to add on economic analysis after the trial has been completed.

The assumptions in the trial and the measures of outcomes help to predetermine what form of economic analysis will be appropriate.

Despite what some people think and others would have us believe, placebo-controlled trials may still have economic analysis integrated into their design. Why is this? It would give a benchmark measure of the economic merits of the 'active' intervention. It would also provide valuable experience and a real example of the practical issues relating to economic data collection and analysis. However, if you had a trial with economics of A versus placebo, and A was found to be more cost-effective than placebo, and another trial with B versus placebo, and B was found to be more cost-effective than placebo, can the economic merits of A be compared with those of B? That is a question which has yet to be more formally answered.

As noted above, economic analysis usually occurs, if it occurs at all, after the trial has been completed. Reality increasingly shows that this late approach involves the same problems and risks as the practice of collecting patient and clinical data without first having sought the advice of a statistician. *See* **Advantages of evidence from clinical trials; Analytic perspective; Causes of delay and failure to complete a clinical trial; Comparing research methods; Disadvantages of evidence from**

Table 21 Economic analysis and clinical trials: issues to consider

Assessing whether an economic analysis should be conducted alongside a trial

Is the trial well designed and capable of giving an unbiased and unambiguous answer to a clearly defined clinical question?

Are the two or more interventions of greatly different cost likely to be widely applied?

Are there critical aspects of economic benefit that are not being fully explored by the trial (e.g. trade-offs between efficacy and side-effects)?

Is current practice one of the alternatives being compared?

Is the trial being conducted in a typical setting, and will the results be generalisable?

Will the addition of economic data collection seriously overburden investigators or patients?

Forms of economic evaluation

Cost-minimisation analysis: assumes that the all-important outcomes of the alternatives being studied are the same, or not significantly different

Cost-effectiveness analysis: outcomes from the interventions are not equal. Outcomes are measured in natural units (e.g. cholesterol level, lumbar flexion, stroke occurrence, number of lives saved)

Cost-benefit analysis: outcomes from the interventions are not equal. Outcomes are measured in monetary units (e.g. what is the monetary value of saving a life from regimen A compared to regimen B?)

Cost-utility analysis: outcomes are not the same. Outcomes are measured in terms of utility

Deciding which of the four forms of economic evaluation to use

Is the hypothesis of the trial that two or more interventions will be equivalent? Try cost-minimisation.

Is the hypothesis that the outcomes are not the same, but are measured in natural units? Try cost-effectiveness analysis.

Is the hypothesis that the outcomes are not the same, but are measured in monetary units? Try cost-benefit analysis.

Is the hypothesis that the outcomes are not the same, but are measured in units of utility? Try cost-utility analysis.

Deciding on economic data collection needs: questions to attend to

Costs

What costs do you need to collect?

How can they be collected?

When can they be collected?

How do the costs vary between settings?

Who actually incurs these costs (e.g. the hospital, doctor, social services, patient)?

When are the costs incurred?

continued overleaf

Table 21 continued

Outcomes
  What outcomes are being measured?
  How are they being measured?
  When are they being measured?
  Who is measuring them?
  When do the outcomes arise?
  How do the outcomes vary across settings or patients?
  How do proxy or surrogate outcomes relate to final outcomes?

Do you need qualitative as well as quantitative analysis?
  If so, what is being analysed or measured, where, when, how and by whom?

What analytic perspective are you taking?
  For example, are you working out from the clinician's perspective, the patient's perspective or a
  wider societal perspective?

  What allowances are being made for imprecision, missing data and uncertainty?

  What allowances are being made for differences in the time profiles of the costs and outcomes?

What effects do you need to consider for the statistics?
  For example, effects on power, sample size or interim analysis

*What adjustments need to be made to make the trial applicable to the clinical and economic setting of
practitioners?*

What are the ethical implications of bringing in economic considerations?

---

clinical trials; European Union Directive on clinical trials of medicinal products for humans; Fate of research studies; Local research ethics committee; Multicentre research ethics committee; National Institute for Clinical Excellence; Outcomes pyramid; Primary outcome; Primary research question; Problems with regard to putting evidence into practice; Reasons given by the investigator for a study being abandoned or in abeyance; Reasons given by the investigator for a study never being started; Research governance in the NHS; Research questions and research methods; Secondary outcome; Types of research questions; Value-for-money table.

○ Altman DG (1994) The scandal of poor medical research. *BMJ*. **308**: 283–4.

○ Briggs A (2000) Economic evaluation and clinical trials: size matters. *BMJ*. **321**: 1362–3.

○ Craig A-M and Kennedy L (2001) Health economic considerations for early drug discovery. *Drug Discov World*. **Summer**: 57–61 (www.ddd-online.com).

○ Drummond M (1994) *Economic Analysis Alongside Controlled Trials*. Department of Health, London.

○ Earl-Slater A (1999) *Dictionary of Health Economics*. Radcliffe Medical Press, Oxford.

○ Earl-Slater A (2002) Critical appraisal of clinical trials: economic analysis and clinical trials. *J Clin Govern*. In press.

○ Strobl J, Cave E and Walley T (2000) Data protection legislation: interpretation and barriers to research. *BMJ*. **321**: 890–2.

Effect

An effect is a consequence – a result of something. Whether or not the trial analysts can determine more precisely what that 'something' is depends on many factors. Whether they can prove causality is a subtle but important challenge for analysts. Remember that evidence of no effect is not the same as no evidence of an effect. *See* **Association; Causal relationship; Effect modifiers; Statistical test diagram; Systematic review**.

Effect modifiers

Effect modifiers are those factors that can or do alter the effect of an intervention.
   For example:

• the effect of a bronchodilator for asthma is likely to be reduced in asthmatic patients who also have peptic ulcers (whether or not the ulcers are known to exist)

• some anti-obesity drugs allegedly modify the effects of warfarin.

See **Causal relationship; Confounding factor; Effect; Factor analysis**.

Effect size

The effect size is simply the size of the effect that occurs in a trial. It may or may not be directly caused by the intervention in the trial. *See* **Effect; Effect modifiers; Funnel plot; Primary outcome**.

Effectiveness trial

An effectiveness trial is a clinical trial that is said to approximate to reality (i.e. clinical practice). It is sometimes called a pragmatic trial. Its main limitation is that the area of reality it seeks to approximate may not in fact be common practice. *See* **Clinical trial; Duhem's irrefutability theory; Efficacy trial; Falsificationism; Lakatosian research programme; Preferential trial; Questions to ask before getting involved in a clinical trial**.

Efficacy

Efficacy is the degree to which an intervention does what it is intended to do under ideal conditions. *See* **Effectiveness trial; Efficacy trial; Randomised controlled trial**.

Efficacy trial

An efficacy trial is a clinical trial that is said to take place under ideal conditions (ideal in the sense of control, monitoring and assessment). The term is sometimes used to categorise all clinical trials that are stylised and which do not approximate to the reality of clinical practice. *See* **Advantages of evidence from clinical trials; Clinical trial; Efficacy; Effectiveness trial; Gold standard; Pragmatic clinical trial; Randomised controlled trial.**

Elasticity

Elasticity is a measure of the responsiveness of one factor to changes in another (e.g. the change in cancer cell growth in response to changes in the administration of a medication). *See* **Dose comparison trial; Dose response; Sensitivity analysis.**

Eligibility

Eligibility means being suitable to be chosen. *See* **Case finding; Consent; Eligibility criteria.**

Eligibility criteria

Eligibility criteria are the same as entry criteria. *See* **Entry criteria; Exclusion criteria.**

Endpoint

An endpoint is a clearly defined point of focus for the clinical trial. For example, the 5-year survival rate is a common endpoint in breast cancer treatment trials.

It is vital for the running and credibility of the trial to include valid and measurable endpoints, and to explain the choice. *See* **Data dredging; Primary endpoint; Surrogate endpoint.**

Entry criteria

Entry criteria are the factors that allow a person to become part of a particular clinical trial.

These criteria could be based on various grounds, including the following:

- medical grounds
- scientific grounds
- administrative grounds
- age
- race

- gender

- location.

Some examples of entry criteria are listed below.

- Dammers and colleagues reported on a study of the effectiveness of a methylprednisolone injection in patients with carpal tunnel syndrome. Their entry criteria specified that patients had to be over 18 years of age, and had to have had signs and symptoms of carpal tunnel syndrome for 3 months or more, confirmed by electrophysiological tests. Patients who had already been treated for carpal tunnel syndrome were excluded.

- Jacobs and colleagues reported on a randomised placebo-controlled trial with a 3-year follow-up to determine whether interferon beta-1a reduced the incidence of clinically definite multiple sclerosis in patients with a first confirmed demyelinating event. Entry criteria were age 18–50 years, first acute clinical demyelinating event confirmed by magnetic resonance imaging, involvement of the optic nerve, spinal cord, brainstem or cerebellum, two or more clinically silent brain lesions 3 mm or more in diameter, and symptom onset less than 14 days after corticosteroid treatment and less than 27 days after randomisation.

- Leone and colleagues reported on a randomised placebo-controlled trial with a 2-week follow-up on the effectiveness of verapamil as prophylaxis for episodic cluster headache. Entry criteria included outpatients with a diagnosis of episodic cluster headache (International Headache Society criteria) with one or more previous clusters lasting one or more months, and who had been in a cluster period for no more than 10 days and had an expected duration of the remainder of the cluster period of 20 days or more.

- Rovers and colleagues reported on a randomised unblinded controlled trial with 12-month follow-up of children with persistent otitis media with effusion. They wanted to determine the effect of ventilation tubes on quality of life at age 1–2 years. Entry criteria included children who had persistent otitis media with effusions confirmed by tympanometry and otoscopy.

See **Consent; Eligibility criteria; Equipoise; Exclusion criteria; Generalisability of trial results; Inclusion criteria; Uncertainty.**

○ Dammers JW, Veering MM and Vermeulen M (1999) Injection with methylprednisolone proximal to the carpal tunnel: randomised double-blind trial. *BMJ*. **319**: 884–6.

○ Jacobs LD, Beck RW, Simon JH *et al.* and the CHAMPS Study Group (2000) Intramuscular interferon beta-1a therapy initiated during first demyelinating event in multiple sclerosis. *NEJM*. **343**: 898–904.

○ Leone M, D'Amico D, Frediani F *et al.* (2000) Verapamil in the prophylaxis of episodic cluster headache: a double-blind study versus placebo. *Neurology*. **54**: 1382–5.

○ Rovers MM, Krabbe PF, Straatman H *et al.* (2001) Randomised controlled trial of the effect of ventilation tubes on quality of life at age 1–2 years. *Arch Dis Child*. **84**: 45–9.

Equipoise

Equipoise has been defined as a group's position of genuine uncertainty or indifference.

If as a group you are in a position of equipoise with regard to treatment options for a particular patient, then this really means that you as a group have no prior knowledge, evidence or understanding of what option would be best for that patient.

If your group is not in a position of equipoise (i.e. it has an idea that one option would be better than another for a particular patient in hand), then the option must be recommended to the patient unless there are other reasons for not recommending it.

Being in a position of equipoise means that subject entry is possible in a clinical trial. If the group is not in a position of equipoise for a particular patient, that patient should not be entered into the trial.

Some authors suggest that equipoise only applies to groups of people and not to individuals. However, breaking this down means that each individual in the group must be in a position of equipoise before they invite the patient into the trial. If the term equipoise does apply to a group, this may create legal, ethical and professional difficulty in attributing responsibility. Why is this? It is usually the consultant or doctor who is ultimately responsible for the welfare of the patient, and not the group.

Another issue that has yet to be resolved is the fact that different people attach different meanings and interpretations to the term equipoise in healthcare. For example, Professor Lilford has argued that equipoise and uncertainty are not mutually exclusive. Professor Richard Lilford's and David Sackett's writings on the matter are particularly helpful here.

If you see the term equipoise, ask the following questions.

- What does it mean?

- To whom does it apply?

- How did they get into that position (i.e. their evidence base and reasoning)?

See **Bayesian analysis; Clinical trial; Declaration of Helsinki; Due process; Evidence-based medicine; Randomisation; Uncertainty.**

○ Bradford Hill A (1963) Medical ethics and controlled trials. *BMJ.* **2**: 1043–9.

○ Edwards SJL, Lilford RJ, Braunholtz DA *et al.* (1998) Ethical issues in the design and conduct of randomized controlled trials. *Health Technol Assess.* **2**: 1–130.

○ Freedman B (1987) Equipoise and the ethics of clinical research. *NEJM.* **317**: 141–5.

○ Lilford RJ and Jackson G (1995) Equipoise and the ethics of randomisation. *J R Soc Med.* **88**: 552–9.

○ Lilford RJ and Djulbegovic B (2001) Equipoise and uncertainty are not mutually exclusive. *BMJ.* **322**: 795.

○ Sackett DL (2001) There is another exchange on equipoise and uncertainty. *BMJ.* **322**: 795.

○ Sackett DL (2000) Equipoise, a term whose time (if ever it came) has surely gone. *Can Med Assoc J.* **163**: 835–6.

○ Weijer C, Shapiro S, Glass K and Enkin M (2000) For and against: clinical equipoise and not the uncertainty principle is the moral underpinning of the randomised controlled trial. *BMJ.* **321**: 756–8.

Equipotent dose

An equipotent dose is either:

• a dose of one medicine that produces the same response as another medicine *or*

• two different doses of one particular medicine that produce the same effect.

See **Dose comparison trial; Equivalence trial.**

Equivalence trial

Equivalence trials seek to determine whether particular interventions are equivalent (*see* Figure 24).

Equivalence is often in terms of bioavailability, but it could relate to any outcome in the clinical trial (e.g. lives saved, strokes avoided, ulcer healing rate). Figure 24 provides a simple illustration of this.

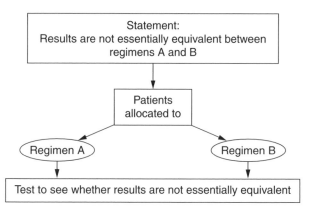

Figure 24 Equivalence trial.

For example:

• Zhu and colleagues conducted a bioequivalence cross-over trial of two sertraline tablet formulations in healthy male volunteers after a single dose of administration

- Weins and Iglewicz reported on a design and analysis of three treatment equivalence trials
- Schnitzer and colleagues reported on the therapeutic equivalence of alendronate 70 mg once weekly and alendronate 10 mg daily in the treatment of osteoporosis
- Stewart and colleagues reported on a demonstration of *in-vivo* bioequivalence of a generic albuterol metered-dose inhaler to ventolin.

Predefinition of a trial as an equivalence trial is necessary for a number of reasons, including the following:

- to set up the proper hypothesis (the null hypothesis should be that there is a difference)
- to ensure that the comparison treatments, doses, patient populations and end-points are appropriate
- to allow proper power calculations to be performed
- to ensure that the equivalence criteria are predefined
- to permit appropriate clinical and statistical analysis plans to be prespecified in the trial protocol
- to ensure that the trial matches its objectives.

Key issues to be considered include the following.

- Why is the trial being designed as an equivalence trial?
- On what dimensions will you test the results?
- What is the regimen being compared with? (Is the comparator sensible?)
- What is meant by equivalence (e.g. is there a range of results that would be accepted as showing equivalence, or is it a single number)?
- One regimen could turn out to be better than another. What does this imply for the trial statistics and the acceptability of the results?

Finally, you have to be careful here because each regimen may be equally ineffective, and may not necessarily reflect the best option available. *See* **Clinical trial; Data dredging; Data fishing; Data types; Economic analysis and clinical trials; Hypothesis; Non-inferiority trial; Primary question; Protocol; Statistical test diagram; Statistical tests: ten ways to cheat with statistical tests; Superiority trial.**

○ Corey AE, Agnew JR, Valentine SN *et al.* (2000) Comparative oral bioavailability of azimilide dihydrochloride in the fed and fasted states. *Br J Clin Pharmacol.* **49**: 279–82.

○ European Agency for the Evaluation of Medicinal Products (1999) *Committee for Proprietary Medical Products (CPMP) Points to Consider on Biostatistical/Methodological Issues Arising from Recent CPMP Discussions on Licensing Applications: superiority, non-inferiority and equivalence.* EMEA, London.

○ Schnitzer T, Bone HG, Crepaldi G *et al.* (2000) Therapeutic equivalence of alendronate 70 mg once weekly and alendronate 10 mg daily in the treatment of osteoporosis. *Aging (Milano).* **12**: 1–12.

○ Stewart BA, Aherns RC, Carrier S *et al.* (2000) Demonstration of *in-vivo* bioequivalence of a generic albuterol metered-dose inhaler to ventolin. *Chest.* **117**: 714–21.

○ Weins BL and Iglewicz B (2000) Design and analysis of three treatment equivalence trials. *Control Clin Trials.* **21**: 127–37.

○ Zhu CJ, Wu JF, Qu ZW *et al.* (1999) Bioequivalence evaluation of two sertraline tablet formulations in healthy male volunteers after a single-dose administration. *Int J Pharmacol Ther.* **37**: 120–4.

Error

An error is a blunder, indiscretion, mistake, oversight or faux pas. Errors are made without motive or consciousness. Lies, deceit and deceptions occur because of a motive. *See* **Bias; Data dredging; Statistical tests: ten ways to cheat with statistical tests.**

Ethical considerations in a randomised clinical trial

More than 30 years ago Bradford Hill set out a small, important and powerful set of ethical considerations with regard to randomised trials.

These ethical considerations remain valid today and still need to be addressed. You should be able to address each one either before you enter into a trial or before you enter a patient into a trial. You should also consider these issues when putting trial evidence into practice.

Table 22 shows an adaptation of the Bradford Hill ethical considerations.

Table 22 Ethical considerations

1 Is the proposed intervention safe for the patient (i.e. unlikely to cause them harm)?
2 What patients may be brought into the controlled trial?
3 What patients may be allocated randomly to any of the arms of the trial?
4 Can a treatment be withheld from a patient, ethically, in the trial?
5 Is it ethical to use a placebo?
6 Is it ethical for the trial to be in any way masked/blinded?

Probably the best way for you to delve into the intricacies of Table 22 is as follows. Find the published evidence for a particular product, read the papers closely and find out whether they answer each of the ethical issues listed above satisfactorily (e.g. do the authors justify the use of a placebo in the trial?).

It has been strongly argued that it is unethical to conduct poor research (e.g. with flawed design, wrong endpoints, inappropriate patient selection), as it absorbs resources and patients' and practitioners' goodwill, exposes patients to unnecessary risks and may deprive them of an effective therapy.

There are also ethical issues that arise with regard to the participation of patients in trials. Once the product is licensed on the market, some patients may not:

- be allowed to continue on the product

- gain access to the product locally

- be able to pay, or get third-party payment, for the medication that they need.

See **Belmont Report; Clinical trial; Declaration of Helsinki; Equipoise; Ethical issues; Local research ethics committee; Multicentre research ethics committee; Randomisation; Research governance in the NHS.**

○ Altman DG (1994) The scandal of poor medical research. *BMJ.* **308**: 283–4.

○ Boyd KM, Higgs R and Pinching AJ (1997) *The New Dictionary of Medical Ethics.* BMA Books, London.

○ Hill AB (1951) The clinical trial. *Br Med Bull.* **7**: 278–82.

○ Hill AB (1977) *A Short Textbook of Medical Statistics* (10e). JP Lippincott Co., Philadelphia, PA.

○ Singer PA (2000) Recent advances: medical ethics. *BMJ.* **321**: 282–5.

○ Strobl J, Cave E and Walley T (2000) Data protection legislation: interpretation and barriers to research. *BMJ.* **321**: 890–92.

Ethical issues

Ethical issues are a collection of subjective principles or rules of conduct. They arise from a reflective inquiry into how people should think or behave, with a view to formulating norms of conduct and evaluation of character.

Table 23 lists some key terms and their meaning.

Table 23 Ethical issues and meaning

Ethical term	Meaning
Beneficence	Attempting to do good
Non-maleficence	Not inflicting harm
Autonomy	Self-determination in terms of freedom of: • will • thought • action
Justice	Action that is fair and just

See **Accountability; Analytic perspective; Belmont Report; Declaration of Helsinki; Ethical considerations in a randomised clinical trial; Local research ethics committee; Morality; Multicentre research ethics committee; Research governance in the NHS.**

○ Beauchamp T and Childress J (1994) *Principles of Biomedical Ethics*. Oxford University Press, Oxford.

○ Boyd KM, Higgs R and Pinching AJ (1997) *The New Dictionary of Medical Ethics*. BMJ Publishing Group, London.

○ Edwards SJL, Lilford RJ, Jackson JC *et al*. (1998) The ethics of randomised controlled trials: a systematic review. *Health Technol Assess*. **2**: 1–128.

○ Edwards SJL, Lilford RJ and Hewison J (1998) The ethics of randomised controlled trials from the perspective of patients, the public and healthcare professionals. *BMJ*. **317**: 1209–12.

○ Gillon R (1995) Defending the 'four principles approach' to biomedical ethics. *J Med Ethics*. **21**: 323–4.

○ Singer PA (2000) Recent advances: medical ethics. *BMJ*. **321**: 282–5.

○ Strobl J, Cave E and Walley T (2000) Data protection legislation: interpretation and barriers to research. *BMJ*. **321**: 890–2.

○ Working Group of the Royal College of Physicians' Committee on Ethical Issues in Medicine (1994) Independent ethical review of studies involving personal medical records. *J R Coll Phys Lond*. **28**: 439–43.

European Union Directive on clinical trials of medicinal products for humans

For a long time (too long according to some) there has been no legal text at the European level relating specifically to the conduct of clinical trials in European member states. Individual countries do of course have their own quality assurance and regulatory systems, and there is the International Conference on Harmonisation enterprise.

The European Parliament and Council adopted the Directive on 4 April 2001. This Directive lays down a series of provisions with respect to the conduct of clinical trials on human subjects involving medicinal products. As it was published in the *Official Journal of the European Communities* in May 2001 it has therefore now, as they say, 'entered into force'.

In general, the Directive applies without prejudice to member states' provisions on the protection of clinical trial subjects if they are more comprehensive than the provisions that are laid down by the Community legislation. These require Member States, if they have not already done so, to adopt detailed rules to protect individuals who are unable to give their consent.

The developments so far are as follows.

- *May 1996*: the European Commission presented its first preliminary proposal for a Directive. This would be a Directive of the European Parliament and of the Council of Ministers on the approximation of provisions laid down by law, regulation or administrative action relating to the implementation of good clinical practice in the conduct of clinical trials on medicinal products for human use.

- *February 1997*: a second preliminary proposal was released for comment.

- *September 1997*: a final proposal (COM(97)369) was presented by the Commission.

- *January 1998*: the Economic and Social Committee gave its opinion on the proposal.

- *November 1998*: the European Parliament proposed several amendments.

- *April 1999*: the European Commission released an Amended Proposal (COM (1999)193).

- *November 1999*: the European Council considered the Amended Proposal. Council could not reach agreement.

- *May–June 2001*: Directive was published.

Member states are required to adopt and publish legislation that complies with the Directive before 1 May 2003 with a view to their application no later than 1 May 2004. As it currently stands, the Directive explains procedures that must be followed for:

- clinical trials on incapacitated adults who are not able to give informed consent

- ethics committees which must prepare opinions before a clinical trial commences

- detailed guidance on the application format and documentation to be submitted in application for an ethics committee opinion

- adoption of single opinions for multicentre clinical trials limited to the territory of a single member state

- commencement of a clinical trial

- conduct of a clinical trial

- exchange of information

- suspension of the trial or infringements

- notification of adverse events

- notification of serious adverse reactions

- guidance concerning reports

- adaptation to scientific and technical progress

- manufacture and import of investigational medicinal products

- verification of compliance of investigational medicinal products with good clinical and manufacturing practice

- labelling

- committee procedures.

Please refer to the *Official Journal* for more details on the exact text of the Directive.

The Directive does not apply to the following:

- non-intervention trials

- the hundreds of trials involving interventions that are not medicines (e.g. trials on healthcare technologies, surgery, counselling, healthcare organisations, physiotherapy, psychotherapy, acupuncture, patient education, career support trials and information advice trials, (such as trials of different ways in which pharmacists may present advice to patients)

- trials outside the EU.

Serious concerns are still being raised about the Directive. These include concerns about the following:

- inadequate protection for vulnerable groups such as the elderly, a concern that was raised by The Netherlands in December 2000 and that is still not being fully or properly addressed

- as it is a Directive and not a Regulation, its effectiveness relies heavily on its actual application in individual member states – there will not be a single harmonised system unless all member states line up together and work in practice in exactly the same manner

- the risks of serious delays to starting up trials involving biotechnology

- whether and why stem, gene and human tissue trials are excluded

- whether the Directive will mean more delays in bringing certain new products on to the market

- which professions can be the lead investigator

- transparency of the trial sponsors, their degree of control over the trial and their ethical behaviour

- academic researchers have expressed concern about being marginalised by the Directive

- patient advocates who are concerned about lack of patient input into the trial plan and dissemination

- the opaqueness of the benefits of adopting the Directive to trial sponsors and ethical committees

- the ambiguity with regard to who bears the burden of the costs to be incurred in aligning to the Directive

- the consultation that is required before a trial is stopped

- which trials are going to be caught in the Directive

- the legality, practicality, transparency, data protection and accessibility of the new European database to which immediate entries have to be made of unexpected adverse reactions

- how currently planned trials over the next 3 years are to proceed if countries are going to be changing their systems by May 2004

- the lack of an effective requirement for publication of the trial protocol or results

- whether and how the Directive and member states' movements to adopt it are going to be harmonised with other good clinical practice rules and requirements

- how the Directive will apply to the many international trials (trials involving EU and non-EU countries, e.g. the USA, Japan)

- why the Directive only applies to medicines for human consumption

- where the evidence base is to support the Directive.

No doubt these concerns and others will be amplified and crystallised as individual member states change their systems to come into line with the Directive, and as more people delve deeper and see more clearly into the practical implications of the Directive. *See* **Accountability; Clinical trial; Due process; Economic analysis and clinical trials; Local research ethics committee; Multicentre research ethics committee; Research governance in the NHS; Research questions and research methods; Transparency**.

○ Earl-Slater A (2001) The European Union's Clinical Trials Directive. *J Roy Soc Med*. **94**: 557–8.

○ EC Directive (2001/20) On the approximation of the laws, regulations and administrative provisions of the Member States relating to the Implementation of Good Clinical Practice in the Conduct of Clinical Trials on Medicinal Products for Human Use. *Official J Euro Comm*. **May**: 0034–0044.

○ European Science Foundation (2001) *Co-ordination of Public Funding for European Clinical Trials*. European Science Foundation Policy Briefing.

○ European Science Foundation (2001) *Harmonisation of Clinical Trials: administrative constraints*. European Science Foundation Policy Briefing.

○ Joint Pharmaceutical Analysis Group (2001) Implications of the new clinical trials directive. *Pharma J*. **267**: 26–7.

○ Strobl J, Cave E and Walley T (2000) Data protection legislation: interpretation and barriers to research. *BMJ*. **321**: 890–2.

○ Watson R (2001) New EU rules might hinder research. *BMJ*. **322**: 385.

Event

An event is an occurrence (it is more often called an effect). It may or may not be what was expected in a trial. *See* **Adverse event; Effect; Outcome; Primary outcome; Transparency; Unanticipated adverse effect; Unanticipated beneficial effect**.

Evidence-based medicine

Evidence-based medicine is the systematic, explicit, conscientious and judicious use of evidence when making a decision.

Your decision is grounded on a collection of issues, including the following:

- the published evidence

- your understanding of it

- your experience

- the context of your work

- the context of the particular patient with whom you are working.

To help to develop evidence-based medicine, you must be able to:

- formulate the question to be tackled

- identify the evidence

- critically appraise the evidence

- distil the essence from the evidence

- determine how the evidence relates to practice

- identify how the evidence can be integrated into practice.

See **Accountability; Advantages of evidence from clinical trials; Analytic perspective; Case–control study; Clinical trial; Cohort study; Critical appraisal; Data-display formats; Disadvantages of evidence from clinical trials; Due process; Hierarchies of evidence; Meta-analysis; Observation study; Paradigm shift; Research governance in the NHS; Statistical test diagram; Systematic review; Transparency; Ways of presenting results.**

○ Barton SW (2000) *Clinical Evidence*. BMJ Books, London.

○ Bond C (2000) *Evidence-Based Pharmacy*. Pharmaceutical Press, London.

○ Cochrane Centre (2001) *The Cochrane Reviewers Handbook*. Cochrane Centre, Oxford.

○ Dunn G and Everitt B (1995) *Clinical Biostatistics: an introduction to evidence-based medicine*. Edward Arnold, London.

○ Glaziou PP and Irwig LM (1995) An evidence-based approach to individualising treatment. *BMJ*. **311**: 1356–9.

○ Li Wan Po A (1998) *Dictionary of Evidence-Based Medicine*. Radcliffe Medical Press, Oxford.

○ McColl A, Smith H, White P and Field J (1998) General practitioners' perceptions of the route to evidence-based medicine: a questionnaire survey. *BMJ*. **316**: 361–5.

○ Prescott K, Lloyd M, Hannah-Rose D *et al.* (1997) Promoting clinically effective practice: general practitioners' awareness of sources of research evidence. *Fam Pract*. **14**: 320–3.

○ Risdale L (1996) Evidence-based learning for general practice. *Br J Gen Pract.* **46**: 503.

○ Rosenberg WM and Donald A (1995) Evidence-based medicine: an approach to clinical problem-solving. *BMJ.* 310: 1122–6.

○ Sackett DL, Rosenberg WM, Gray JA *et al.* (1996) Evidence-based medicine – what it is and what it isn't. *BMJ.* **312**: 71–2.

○ Stevens A, Abrams K, Brazier J, Fitzpatrick R and Lilford R (eds) (2001) *The Advanced Handbook of Methods in Evidence-Based Healthcare.* Sage Publishing, London.

Exclusion criteria

Exclusion criteria are those rules which, when applied, stop a person from taking part in a clinical trial.

Reasons for exclusion can be based on the following grounds:

- medical
- scientific
- administrative
- finance
- age
- race
- gender.

For example, in a study by Ettinger and colleagues to determine whether raloxifene reduces the rate of vertebral and non-vertebral fractures in postmenopausal women with osteoporosis, patients with the following conditions were excluded from the trial:

- other bone disease
- postmenopausal symptoms
- abnormal uterine bleeding
- a history of breast or endometrial cancer
- a history of thromboembolic disorder
- other cancers
- treated endocrine disorders except for type 2 diabetes or hypothyroidism
- renal lithiasis
- abnormal hepatic or renal function
- untreated malabsorption
- consumption of more than four drinks of alcohol per day.

Listed below are some of the key issues to ask about exclusion criteria.

- What are the exclusion criteria?
- Are they clearly and completely set out in the trial report?
- Are they justified?
- Where is the evidence to support each exclusion criterion?
- How do they relate to excluding patients in clinical practice? Do you use the same criteria?
- What implications do the exclusions have for taking the trial results into practice?

See **Eligibility; Eligibility criteria; Equipoise; Generalisability of trial results; Inclusion criteria.**

○ Chalmers TC (1990) Ethical implications of rejecting patients for clinical trials. *JAMA*. **263**: 865.

○ Ettinger B, Black DM, Mitlak BH *et al.* (1999) Reduction of vertebral fracture risk in postmenopausal women with osteoporosis treated with raloxifene. Results from a 3-year randomized clinical trial. *JAMA*. **282**: 637-45.

Experimental group
This is the group that receives the experimental intervention of interest in the clinical trial (sometimes also called the 'cases'). *See* **Clinical trial; Control group; Experimental study.**

Experimental study
Experimental studies are those in which events can be deliberately influenced and subject to analysis. *See* **Clinical trial; Experimental group; Observational study; Randomised controlled trial.**

Explanatory trial
An explanatory trial is a clinical trial that is designed primarily to explain *how* a particular phenomenon works. *See* **Efficacy trial; Efficiency trial; Mega-trial; Pilot trial.**

Exploratory data analysis
Exploratory data analysis is another more polite and palatable term for data dredging. *See* **Data dredging.**

Expose

To expose means to lay open to risk. Exposure occurs in all clinical trials as, by definition, a clinical trial is an experiment and experiments have risks attached to them. Patients are also laid open to risk in clinical practice, as all decisions expose patients to some form of risk. *See* **Clinical trial; Declaration of Helsinki.**

External validity of clinical trial results

When you see the results of a clinical trial you will soon find out that the trial has been conducted under certain conditions. What you really want to know is how the trial and its results relate to your practice. Therefore you have to compare the trial with your practice, say, in the primary care group. Of course there will be differences between the trial and practice, but the key question is how important those differences are.

Once you have this information, you can determine how valid and relevant the clinical trial results are to your practice. Remember though, that what you do in your practice may differ from what a colleague does in their practice, even within the same primary care group or trust. Therefore the external validity of clinical trial results will depend on the specific area of reality you are looking at in the health service.

By definition, therefore, the external validity of clinical trial results is the extent to which the results of that trial are valid in another place or at another time.

Sometimes the external validity of results is called the generalisability, trans-ferability or applicability of trial results. *See* **Advantages of evidence from clinical trials; Analytic perspective; Efficacy; Evidence-based medicine; Fixed-effects model; Internal validity of results; Meta-analysis; Problems with regard to putting evidence into practice; Questions to ask before getting involved in a clinical trial; Random effects model; Systematic review.**

○ Earl-Slater A (2001) Critical appraisal of clinical trials: barriers to putting evidence into practice. *J Clin Govern.* **6**: 279–82.

○ Lilford RJ, Pauker SG, Braunholtz DA and Chard J (1998) Getting research findings into practice: decision analysis and implementation of research findings. *BMJ.* **317**: 405–9.

Factor analysis

Factor analysis is the study of the key elements in a clinical trial. It is sometimes called principal component analysis for the simple reason that it looks at the principal components of the study. *See* **Clinical trial; Interim analysis; Primary outcome**.

Factorial trial

In general, a factorial trial is a type of clinical trial in which treatments are compared with each other, in combination, and with a control. Figure 25 illustrates this.

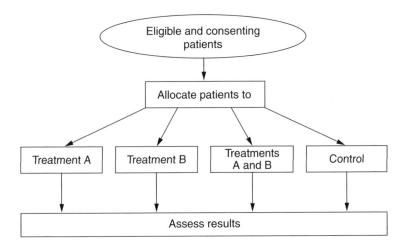

Figure 25 Factorial trial.

For example:

- in a factorial trial of nicotine replacement (A) and counselling (B), patients would be allocated to nicotine replacement alone (A), counselling alone (B), both together (A and B) or neither (placebo/control)

- the Collaborative Group of the Primary Prevention Project reported on a randomised, unblinded, 2×2 factorial trial with a mean follow-up of 3.6 years to see how effective treatment with aspirin and vitamin E was in preventing cardiovascular events in patients with one or more cardiovascular risk factors but no history of cardiovascular disease

- Green and colleagues reported on a randomised, single-blind, placebo-controlled 2×2 factorial trial to see whether in healthy adults a daily dose of sunscreen or beta-carotene supplements prevented skin cancer

- the Heart Outcomes Prevention Evaluation Study used a randomised, triple-blind controlled 2×2 factorial trial to assess whether in adults who are at high risk for cardiovascular events, ramipril or vitamin E reduce cardiovascular events (interestingly, they published two separate reports on the trial).

The main advantage of this type of trial is that you can compare the individual effects of each intervention relative to the combined intervention and to the control/placebo. *See* **Active control trial**; **Adaptive–adoptive trial**; **Clinical trial**; **Cluster randomised trial**; **Combination trial**; **Confounding factor**; **Control**; **Multiple outcomes**; **Placebo**; **Placebo-controlled trial**; **Randomised controlled trial**; **Sequential trial**; **Value-for-money table**.

○ Collaborative Group of the Primary Prevention Project (2001) Low-dose aspirin and vitamin E in people at cardiovascular risk: a randomised trial in general practice. *Lancet*. **357**: 89–95.

○ Green A, Williams G, Neale R *et al.* (1999) Daily sunscreen application and betacarotene supplementation in prevention of basal-cell and squamous-cell carcinomas of the skin: a randomised controlled trial. *Lancet*. **354**: 723–9.

○ Heart Outcomes Prevention Evaluation Study Investigators (2000) Effects of an angiotensin-converting-enzyme inhibitor, ramipril, on death from cardiovascular causes, myocardial infarction and stroke in high-risk patients. *NEJM*. **342**: 145–53.

○ Heart Outcomes Prevention Evaluation Study Investigators (2000) Vitamin E supplementation and cardiovascular events in high-risk patients. *NEJM*. **342**: 154–60.

Falsificationism

Falsificationism is the belief that the validity of a theory depends on whether or not it is falsified by empirical evidence.

- In simple falsification the theory is discarded if it is falsified by one empirical test.

- In sustained falsification the theory is discarded if it is falsified by more than one empirical test.

Theories are provisionally accepted until they have been falsified. Falsificationism is used in areas such as systematic reviews, evidence-based decision making, clinical practice, clinical trials and meta-analysis. *See* **Duhem's irrefutability theory**; **Hypothesis**; **Lakatosian hard-core, protective belt**.

Fate of clinical research

Figure 26 illustrates the fate of clinical trials research pyramid. It runs from the base initial idea for the trial up to its highest point, namely influencing clinical practice. There are various stages in between these extremes, as highlighted in the diagram.

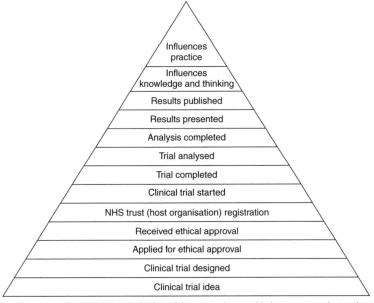

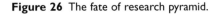

Whilst we identify clinical trials in the fate of the research pyramid above, you can in practice change the terminology of the pyramid to reflect the fate of any other method of research. The only steps that may then be missed out in the current pyramid is if the research does not need ethics approval. The essence of the pyramid essentially stays the same.

Figure 26 The fate of research pyramid.

Reading the pyramid from the base upward, the impression is gained that there are many more clinical trial ideas than there are clinical trials designed. Moving further up the pyramid we see that not all trials that are designed receive ethical approval. This is not necessarily bad news, as failure to obtain research approval can signal concerns about the research idea and methods. The issue, however, is that there is no comprehensive database of research application failures and reasons for failure, and therefore no memory or databank from which other researchers and research approval committees can learn.

For various reasons, not all trials that are started are completed, and not all of those that are completed are analysed, presented or published. Some of those that are analysed are presented to licensing authorities in confidence as part of the application for a market licence. If a licence is required and given, then the product can go on to the market. As yet the Medicines Control Agency in the UK, as a licensing authority for medicines, does not require that the trials supporting the licence application be published as part of the condition of giving the product market approval. In contrast, if the applicant for a market licence goes through the pan-European medicines licensing system to obtain approval to go on to all EU markets, the licensing agency's summary interpretation of the trial evidence is published on the Internet in the form of a public assessment report. Should licensing agencies be required to publish the evidence on which they base their decisions as well as their summaries of the evidence and their decisions?

Some health technology manufacturers are subjecting their products to clinical trials, as the results of these suggest more 'scientific kudos' if their product is shown to be beneficial under trial conditions. These companies should be encouraged to publish their trial protocols and their results.

In general, then, it can be argued that protocols and results of experiments, which is in essence what clinical trials are, should be published at least on the Internet. The trial protocol and the trial results should be available to everyone, as the publication of trial protocols and results allows and enables open, independent and structured appraisal of the trial. It allows the methods and results to be set out on public record for retrieval and inspection, and it can permit easier access at any time, as the publication of trial methods and results allows easier access than asking the trialists or trial sponsors for the otherwise unpublished trial information, or the sponsor for relevant 'data on file'. The publication of trial protocols and results also helps forward planning.

Although the highest point in the pyramid is taken by trials that influence practice, remember that many factors affect clinical practice in a complex way, interpretation of results from clinical trials being just one of the possible influences.

While we have said that the pyramid applies to clinical trials, it also applies to all other forms of research. You can use it as a kind of checklist. For example, if a doctor states that the results of a particular clinical trial influenced her decision, then both she and you can use the pyramid and ask some questions related to the lower levels in the pyramid. *See* **Advantages of evidence from clinical trials; Causes of delay and failure to complete a clinical trial; Disadvantages of evidence from clinical trials; Reasons given by the investigator for a study being abandoned or in abeyance; Reasons given by the investigator for a study never being started; Research questions and research methods.**

○ Earl-Slater A (2002) Research governance and the fate of research. *Br J Clin Gov.* **7**: 57–62.

○ Easterbrook PJ and Mathews DR (1992) Fate of research studies. *J R Soc Med.* **85**: 71–6.

○ Prescott RJ *et al.* (1999) Factors that limit quality, number and progress of randomised controlled trials. *Health Technol Assess.* **3**: 1–137.

Feasibility trial

A feasibility trial is a clinical trial which seeks to determine the following:

• the ability to identify appropriate patients

• the ability to recruit appropriate patients

- the ability to recruit appropriate healthcare professionals
- the viability of a particular process, system of monitoring, recording or coding.

Sometimes a feasibility trial is called a pilot trial. *See* **Case finding; Demonstrative trial; Equivalence trial; Explanatory trial; Mega-trial; Pilot trial**.

Feedback trial

A feedback trial is a clinical trial in which all preliminary findings are relayed shortly after they have been analysed in the trial. Many pharmaceutical companies use feedback trials of chemical compounds to signal the progress of their work. This information is often fed into finance meetings to show how the investment is doing, and possibly to encourage more investment to facilitate further study. Whether the information becomes public remains unclear. However, reality shows that it depends on who is sponsoring the trial, their motives and the trial results. *See* **Accountability; Clinical trial; Due process; Efficiency trial; Feasibility trial; Interim analysis; Pilot trial; Research governance in the NHS; Transparency**.

Field trial

A field trial is a clinical trial that takes place outside the normal confines of a clinic. *See* **Efficacy trial; Efficiency trial**.

Fixed-effects model

Used in the context of meta-analysis, a fixed-effects model is a statistical model stipulating that the units of analysis, e.g. people in a trial in the meta-analysis, are the ones of interest. They therefore constitute the entire population.

Consider two sources of variation: you can have variations within a study and you can have variations between the studies in a meta-analysis. In a fixed-effects model only the former, variations within studies, influences the uncertainty of the results (and hence the confidence intervals). The confidence intervals of a fixed-effects model are narrower, less conservative, than the confidence intervals in a random-effects model.

Suppose we considered the 'study centre' as a factor in the analysis. Then, in a fixed-effects model, the meta-analytic results are only applicable to those centres that took part in the trials.

Tests of heterogeneity are used to help determine the choice of model. Recent innovations and developments in research methodology have introduced us to two other genres of models: mixed-effects models and Bayesian-effects models.

See **Bayesian analysis; Duhem's irrefutability theory; Error; External validity of clinical trials; Generalisability of trial results; Lakatosian's hard-core, protective belt; Meta-analysis; Random-effects model**.

○ Cooper H and Hedges LV (1994) *The Handbook of Research Synthesis*. Russel Sage Foundation, New York.

○ Egger M, Davey Smith G and Phillips AN (1997) Meta-analysis: principles and procedures. *BMJ*. **315**: 1533–7.

○ Fleiss JL (1993) The statistical basis of meta-analysis. *Stat Meth Med Res*. **2**: 121–45.

Fixed-size trial

A fixed-size trial is one that recruits patients into arms of the trial until the required number of patients are in the trial. *See* **Closed sequential trial; Power calculation; Sequential trial.**

Focus group

This is a research method in which a collection of people are interviewed on what they think about a particular issue while interacting in small groups.

Focus groups can be used to:

- facilitate group dynamics to stimulate discussion

- gain insight

- generate ideas and information with a view to testing the hypothesis

- seek expert views on future influences on the topic under consideration.

Focus group discussions could (and some argue should), with permission, be tape recorded. The tapes can then be transcribed, analysed and reflected on in more detail.

The advantages of focus groups include the following:

- facilitating open discussion of sensitive or personal topics

- exploring what people think

- identifying how people articulate their thoughts

- revealing the foundation of people's thoughts

- identifying the range of views and knowledge

- signalling areas of common ground and divergence

- revealing subgroup themes

- not being restricted to those who can read or write.

Possible limitations of focus groups include the following:

- mixing people from different sectors, resulting in much time being spent learning about the topic under consideration

- positioning of group members

- dominance

- dealing with dropouts from the exercise.

See **Delphi technique; Problems with regard to putting research evidence into practice; Qualitative research; Research questions and research methods.**

○ Barbour RS (2001) Checklists for improving rigour in qualitative research: a case of the tail wagging the dog? *BMJ.* **322**: 1115–17.

○ Giacomini MK (2001) The rocky road: qualitative research as evidence. *Evidence-Based Med.* **6**: 406.

○ Greenhalgh T and Taylor R (1997) Papers that go beyond numbers (qualitative research). *BMJ.* **315**: 740–3.

○ Kitzinger J (1995) Introducing focus groups. *BMJ.* **311**: 299–302.

○ Pope C and Mays N (eds) (2000) *Qualitative Research in Health Care.* BMJ Books, London.

Follow-up

Follow-up is the assessment of a patient or group of patients after a particular point in time.

Examples include the following.

- In a trial on adding tamoxifen to lumpectomy and radiation therapy in women with non-invasive ductal carcinoma *in situ*, Fisher and colleagues had a 74-month median follow-up.

- In a trial of labour pain treated with cutaneous injections of sterile water, women who were in the first stage of labour were studied at 10, 45 and 90 minutes after treatment.

- The GISSI–Prevenzione Investigators study of patients with recent myocardial infarction used a 42-month follow-up.

- Beral and colleagues published the results of a 25-year follow-up of a cohort of 46 000 women from the Royal College of General Practitioners oral contraception study.

- Jolly and colleagues published the results of a randomised control trial of follow-up care in general practice of patients with myocardial infarction and angina.

- Talley and colleagues studied the eradication of *Helicobacter pylori* in functional dyspepsia using a randomised double-blind placebo-controlled trial with a 12-month follow-up.

- Hart and colleagues used a 21-year follow-up of alcohol consumption and mortality from all causes, coronary heart disease and stroke in a cohort of Scottish men.

Too short a follow-up period may mean that the full effects of the intervention have not yet become established, whereas too long a follow-up period may mean that patients are difficult to find and that other factors have played a role in their changed condition. *See* **Long term**; **Short term**.

○ Fisher B, Gignam J, Wolmark N *et al.* (1999) Tamoxifen in treatment of intraductal breast cancer: National Surgical Adjuvant Breast and Bowel Project B-24 randomised controlled trial. *Lancet*. **353**: 1993–2000.

○ GISSI-Prevenzione Investigators (1999) Dietary supplementation with n-3 polyunsaturated fatty acids and vitamin E after myocardial infarction: results of the GISSI-Prevenzione trial. *Lancet*. **354**: 447–55.

○ Martensen L and Wallin G (1999) Labour pain treated with cutaneous injections of sterile water: a randomised controlled trial. *Br J Obstet Gynaecol*. **106**: 633–7.

Food and Drug Administration (FDA)

This is a US government agency which reviews and approves clinical studies and the licensing of drugs for human consumption in the USA. The FDA also has regulatory powers with regard to post-marketing surveillance, the advertising of medicines, medical devices, foods, food additives, cosmetics, and veterinary and animal health products. It can demand further clinical studies on a particular product, and grant, revoke, amend, refuse or rescind a market licence. It also has an inspectorate role with regard to products, manufacture facilities, processes, shipments, storage, labelling and advertising. The FDA can demand product withdrawal and closing down of facilities, it can require corrections to be made and, through the courts, violators can be fined or even imprisoned. *See* **Accountability**; **Due process**; **Institutional review board**; **Medicines Control Agency**; **Transparency**.

Funnel plot

Suppose that elected members from primary and secondary care get together every month to review the evidence concerning a particular product. Each paper on the product is analysed according to a structured set of questions.

Two important questions arise.

• What was the size of the samples used?

• What was the size of the effects achieved?

A funnel plot is a graphical method of representing, say, the size of the sample and the size of the effect as seen in different studies. If there are any gaps in the funnel, or if the funnel is not symmetrical, then there is said to be publication bias.

Figure 27 shows an 'ideal' funnel plot.

If the analysis is performed on published material, then in the absence of publication bias, a plot of the sample size versus the size of the effect should look like an inverted funnel because, it has been argued:

• studies with small sample sizes are expected to be quite variable

• studies with larger sample sizes are expected to show less spread

• the mean size of the effect should be the same regardless of sample size.

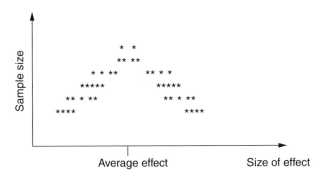

Figure 27 Funnel plot.

Funnel plots have been used, arguably, to help to detect publication bias, where a gap on one side of the funnel or asymmetry in the funnel plot, would suggest that some studies have not been published or located. In fact, more detailed analysis of the gap may indicate that certain studies have not even been conducted! There is no empirical evidence to demonstrate what funnel plots can show, and their logic has been questioned. Thus whether these plots do help to detect publication bias *per se* remains the subject of ongoing debate.

Three issues need to be kept in mind.

- Funnel plots do not always state whether the same intervention was provided in each study (they should, but always check them out).

- Funnel plots do not always make clear differences in the types of people, clinics or clinicians who were involved in the trials.

- Exactly what funnels plots do show is currently the subject of renewed debate.

See **CONSORT; Data-display format; L'Abbe plot; Meta-analysis; Pooled analysis; Systematic review**.

○ Bandolier (2000) Funnel plots and heterogeneity. *Bandolier*. **November**: 81–5.

○ Bowling A (1997) *Research Methods in Health*. Open University Press, Buckingham.

○ Gavaghan DJ, Moore RA and McQuay HJ (2000) An evaluation of homogeneity tests in meta-analysis in pain using simulations of individual patient data. *Pain*. **85**: 415–24.

○ Lewis S and Clarke M (2001) Forrest plots: trying to see the wood and the trees. *BMJ*. **322**: 1479–80.

○ Light RJ and Pillemer D (1984) *Summing Up*. Harvard University Press, Cambridge, MA.

○ Stevens A, Abrams K, Brazier J, Fitzpatrick R and Lilford R (eds) (2001) *The Advanced Handbook of Methods in Evidence-Based Healthcare*. Sage Publishing, London.

○ Tang J and Liu JI (2000) Misleading funnel plot for detection of bias in meta-analysis. *J Clin Epidemiol*. **53**: 477–84.

G

Gambler's fallacy

This is the idea that if a chance event has not yet happened, it is bound to occur soon.

GCP European Clinical Trials Directive

See **European Union Directive on clinical trials of medicinal products for humans**.

Generalisability of trial results

Generalisability of trial results relates to how readily the results of a particular clinical trial can be applied to other situations (sometimes also called external validity of trial results or 'applicability'). *See* **External validity of trial results; Fate of clinical research; Fixed-effects model; Internal validity of trial results; Random-effects model**.

○ Lilford RJ, Pauker SG, Braunholtz DA and Chard J (1998) Getting research findings into practice: decision analysis and implementation of research findings. *BMJ*. **317**: 405–9.

○ Rosser WM (1999) Application of evidence from randomised controlled trials to general practice. *Lancet*. **353**: 661–4.

○ Rothwell PM (1995) Can overall results of clinical trials be applied to all patients? *Lancet*. **345**: 1616–19.

Gold standard

A gold standard is an 'ideal' measure, technique or result against which all other measures, techniques or results can be compared.

Some people consider randomised double-blind placebo-controlled trials to be the gold standard source of evidence. However (and here is a paradox for you to muse over), there is in fact no robust evidence to support that view.

Sometimes a gold standard is not 'ideal' – it may just be something that is used as the benchmark. *See* **Benchmarking; Randomised controlled trial; Systematic review**.

○ Britton A, McKee M, Black N *et al.* (1998) Choosing between randomised and non-randomised studies: a systematic review. *Health Technol Assess*. **2**: 1–119.

○ Earl-Slater A (2001) Critical appraisal of clinical trials: critical appraisal and hierarchies of the evidence. *J Clin Govern*. **6**: 59–63.

Good clinical practice

Sets of standards aim to identify, support and promote good clinical practice (GCP). There are various sets of good clinical practice around, which are still being developed, and none are set in stone. Many of those readers who have been involved in clinical trials for American pharmaceutical companies will be aware of the GCP systems in the USA, a country that is sometimes regarded as the originator and leader of GCP.

The key tasks for you are as follows:

- to take these sets of standards seriously

- to identify which sets apply to the trial in which you are interested or involved

- to determine to what extent they have been followed in a particular trial.

See **Audit; Benchmarking; Declaration of Helsinki; European Union Directive on clinical trials of medicinal products in humans; International Conference on Harmonisation; Medical Research Council Guidelines for Good Practice in Clinical Trials; Research governance in the NHS.**

Grey literature

Grey literature is material that is not:

- generally available

- published in large quantities

- readily distributed

- generally indexed in public-domain reference systems

- necessarily peer reviewed.

For example, it could include the following:

- company reports

- committee reports

- political papers

- civil servant and quasi-government reports

- non-governmental organisations' reports

- proceedings of conferences, workshops or symposia

- oral or poster information presented at conferences, workshops or symposia

- briefing papers presented at finance or clinical meetings
- reports used when applying for a market licence (e.g. with regard to medicines, most drug companies have large banks of grey literature which they usually refer to as 'data on file').

The quality of the evidence in the grey literature has yet to be formally established. In my experience, most people who have grey literature or have produced it will be happy to share it with you provided that you state exactly why you want it and what you will do with it. *See* **Systematic review**.

Group randomisation

Group randomisation occurs when patients are classified into groups and then each group is randomly allocated to a particular arm of the trial (*see* Figure 28).

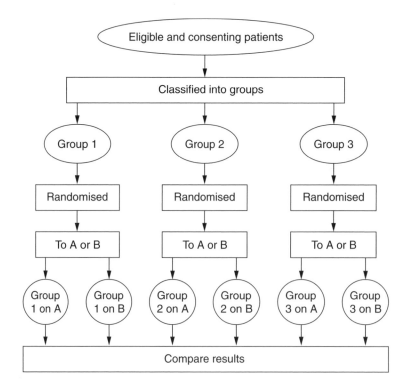

Figure 28 Group randomisation.

For example, the groups may be specified in terms of the patient's hospital ward, birth cohort, gender, condition, age, clinic of attendance, GP practice list, geographical area or previous medical history. Figure 28 gives an example of three groups and two regimens in trials A or B. In this example we have used a parallel-group randomised trial. We could of course have used other types of trials (e.g. a cross-over group randomisation trial). These are sometimes loosely called cluster trials. *See* **Clinical trial; Cluster randomisation; Cross-over trial; Parallel trial; Randomisation**.

○ Murray DM (1998) *Design and Analysis of Group Randomized Trials*. Oxford University Press, Oxford.

Guideline

A guideline is a collection of statements that can aid decision making.
 Recently published articles dealing with guidelines include the following:

- computer and manual reminders for compliance with a mental health clinical practice guideline

- an evaluation of the effectiveness of national guidelines and local protocols in improving hospital care for women with menorrhagia or urinary incontinence

- a randomised comparison of the effect of non-specific versus specific guidelines on physician decision making

- the effects of a clinical practice guideline and practice-based evaluation on detection and outcome of depression in primary care (the Hampshire Depression Project randomised controlled trial).

See **Algorithm; Care path; Clinical path analysis; Evidence-based medicine; Guidelines, clinical trials and change; Multilevel modelling; Protocol; Transparency**.

○ Cannon DS and Allen SN (2000) A comparison of the effects of computer and manual reminders on compliance with a mental health clinical practice guideline. *J Am Med Inform Assoc.* **7**: 196–203.

○ Chadha Y, Mollison J, Howie F *et al*. (2000) Guidelines in gynaecology: evaluation in menorrhagia and in urinary incontinence. *Br J Obstet Gynaecol.* **107**: 535–43.

○ Shekell PG, Kravitz RL, Beart J *et al*. (2000) Are nonspecific practice guidelines potentially harmful? A randomized comparison of the effect of nonspecific versus specific guidelines on physician decision making. *Health Serv Res.* **34**: 1429–48.

○ Thompson C, Kinmonth AL, Stevens L *et al*. (2000) Effects of a clinical-practice guideline and practice-based evaluation on detection and outcome of depression in primary care: Hampshire Depression Project randomised controlled trial. *Lancet.* **355**: 185–91.

Guidelines, clinical trials and change

One aspect of the clinical trial business, and indeed a growing factor in our clinical practice, is the existence of guidelines.

Is there a relationship between the guideline development strategy and the likelihood of change? Figure 29 suggests that the further away local people are from the guideline development strategy, the less likely it is that they will change practice.

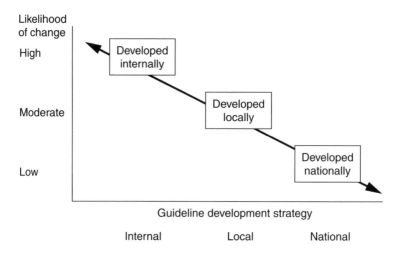

Figure 29 Guidelines and change.

Figure 29 suggests that guidelines developed nationally – the top-down approach – will have a low likelihood of changing actual practice, whereas those developed internally – the bottom-up approach (e.g. in your hospital or in your practice) – have a greater likelihood of effecting change.

Of course, healthcare systems have in place other factors that may help or hinder, command and control or impel the use of guidelines. In an increasingly litigious healthcare arena, guidelines can be used in legal defence or attack. The fact is that pleading ignorance of a guideline is not a robust defence, so even if you are not involved in or not using certain guidelines, knowledge of them may be expected as standard practice. To complicate matters further, but to make them more realistic, not every patient will fit into any particular guideline.

There is nothing in Figure 29 to suggest anything about the quality of the guidelines. Are internally developed guidelines of lower quality than those developed nationally? There is no robust evidence to support this view.

In terms of clinical trials, then, one reason why they may quite often fail to change local practice is because of the lack of local ownership or attachment. The idea is that the likelihood of change is greater in an organisation that has been involved in or linked with the trial than in one that has not. Various strategies can be used to increase local ownership of and attachment to the trial (e.g. multicentre trials, dissemination of trial progress, peer group meetings).

Change is also dependent on the results of the trial, so while more local ownership and attachment may be necessary drivers of change in clinical practice, they are not the only ingredients to consider. *See* **Clinical practice guidelines; Evidence-based medicine; Guideline; Problems with regard to putting evidence into practice**.

○ Earl-Slater A (2001) Critical appraisal of clinical trials: barriers to putting trial evidence into clinical practice. *J Clin Govern.* **6**: 279–82.

○ Hurwitz B (1999) Legal and political considerations of clinical practice guidelines. *BMJ.* **318**: 661–4.

○ Sackett D and Oxman A (1999) Guidelines and killer Bs. *Evidence-Based Med.* **4**: 100–1.

○ Scottish Intercollegiate Guidelines Network (SIGN) (1999) *Guidelines: an introduction to SIGN methodology for the development of evidence-based clinical guidelines.* SIGN, Edinburgh.

○ Shaneyfelt TM, Mayo-Smith MF and Rothwangl J (1999) Are guidelines following guidelines? The methodological quality of clinical practice guidelines in the peer-reviewed medical literature. *JAMA.* **281**: 1900–5.

○ Woolf SH, Grol A, Hutchinson A *et al.* (1999) Potential benefits, limitations and harms of clinical guidelines. *BMJ.* **318**: 527–30.

H

Halo effect

The Halo effect occurs when a person's performance in a clinical trial is over-rated. *See* **Baseline; Bias; Hawthorne effect; Health gain; Hello–goodbye effect**.

Hawthorne effect

When people are under study, observation or investigation, this very fact can have an effect on them and on the results of the study. This is known as the Hawthorne effect.

In a clinical trial, a Hawthorne effect can be positive, negative, or a mixture of both (and therefore not necessarily detected).

The Hawthorne effect was first noted in the results of studies by Elton Mayo and others at the Western Electric Plant, Hawthorne, USA, in the 1920s and 1930s. They studied the effects on productivity of improving lighting in one part of a factory and not changing the lighting in another part. It was found that productivity improved in both parts of the factory. The improved productivity in the part of the factory where the lighting did not change was attributed to what is now called the Hawthorne effect.

The original data have since been re-analysed, and it is not so clear whether the original results hold up. Nevertheless, the concept is established – the very fact that people are under study, observation or investigation can have an effect on them and on the results. *See* **Baseline; Halo effect; Hello–goodbye effect**.

○ de Amici D, Klersy C, Ramajoli F, Brustia L and Politi P (2000) Impact of the Hawthorne effect in a longitudinal clinical study. The case of anesthesia. *Control Clin Trials*. **21**: 103–14.

Health

In 1948 the World Health Organization defined health as 'A state of complete physical, mental and social well-being, and not merely the absence of disease or infirmity'. Thus health is not just determined by healthcare. *See* **Baseline; Health gain; Quality of life**.

Health gain

Health gain is an improvement in a person's health. In clinical trials, health gain can be assessed in terms of the following:

- how the patient was at the start of the trial compared with how they are at the end

- how much worse the patient would have been if they did not receive the intervention

- the well-being of other patients.

Therefore health gain could be measured in terms of the patient's previous position, the position they could have been in, or the position of other patients. *See* **Baseline; Health; Matched pairs; Outcomes pyramid; Primary outcome; Surrogate endpoint**.

Hello–goodbye effect

This is part of the psychodynamics of some people, whereby they initially present themselves in the worst possible light in order to become eligible for treatment, and then after treatment present themselves in the best possible light in an attempt to signal substantial gain in their condition. If uncorrected, the health gain of the patient will be overestimated. The hello–goodbye effect is a serious threat to the validity of clinical studies, meta-analyses and policy making. *See* **Audit; Baseline; Bias; Halo effect; Health gain; Meta-analysis; Outcomes pyramid**.

Heterogeneity

Heterogeneity means difference.

In clinical trials we can have heterogeneity in the following:

- methods

- interventions

- patient characteristics

- entry and exclusion criteria

- care paths

- statistical tests used

- outcomes

- time in the trial

- time in follow-up assessment

- context.

For example:

- there are over 40 types of portable blood test equipment on the market today
- there are over ten ACE inhibitors on the market
- there are more than five COX-2 inhibitors on the market
- trials on the same disease often have different entry and exclusion criteria
- results obtained from similar trials often vary
- implementation of results from the evidence base varies across the country.

If it is not properly accounted for, heterogeneity can seriously impair the validity of the results. *See* **Evidence-based medicine; Funnel plot; Homogenous product; Meta-analysis; Pooled analysis; Systematic review**.

Heterogeneous product
A product which is different, or perceived to be different, from another product is a heterogeneous product. *See* **Heterogeneity; Homogeneous product**.

Hierarchies of the evidence
Given the variety of methods of collating the evidence, and the volume of literature to be addressed, some people use summary codes which are said to reflect the quality of the evidence. These summary codes can be called hierarchies of the evidence. By definition, a hierarchy of the evidence is a table that ranks the value of the evidence.

There are many hierarchies of the evidence, some of which are deceptively simple, while others are incredibly complex. Their *raison d'être* is generally the same, namely to rank the evidence, but their construct, validity, reliability, applicability and usefulness can differ.

Three hierarchies of evidence are provided as examples and for discussion.

Table 24 shows an example of a hierarchy based solely on the nature of the study. Thus at the top of the league table one would put most emphasis on meta-analysis – a technique that seeks to establish a summary statistic of the studies under consideration. At the other end of the table lies 'expert opinion', which some consider to be the weakest form of evidence (but of course it really depends on how the expert developed their 'opinion'!).

Table 24 Hierarchy of evidence

Grade of evidence	Source of evidence
1	Meta-analysis of various clinical trials
2	Systematic review of clinical trials
3	Randomised controlled trials
4	Case–control studies
5	Cohort studies
6	Expert opinion

Table 25 provides another example of a hierarchy of evidence.

Table 25 More sophisticated hierarchy of evidence

Grade of evidence	Source of evidence
I	Well-designed randomised controlled trial
II-1a	Well-designed controlled trial with pseudorandomisation
II-1b	Well-designed controlled trial with no randomisation
II-2a	Well-designed prospective cohort study with concurrent controls
II-2b	Well-designed prospective cohort study with historical controls
II-2c	Well-designed retrospective cohort study with concurrent controls
II-3	Well-designed retrospective case–control study
III	Large differences from comparisons between times and/or places, with and without intervention
IV	Opinions of respected authorities based on clinical experience, descriptive studies and reports of expert committees

A third hierarchy (*see* Table 26) uses a more descriptive terminology to help to classify the evidence. On the face of it, the categories in this hierarchy do not impose strict rules on what should be included in each area. A further advantage is that the hierarchy runs from clear evidence of benefit, through no evidence of benefit, to insufficient evidence. This is very useful because there is a serious distinction to be made, and it needs to be remembered that the term *'no evidence of benefit'* is not the same as *'evidence of no benefit'*. The hierarchy shown in Table 26 is novel in that it includes negatives (i.e. evidence of harm). In summary, this hierarchy covers the wider range of the results of the evidence, and it does not rely primarily on the source of evidence.

Table 26 The state of the clinical evidence

Term	Meaning
Evidence that products are beneficial	Interventions whose effectiveness has been demonstrated by clear evidence from controlled trials
Evidence that products are likely to be beneficial	Interventions for which the effectiveness is less well established than for those classified as 'beneficial'
Evidence of a trade-off between benefits and harm	Interventions for which clinicians and patients should weigh up the beneficial and harmful effects according to individual circumstances and priorities
Unknown effectiveness	Interventions for which there are currently insufficient data, or data of insufficient quality
Products are unlikely to be beneficial	Interventions which lack effectiveness are less well established than for those classified as 'likely to be ineffective or harmful' (see below)
Evidence that products are likely to be ineffective or harmful	Interventions whose effectiveness or harmfulness has been demonstrated by clear evidence

This hierarchy was initially developed under the Cochrane enterprise and is currently being used, for example, in the *British Medical Journal*'s co-developed publication, *Clinical Evidence*, which is a twice-yearly summary of some of the evidence on particular clinical issues.

If we delve deep enough into any particular study or collection of studies, and then sit down with our patient, we may very often categorise the evidence as 'evidence of a trade-off between benefits and harm'. In reality we have to consider trade-offs between risks and benefits for almost everything we do for and with patients. Thus if most of the evidence really falls into that category, then the hierarchy is insufficiently sensitive or specific.

Remember that any hierarchy is only a suggestion as to how to grade the evidence, and as yet there is no robust published research on which hierarchy is most useful to decision makers in any particular circumstance. Hierarchies are not problem free, nor are they all equally useful in any one case. As with any other league-table system, there is no consensus as to which hierarchy is superior. For example, Britton and colleagues argued that good-quality non-randomised studies could be more robust than poor-quality randomised control trials. Schulz *et al.* have provided empirical evidence that inadequate methodological approaches in clinical trials are associated with bias.

One important issue to consider is to what extent hierarchies help or hinder the decision makers' appreciation of the quality of the evidence. You also require a critical appraisal of the different hierarchies of the evidence.

Finally, you should never under any circumstances slavishly adopt or accept a hierarchy or grade of evidence. Ask about the following:

- the grading system

- who developed it

- why it was developed (as opposed to using a hierarchy that already existed)

- the existence of any independent evidence to support the grading system

- its sensitivity (e.g. can it distinguish between poor-quality randomised controlled trials and good-quality randomised controlled trials?), validity and reliability (if someone else used the grading system on the same literature to answer the same question, would they come to the same conclusion?)

- yourself, if it seems to be intuitive (if it looks too good to be true, it probably is!).

See **Advantages of evidence from clinical trials; Benchmarking; Case–control study; Clinical trial; Cohort analysis; Evidence-based medicine; Gold standard; Meta-analysis; Pseudorandomisation; Quasi-randomised controlled trial; Randomised controlled trial; Systematic review.**

○ Barton S (2000) Which clinical studies provide the best evidence? *BMJ.* **321**: 255–6.

○ Benson K and Hartz AJ (2000) A comparison of observational and randomised controlled trials. *NEJM.* **342**: 1878–86.

○ Britton A, McKee M, Black N *et al.* (1998) Choosing between randomised and non-randomised studies: a systematic review. *Health Technol Assess.* **2**: 1–119.

○ Concato J, Shah N and Horwitz RI (2000) Randomized, controlled trials, observational studies and the hierarchy of research designs. *NEJM.* **342**: 1887–92.

○ Earl-Slater A (2001) Critical appraisal of clinical trials and hierarchies of the evidence. *J Clin Govern.* **6**: 59–63.

○ Lindbaek M and Hjortdahl P (1999) How do two meta-analyses of similar data reach opposite conclusions? *BMJ.* **318**: 873–4.

○ Schulz KF, Chalmers I, Haynes RJ and Altman DG (1995) Empirical evidence of bias: dimensions of methodological quality associated with estimates of treatment effects in controlled trials. *JAMA.* **273**: 408–12.

Historical control

A historical control is a patient of a previous period.

For example, you could:

- use previous patients of the orthopaedics outpatient department and compare them with current patients under a new outpatient regimen

- compare patients in the new chest clinic with those previously attended to by the hospital

- compare patients attending a quick and early cancer diagnosis clinic with those who used a previous service.

Issues to think about include the following:

- the mixing of retrospective and prospective studies

- factors other than treatments (e.g. organisation) may influence results

- there may be a tendency for historical controlled trials to yield more optimistic results than randomised controlled trials.

See **Clinical trial; Randomised controlled trial**.

○ Sacks H, Chalmers TC and Smith H (1982) Randomized versus historical controls for clinical trials. *Am J Med.* **72**: 233–40.

History of clinical trials

For those who are interested in the history of clinical trials, trials in education and trials in social care, a good place to start is the Royal College of Physicians of Edinburgh website pages on 'controlled trials from history' (www.rcpe.org).

You will find the following on the College's website pages:

- an account of how the casting of lots has been used in human societies faced with choices under uncertainty

- control of selection biases

- control of observer biases

- images from trial records

- a bibliography of articles and books relevant to the historical aspects of trials

- a collection of other references to trial records

- a 'what's new' section listing recent additions and improvements to the website.

See **National Research Register**.

Homogeneity

Homogeneity means similarity. *See* **Heterogeneity**.

Homogeneous product

A product which is not different, or not perceived to be different, from another is said to be a homogeneous product. This means that there is some standardisation, or perception of standardisation, of the goods or services in question. *See* **Heterogeneous product; Homogeneity; Meta-analysis**.

Hypothesis

A hypothesis is a statement that can be tested by clinical research, observation, and analysis. *See* **Alternative hypothesis; Duhem's irrefutability theory; Falsificationism; Hypothesis testing; Lakatosian research programme; Null hypothesis.**

Hypothesis testing

Hypothesis testing is the practice of testing a hypothesis in order to determine its acceptability. *See* **Hypothesis; Hypothesis test decisions.**

Hypothesis test decisions

Once you have set a hypothesis and analysed the results, four issues arise (*see* Table 27).

Table 27 Hypothesis test decisions

Decision		Reject H_o	Do not reject H_o
Truth	H_o	Type 1 error	Right decision
	H_1	Right decision	Type 2 error

There are two right decisions, namely not rejecting the null hypothesis when it is true, and rejecting the null hypothesis if the alternative hypothesis is true. There are two errors. A type 1 error occurs when you reject a true null hypothesis, and a type 2 error occurs when you do not reject the null hypothesis when the alternative hypothesis is true.

Research methodology and philosophy suggest that matters are more complicated than this. *See* **Duhem's irrefutability theory; Falsificationism; Hypothesis; Lakatosian research programme; Type 1 error; Type 2 error.**

I

Iatrogenic disease
An iatrogenic disease is a disease that is said to occur as a result of an intervention. *See* **Adverse effect; Side-effect.**

Inactive
Something that is inactive is inert, and it cannot produce a treatment effect. *See* **Placebo.**

Individual patient trial
This is a clinical trial that involves just one patient (also called an N-of-1 trial or N1 trial).

The advantages of such trials include their relative speed of accomplishment and ease of analysis. Disadvantages include the lack of a control and a lack of generalisibility. *See* **Clinical trial; Generalisability of trial results; Number-of-1 trial.**

ICD
ICD is an acronym for International Classification of Diseases. *See* **International Classification of Diseases.**

ICH
ICH is an acronym for the International Conference on Harmonisation of Technical Requirements for Registration of Pharmaceuticals for Human Use. *See* **International Conference on Harmonisation.**

Incidence
The incidence is the number of new cases that occur in a given period (e.g. today, this week). The incidence (I) is usually calculated as follows:

$$I = \frac{\text{Number of new cases occurring during the time period}}{\text{Number of individuals exposed to the risk during the time period}} \times 1000$$

The incidence is a direct estimate of the probability of developing the event of interest (e.g. a disease or a side-effect of medication).

A recently published example includes a determination of the incidence of neurological disorders in a prospective community-based study of neurological disorders in the UK. *See* **Prevalence**.

○ Hawkes ND, Swift GL, Smith PM and Jenkins HR (2000) Incidence and presentation of coeliac disease in South Glamorgan. *Eur J Gastroenterol Hepatol.* **12**: 345–9.

○ MacDonald BK, Coekerell OC, Sander JW and Shorvon SD (2000) The incidence and lifetime prevalence of neurological disorders in a prospective community-based study in the UK. *Brain.* **123**: 665–76.

Inclusion criteria
Another term for entry criteria. *See* **Entry criteria; Exclusion criteria**.

Incomplete treatment option design
Suppose that a clinical trial involves combinations of radiology and anaesthesia, namely two radiological interventions, A and B, and two anaesthetics, X and Y. If the trial reports on AX, AY and BX combined interventions, then we have an incomplete treatment option design, because option BY is missing from the trial (*see* Figure 30).

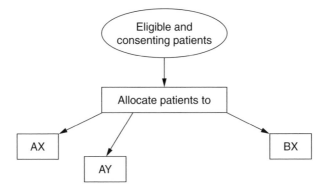

Figure 30 Incomplete treatment design.

Figure 30 makes it look obvious that something is missing from the trial (there are no BYs).

However, very often in the complexities of clinical trial reports and papers, it is not so clear that something is missing. The simplest way to work out what is going on is to draw a diagram for the particular trial in which you are interested.

When you see combinations of interventions you should:

• find out whether any explanation is given in the report for the combinations

• always look to see what possible combinations are missing

- check whether any explanation is given for missing combinations

- ask if the order of the interventions matters.

See **Due process; Multicentre research ethics committee; Order effects; Research governance in the NHS; Statistical tests: ten ways to cheat with statistical tests; Transparency.**

Independence
Events are independent if knowing the value of one tells us nothing about the value of another. *See* **Association; Causal relationship.**

Induction period
This is the period of time between exposure to a risk and onset of the disease.
   Examples of conditions that have an induction period include the following:

- cardiovascular disease

- cancers

- ulcers

- central nervous system diseases.

See **Latent period.**

Inference
Inference involves taking evidence from a sample, analysing it and then drawing 'conclusions' about a larger group.
   See **Generalisability of trial results; Meta-analysis; Sampling; Systematic review.**

Informed consent
Informed consent is voluntary agreement by a person to participate in a clinical trial after they have been made aware of all the relevant details. If the person has a power of attorney, then the power of attorney can give or refuse consent.
   Some studies have suggested that the more information that is given to a patient and the more time that the patient has to reflect on this information, the less likely it is that consent will be given.
   Other research has shown that the more information that is provided, the more uncertainty exists in the mind of the patient. Yet some work has shown the opposite – that more information leads to more certainty.
   In reality, there is probably an optimal level of information for each patient. The problem is that you will never really understand what that optimal level is, as it will

be case-, time- and context-specific. This does not mean that you should ignore the problems in informing patients prior to clinical trial, but rather that you have to take extra care to ensure that each patient is comfortable with the information and their understanding of the issues, and has no unnecessary uncertainties.

Given recent cases involving issues of informed consent (e.g. in hospitals in North Staffordshire, Manchester, Leeds and Bristol in England, as well as cases in France, America and Australia), these issues are quite rightly being seriously debated in professional, political and legal domains. *See* **Assent; Belmont Report; Consent; Data-monitoring committee; Declaration of Helsinki; Equipoise; Ethical issues; Questions to ask before getting involved in a clinical trial; Research governance in the NHS; Transparency.**

○ Edwards SJL, Lilford RJ, Thornton J and Hewison J (1998) Informed consent for clinical trials: in search of the 'best' method. *Soc Sci Med.* **47**: 1825–40.

○ Tobias J and Doyal L (2000) *Informed Consent: respecting patients in research and practice.* BMJ Books, London.

Institutional review board

Very common in the USA, an institutional review board (IRB) is an independent group of healthcare professionals from the institution where the trial is taking place and members of the local community. The board usually consists of physicians, statisticians, community advocates and others whose task is to ensure that the trial is ethical and that the rights of the study subjects are protected. The board has the power to scrutinise all trial activities, such as protocol design, trial recruitment, advertising, investigators' practices, risk management and data handling. The IRB also has to ensure that the trial is following the appropriate Food and Drug Administration regulations. Every clinical trial in the USA must be approved and monitored by an institutional review board. Indeed, institutions and groups that conduct or support trials in the USA are compelled by Federal law to have such a board. The practices of the IRBs themselves are subject to investigation and supervision by the trial regulators (Federal or State).

This is not to suggest that IRBs are 'problem free' or that they should be set in stone. The US Office of the Inspector General issued a report in June 1998, entitled *Institutional Review Board: A Time For Reform*, arguing that:

• the research atmosphere had changed significantly in recent years, as the number and complexity of clinical trials had increased dramatically

• IRBs were forced to do too much, too fast and with too little expertise

• IRBs did not provide enough ongoing review and, as a result, did not have a clear picture of how the informed consent process worked

• neither IRBs nor investigators were adequately trained

• not enough attention was given to evaluating the effectiveness of IRBs.

The report from the Office of the Inspector General made various recommendations, including the following:

- restructuring US law to give IRBs more flexibility and to make the IRBs more accountable
- strengthening protection for human research subjects
- imposing educational requirements on IRB members
- protecting IRBs from conflicts of interest
- easing workload pressures on IRBs
- revamping the federal oversight process, including a requirement that IRBs register with the government.

In April 2000, the Office of the Inspector General issued a follow-up report and found that 'minimal progress' had been made in implementing its recommendations.

In May 2000, the US Department of Health and Human Services Secretary Donna Shalala announced new efforts to improve subject protection, strengthen government supervision of clinical trials and reinforce the investigators' obligations to comply with federal requirements.

In June 2000, the Office of the Inspector General issued a report entitled *Recruiting Human Subjects: Pressures in Industry Sponsored Clinical Research*, which controversially claimed that the pharmaceutical industry used 'inappropriate' recruitment practices caused by market pressures for fast turnaround times, plus the increased number and complexity of clinical trials.

Not surprisingly, the Office of the Inspector General's reports started and stimulated considerable debate, including US Congressional hearings where a complete overhaul of the clinical trial and IRBs' supervision scheme was called for.

In June 2000, the US Human Research Subject Protection Act 2000 was introduced to the US Congress. This Act, as it stands, will address some but not all of the concerns raised in this area.

In December 2000, Donna E Shalala HHS Secretary announced the appointment of 12 members to the new National Human Research Protection Advisory Committee. Their first meeting, at Bethesda Marriott, Pooks Hill Road, Bethesda, MD, on 20–21 December, aimed to focus on financial arrangements in human research, the revised Declaration of Helsinki, research involving children, institutional review and oversight of non-biological research under the common rule.

Also during early 2001, various testimonies were put forward for consideration by a wide variety of individuals from different organisations with regard to ways to improve research policy, regulation and practice. The Internet is a useful way of keeping up to date with all of these developments.

In summary it can be suggested that:

- the business of conducting and governing clinical research is increasingly complex, of considerable size, dynamic and challenging

- evaluation of IRB competencies and practices should be independent and routine
- good research governance practices should be identified, publicised, replicated and rewarded
- poor research governance practices should be identified, publicised and dealt with
- the business of clinical research oversight and governance needs to become more transparent, rigorous and accountable
- the fate of clinical research needs to be audited.

After all this, you may be wondering why you need to be concerned about IRBs and other such developments in the USA.
The reasons are listed below.

- Many clinical trials are now international, and people are looking to develop more international standards.
- Many clinical trials are sponsored by US pharmaceutical companies, their agents, or US authorities.
- The USA is the largest clinical trial market in the world in terms of number of trials, number of patients involved, number of trial investigators, and the amount of money spent on clinical trials.
- It is easier to find out what is going on in clinical research fields in the USA than it is to find out what is going on in other countries.
- Trials conducted outside the USA wholly or as part of a submission for a US product licence have to adhere to US rules and regulations. Thus most of the research evidence that you see in clinical trial reports will include US centres, and most of the clinical trials with which you may be asked to become involved may be making some overtures to the US market.
- What happens in the USA usually has a bearing on what happens in other countries (i.e. your own country).

The institutional review board (IRB) system and trial regulations can be compared with other systems of research governance and oversight in other countries (e.g. the UK, Italy, France, China, India, Japan, Australia). *See* **Accountability**; **Clinical trial steering committee**; **Data-monitoring committee**; **Due process**; **Interim analysis**; **Local research ethics committee**; **Multicentre research ethics committee**; **Research governance in the NHS**; **Transparency**.

○ Food and Drug Administration (1998) (update) *Guidance for Institutional Review Boards and Clinical Investigators*. Available at http://www.fda.gov/. Department of Health and Human Services. 'Recruiting human subjects'. Office of the Inspector General, June 2000.

Intention

Intention is that which is planned. *See* **Analysis by assigned treatment; Intention-to-treat analysis**.

Intention-to-treat analysis

This is analysis based on what people were initially assigned to in the trial.

Some patients may drop out, withdraw or cross over treatment arms, or receive treatment other than that to which they were assigned. In order to minimise bias resulting from cases like these, all patients for whom we have information are analysed in the groups to which they were allocated.

For example:

- Hjalmarson and colleagues used intention-to-treat analysis to determine whether in patients with symptomatic chronic heart failure, controlled- and extended-release metoprolol succinate reduced mortality, symptoms and hospital admission

- Holman and colleagues used intention-to-treat analysis to study the effectiveness of acarbose in maintaining glycaemic control in patients who were receiving established therapy for type 2 diabetes mellitus

- Langer and colleagues used intention-to-treat analysis to determine whether glyburide is as safe and effective as insulin in women with gestational diabetes mellitus

- Mogensen and colleagues used intention-to-treat analysis to determine the effect of candesartan or lisinopril, or both, on blood pressure and the urinary albumin excretion rate in patients with hypertension, microalbuminuria and type 2 diabetes mellitus

- Ward and colleagues used intention-to-treat analysis to determine whether, in patients with depression, psychological therapy (non-directive counselling or cognitive behavioural therapy) was more effective than usual general practitioner care.

Again, note that in intention-to-treat analysis patients are assessed according to the arm of the trial to which they were originally assigned. There is debate as to whether this technique can be used when patients originally choose which arm of the trial they go into.

At best, intention-to-treat analysis can offer a way of generating more confidence in the study for clinical practice. It can also be used as a benchmark against actual paths followed, and as such it can signal underlying concerns about the trial protocol, patient entry and management issues.

You should at least read the paper by Sally Hollis and Fiona Campbell reporting their survey of published randomised controlled trials on what is meant by intention-to-treat analysis. In their survey of randomised controlled trials reported in four leading medical journals (the *British Medical Journal*, *Lancet*, the *Journal of the American Medical Association* and the *New England Journal of Medicine*), Sally and Fiona found that the intention-to-treat approach was inadequately described in the trials and inadequately applied. *See* **Adjusting for baseline; Analysis by administered treatment; Analysis by assigned treatment; Available case analysis; Care path analysis; Completer analysis; Dropout; Efficacy; Intention; Lost in follow-up; Missing values; Number needed to treat; Preference trial; Protocol; Withdrawal**.

○ Hjalmarson A, Goldstein S, Fagerberger B *et al.* for the MERIT-HF Study Group (2000) Effects of controlled-release metoprolol on total mortality, hospitalizations and well-being in patients with heart failure: the Metoprolol CR/XL Randomized Intervention Trial in Congestive Heart Failure (MERIT-HF). *JAMA*. **283**: 1295–302.

○ Hollis S and Campbell F (1999) What is meant by intention-to-treat analysis? Survey of randomised controlled trials. *BMJ*. **319**: 670–4.

○ Holman RR, Cull CA and Turner RC on behalf of the UK Prospective Diabetes Study Group (1999) A randomised double-blind trial of acarbose in type 2 diabetes shows improved glycemic control over 3 years. *Diabetes Care*. **22**: 960–4.

○ Langer O, Conway DL, Berkus MD *et al.* (2000) A comparison of glyburide and insulin in women with gestational diabetes mellitus. *NEJM*. **343**: 1134–8.

○ McCormack J and Greenhalgh T (2000) Seeing what you want to see in randomised controlled trials. Versions and perversions of UKPDS data. *BMJ*. **320**: 1720–3.

○ Mogensen CE, Neldan S, Tikkanen I *et al.* for the CALM study group (2000) Randomized controlled trial of dual blockade or renin–angiotensin system in patients with hypertension, microalbuminuria and non-insulin-dependent diabetes: the Candesartan and Lisinopril Microalbuminuria (CALM) Study *BMJ*. **321**: 1140–4.

○ Ward E, King M, Lloyd M *et al.* (2000) Randomised controlled trial of non-directive counselling, cognitive-behaviour therapy, and usual general practitioner care for patients with depression. I. Clinical effectiveness. *BMJ*. **321**: 1383–8.

Interim analysis

An interim analysis is the analysis of a clinical trial before its planned completion date.

For example:

• the trial reported by Hjalmarson and colleagues on the effects of controlled-release metoprolol on total mortality, hospitalisations and well-being in patients with heart failure was subject to an interim analysis (the results of which led to a decision to stop the trial)

• in patients with one or more cardiovascular risk factors but no history of cardiovascular disease, the Collaborative Group of the Primary Prevention Project reported on a randomised, unblinded 2×2 factorial trial with a mean follow-up of 3.6 years of aspirin and vitamin E. The trial was stopped early because evidence from two large trials indicated a benefit of aspirin in cardiovascular primary prevention that was borne out by the planned interim analysis in this trial

- in patients with a first confirmed demyelinating event, does interferon beta$_{1a}$ reduce the incidence of clinically definite multiple sclerosis? To address this question, Jacobs and colleagues reported the results of a randomised triple-blinded placebo-controlled trial with a 3-year follow-up. Interim analysis was planned and performed at 6, 12 and 18 months into the trial

- Pitt and colleagues reported on a randomised controlled trial of aggressive lipid-lowering therapy compared with angioplasty in stable coronary artery disease. In their main results they took into account the fact that an interim analysis was performed, and they adjusted their statistics accordingly.

Any clinical trial should include the following:

- clear procedures to be adopted for an interim analysis to take place

- a clear account of how the statistics change to take into account the fact that an interim analysis takes place

- specific details of who should see the interim results

- specific details of who should not see the interim analysis

- precise details of the criteria for stopping a trial on the basis of interim results

- precise detail of the criteria for continuing a trial on the basis of interim results.

Interim analysis is strongly advised in order to establish whether or not the regimens in the trial are producing favourable or unfavourable results. Looking too late at the evidence may mean that some patients continue to receive inferior treatment or suffer otherwise avoidable adverse events. This has to be weighed against the following considerations.

- Looking too early at trial data can give unreliable results (e.g. if there are relatively few patients in the trial).

- If we use a 5% level of significance and perform 20 interim analyses, then on one occasion we shall, just by chance, find statistically significant results.

- Interim analysis can mean that the final analysis of the trial data may require a lower level of significance (1% rather than 5%).

The issue of who should see the results of interim analysis is important. If the doctors see the results, this could affect their recruitment and selection of patients. If the patient sees the results of an interim analysis, this may affect the way in which they respond to the trial. If the patient hears that interim analysis showed that one treatment was better than another, and if they knew or could make educated guesses about what treatment they were on, then they may feel better if they are receiving the 'superior treatment', but worse if they are not.

It is important for trialists and sponsors to get interim analysis right, as the business history case of British Biotech shows. *See* **Bias; Blind; Data-monitoring committee; Early stopping rule; Multicentre research ethics committee; Primary outcome; Primary question; Protocol; Research governance in the NHS; Transparency.**

○ Collaborative Group of the Primary Prevention Project (2001) Low-dose aspirin and vitamin E in people at cardiovascular risk: a randomised trial in general practice. *Lancet.* **357**: 89–95.

○ Comella P, Frasci G, Panza N *et al.* (2000) Randomized trial comparing cisplatin, gemcitabine and vinorelbine with either cisplatin and gemcitabine or cisplatin and vinorelbine in advanced non-small-cell lung cancer: interim analysis. *J Clin Oncol.* **18**: 1451–7.

○ Freidlin B, Korn EL and George SL (1999) Data-monitoring committees and interim monitoring guidelines. *Control Clin Trials.* **20**: 395–407.

○ Hjalmarson A, Goldstein S, Fagerberger B *et al.* for the MERIT-HF Study Group (2000) Effects of controlled-release metoprolol on total mortality, hospitalizations and well-being in patients with heart failure: the Metoprolol CR/XL Randomized Intervention Trial in Congestive Heart Failure (MERIT-HF). *JAMA.* **283**: 1295–302.

○ Jacobs LD, Beck RW, Simon JH *et al.* and the CHAMPS Study Group (2000) Intramuscular interferon beta-1a therapy initiated during a first demyelinating event in multiple sclerosis. *NEJM.* **343**: 898–904.

○ Pitt B, Waters D, Brown WV *et al.* for the Atrovastatin versus Revascularization Treatment Investigators (1999) Aggressive lipid-lowering therapy compared with angioplasty in stable coronary artery disease. *NEJM.* **341**: 70–6.

Internal validity of results

The internal validity of clinical trial results is a measure of the extent to which the results of that trial are valid in that trial. *See* **External validity of results; Fixed-effects model; Systematic review; Validity.**

International Classification of Diseases

The International Classification of Diseases (ICD) is an attempt to standardise records of disease.

It is a list of diseases that have been assigned a four-number code. An international group of experts advised the World Health Organization on coding. The ICD has been subject to continued revision and refinement, and the tenth edition is in common use (ICD-10).

Below is an example of the use of the codes for chronic rheumatic heart disease:

- ICD code I05 covers rheumatic mitral valve disease

- code I05.0 covers mitral stenosis

- code I05.1 covers rheumatic mitral insufficiency

- code I05.2 covers mitral stenosis with insufficiency

- code I05.8 covers other mitral valve disease

- code I05.9 covers mitral valve disease unspecified.

See **Benchmarking**.

○ World Health Organization (1992) *International Statistical Classification of Diseases and Related Health Problems* (10e). World Health Organization, Geneva.

International Conference on Harmonisation

Established in 1990, the International Conference on Harmonisation of Technical Requirements for Registration of Pharmaceuticals for Human Use (ICH) is a series of conferences that brings together, in equal partnership, experts from the pharmaceutical industry and regulatory authorities in Europe, Japan and the USA.

The key objective of the ICH enterprise is to make recommendations on ways to achieve greater harmonisation in the interpretation and application of technical guidelines and requirements for product registration, in order to reduce or obviate the need to duplicate the testing that is performed during the research and development of new medicines. In doing so it seeks to make more efficient the use of human, animal and material resources, and to eliminate unnecessary delay in global development and availability of medicines, whilst simultaneously maintaining safeguards on quality, safety, efficacy and regulatory obligations to protect public health.

The parties to ICH are the European Commission, the European Federation of Pharmaceutical Industries' Associations, the Ministry of Health and Welfare in Japan, the Japan Pharmaceutical Manufacturers Association, the US Food and Drug Administration and the Pharmaceutical Research and Manufacturers of America. The World Health Organization, the European Free Trade Area (represented by Switzerland) and the Canadian authorities are observers for ICH.

ICH runs conferences and workshops, and produces videos and guidelines. With regard to clinical trials, interesting ICH documents that you could look at include the following:

- good clinical practice

- general considerations for clinical trials

- structure and content of clinical study reports

- clinical investigation of medicinal products in the paediatric population

- statistical principles for clinical trials

- choice of control groups in clinical trials

- ethnic factors in the acceptability of foreign clinical data

- dose–response information to support drug registration

- clinical safety data management

- timing of preclinical studies in relation to clinical trials

- common technical document

- stability testing

- impurity testing

- carcinogenicity testing

- genotoxicity testing

- validation of analytical procedures

- clinical investigation of medical products in the paediatric population.

The ICH work is internationally important, and these documents aid the understanding of trials and their application and interpretation nationally, regionally and locally. For more information, see the website (http://www.ifpma.org).

Inter-observer agreement

Inter-observer agreement is the degree to which one person's observation matches another person's observation.

For example:

- Chui and colleagues used a multicentre study of the comparability and inter-rater reliability of clinical criteria for the diagnosis of vascular dementia.

Inter-observer agreement is sometimes called inter-rater reliability. Inter-observer agreement is usually assessed using the kappa statistic. *See* **Intra-observer agreement; Kappa coefficient; William's agreement measure**.

○ Chui HC, Mack W, Jackson JE *et al.* (2000) Clinical criteria for the diagnosis of vascular dementia: a multicentre study of comparability and inter-rater reliability. *Arch Neurol.* **57**: 191–6.

Inter-rater reliability

Another term for inter-observer agreement. *See* **Inter-observer agreement**.

Intervention

The act of interfering, or trying to interfere, with the natural course of events. *See* **Clinical trial**.

Intra-observer agreement

Intra-observer agreement is the degree to which your observation today matches your previous observations. *See* **Inter-observer agreement**.

Investigator

An investigator is someone who is responsible for conducting a trial at one of the trial sites. *See* **Accountability; Assessor; Data-monitoring committee; Medical Research Council Guidelines for Good Practice in Clinical Trials; Principal investigator; Research governance in the NHS.**

Involving consumers in designing, conducting and interpreting randomised controlled trials

Thousands of clinical trials, costing millions of pounds and involving large numbers of people, are taking place at any moment in time.

How many of them have involved consumers in their design, execution or interpretation? What are the costs and benefits of consumer involvement in such aspects of clinical trials? More fundamentally, should consumers be involved in clinical trials in any way? How can they be actively involved? Who should be involved? What are the ethics, logistics and practical problems of having consumer involvement in your clinical trial? At present, these questions remain unanswered.

In using the word 'consumer' I am following the *Consumers in NHS Research* definition:

> patients or potential patients, carers, organisations representing consumers' interests, members of the public who are targets of health promotion programmes and groups asking for research because they believe they have been exposed to potentially harmful circumstances, products or services.

In using the term 'involvement' I am again following the *Consumers in NHS Research* definition:

> the active involvement of consumers in the research process, rather than the use of consumers as the 'subjects of research'.

Probably some of the first real glimpses of light have now been shed on involving consumers in designing, conducting and interpreting randomised controlled trials. In March 2001, Hanley and colleagues reported on a national study of clinical trial co-ordinating centres in the UK to assess the extent to which consumers were involved in the work of clinical trial co-ordinating centres, and the nature of consumers' involvement in randomised trials co-ordinated by these centres.

The positive comments of the investigators are listed in Table 28.

Table 29 lists some other comments from investigators about involving consumers in trials. Hanley and colleagues called them negative comments, but I regard them as additional insights or learning points for improving the involvement of consumers in designing, conducting and interpreting randomised controlled trials.

Although the evidence from Hanley and colleagues relates to investigators' comments from consumer-involvement-specific trials, there is no reason to believe that

Table 28 Positive comments from investigators about involving consumers in trials

Setting the scene
    They were important in helping to refine the questions
    More relevant and clearer questions were asked
    They pushed hard for the trial
    The consumers helped to convince researchers and funders that the trial was possible and ethical
    Useful for developing patient-centred outcome measures
    Provided important insights into how to make the trial work

Informing participants
    They were important in helping to refine information
    They helped to make a complex trial comprehensible to most patients
    The backing and input of the range of relevant consumer groups undoubtedly improved the
    quality of information that was given to potential participants
    The consumers had an impact on the type of information about the trial. The leaflet was
    produced to inform patients fully about risks associated with their treatment
    Consumers were able to increase their knowledge of the rationale for the trial

Recruiting participants
    They provided insights into issues important to the community and patients
    Their participation led to improved recruitment
    They played a pivotal role in providing 'front-line' intelligence on how the trial was being received
    during its development and execution

Advocating for the trial
    A similar US trial was stopped prematurely, and we considered it important to continue with the
    trial

Disseminating information
    They provided a link to consumer networks which helped to publicise the trial

Owning the trial
    They brought a sense of ownership of the concept and design of the trial to all who were
    involved and affected
    They helped to build relationships that have enabled more proactive involvement of consumers in a
    trial that followed on from a particular study

consumer involvement would not be beneficial in any type of research (clinical trial or otherwise). In fact, it needs to be asked whether sponsors of research, including government spending taxpayers' money, their agents, charities, research foundations, health technology manufacturers and pharmaceutical companies investing their profits, who together now spend in excess of £1.5 billion in the UK per year on clinical research, should now mandate that consumer involvement must be a feature of all of the research that it funds hereafter? If so, how? And if not, exactly why not? *See* **Accountability; Analytic perspective; Audit; Causes of delay and failure to complete a clinical trial; Due process; Fate of research studies; Post-marketing surveillance; Problems with regard to putting evidence into practice; Reasons given by the investigator for a study being abandoned or in abeyance; Reasons**

Table 29 Other comments from investigators about involving consumers in trials

There need to be clear guidelines on the remit of a consumers' group so that expectations are not disappointed

The problem is that there is no such thing as a 'consumer representative'. They are individuals who often have totally conflicting viewpoints. Their knowledge and understanding of trials also vary greatly

At the moment there is no obvious impact

The role of the consumer in this particular project was not a major one

The whole process took much longer

The involvement of the community health council somewhat jeopardised the usefulness of the data. Their insistence that patients should not be sent a reminder letter resulted in a low response rate and poor representativeness of our sample

given by the investigator for a study never being started; Research governance in the NHS; Transparency.

○ Altman DG (1994) The scandal of poor medical research. *BMJ*. **308**: 283–4.

○ Chalmers I (2000) A guide to patient-led good controlled trials. *Lancet*. **356**: 774.

○ Edwards SJL, Lilford RJ and Hewison J (1998) The ethics of randomised controlled trials from the perspectives of patients, the public and healthcare professionals. *BMJ*. **317**: 1209–12.

○ Hanley B (1999) *Involvement Works*. Department of Health, London.

○ Goodare H and Smith R (1995) The rights of patients in research. *BMJ*. **310**: 1277–8.

○ Hanley B, Trusdale A, King A, Elbourne D and Chalmers I (2001) Involving consumers in designing, conducting and interpreting randomised controlled trials: questionnaire survey. *BMJ*. **322**: 519–23.

○ NHS Executive (1998) *Research: what's in it for consumers?* NHS Executive, Department of Health, London.

○ Tallon D, Chard J and Dieppe P (2000) Relation between agendas of the research community and the research consumer. *Lancet*. **355**: 2037–40.

○ Thomas P (2000) The research needs of primary care: trials must be relevant to patients. *BMJ*. **321**: 2–3.

J

Jack-knife

The jack-knife is a method of reducing bias when estimating the values of variables.

Suppose that you have 200 cases in a clinical trial. The jack-knife method involves taking samples, omitting one case at a time. You would therefore generate a collection of samples each of size 199 cases. The factor of interest (e.g. average pulmonary function) can then be estimated for each sample. *See* **Bias; Sampling strategies; Statistical test diagram; Statistical tests: ten ways to cheat with statistical tests**.

J-shaped distribution

A J-shaped distribution is a description of data where the data fall and then rise higher after some point in time.

For example, the J-shaped distribution *may* reflect the following:

- the efficacy of some drugs

- the relationship between diastolic blood pressure and risk of mortality from coronary heart disease

- the relationship between alcohol consumption and risk of cardiovascular disease

- the relationship between age and risk of death.

There is some healthy debate in the scientific and clinical trials community as to whether or not the J-shaped distribution does indeed exist in specific areas.

Figure 31 shows an example.

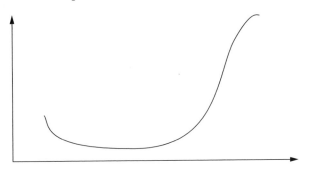

Figure 31 J-shaped distribution.

Kappa coefficient

Very often one needs to assess how one person's view or finding compares with another person's view. One way to do this is by using the kappa coefficient.

The kappa coefficient is a measure of the amount of agreement between people over and above that which would be expected by chance. It applies to dichotomous data.

Kappa coefficients have been used to guide decisions on the following:

- case finding

- patient recall compared with medical chart analysis

- how many patients in the primary care group would be eligible to enter a trial

- diagnostic skills and competences

- clinical governance

- which trial to pursue.

The kappa coefficient (K) is calculated as follows:

$$K = \frac{P_0 - P_c}{\text{Total observed} - P_c}$$

where P_0 is the observed frequency of agreement and P_c is the expected frequency of agreement.

For example, if the amount of observed agreement (P_0) is 0.8, and the expected frequency of agreement (P_c) is 0.2, then the kappa coefficient is:

$$K = \frac{0.8 - 0.2}{1 - 0.2} = 0.75$$

which suggests a good level of agreement (or some have interpreted this as indicating that 75% of agreement between people has not occurred by chance).

Table 30 compares agreement between the patient's recall of using a product and the history of use of the product on the patient's medical record.

Table 30 Comparing agreement between the patient's recall of using a product and the history of use of the product on the patient's medical record

		History of use of the product according to the medical chart		Total
History of use of the product according to the patient		Yes	No	
	Yes	14	7	21
	No	25	171	196
Total		39	178	217

The kappa coefficient is then calculated as follows:

$$K = \frac{(14 + 171) - (196 \times 178)/217}{217 - (196 \times 178)/217} = \frac{185 - 160.8}{217 - 160.8} = 0.43$$

This suggests a moderately low level of agreement between patient recall in interview and inspection of their medical records.

Other studies have used kappa to determine levels of agreement between the following:

- pathologists' diagnoses
- consultants' grade of patients' pain compared with patient's grading of their pain
- medical students' detection of acute pulmonary embolism
- ward nurses' recall of patients' medication compared with medical charts
- pharmacists' listing of contraindications of a commonly used medication for a particular patient compared with the contraindications indicated on the summary product sheet
- certain doctors' clinical decisions about a hypothetical patient compared with what their peers would decide to do for the same 'specified' patient.

The kappa coefficient usually ranges from 0 to 1 (*see* Figure 32).

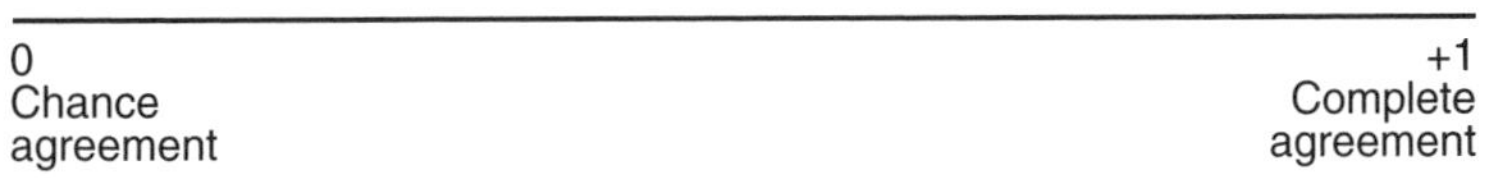

```
0                                                                    +1
Chance                                                         Complete
agreement                                                     agreement
```

Figure 32 Kappa results.

How do you interpret the kappa results? A score of 1 represents excellent agreement, and a score of 0 represents chance agreement. Apart from these two extremes there are no hard-and-fast rules, but in general perhaps a kappa score:

- from above 0 to below 0.2 can be considered to represent a very poor level of agreement

- from 0.2 to below 0.4 can be considered to represent a poor level of agreement

- from 0.4 to below 0.6 can be considered to represent a moderate level of agreement

- from 0.6 to below 0.8 can be considered to represent a good level of agreement

- from 0.8 to below 1.0 can be considered to represent a very good level of agreement.

The kappa coefficient is a measure of the amount of agreement between people over and above that expected by chance. Issues or questions that people addressed could, for example, have included any of the following.

- Does the patient have mild to moderately severe Alzheimer's dementia?

- Does the consultant have grade A interpersonal skills?

- Did the doctor breach the trial protocol?

- How do these patients score on lower back pain?

You really need to look closely at the question that is being addressed in order to help interpret the kappa coefficient.

Some have run kappa below zero to reflect, they say, levels of disagreement. This sounds intuitive, but the logic, mathematics and implications of a value below zero are still being debated and refined. *See* **Case finding; Clinical trial; Data types; Entry criteria; Exclusion criteria; Inter-rater reliability; Primary question; Split-half method; Take-up rate; William's agreement measure.**

L

L'Abbe plot

A L'Abbe plot is a method of displaying the relative results of analysis from several studies. Figure 33 shows what seven reports suggest in terms of the new anaesthetic compared with the anaesthetic most commonly used in the hospital at present. Suppose that A is the new product and B is what the consultants consider to be the best currently used product.

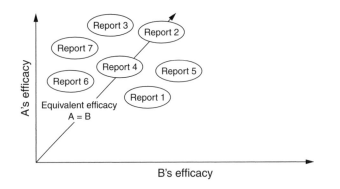

Figure 33 L'Abbe plot on efficacy of new anaesthetic compared with existing regimen.

The new Chief Executive at your local hospital has recently become an ardent believer in evidence-based decision making. She declares that any new non-capital programme of hospital spending above £50 000 per year will be based on a full review of the best evidence.

Results from a clinical trial show that a new anaesthetic reduces the incidence of post-surgical sickness. The surgeons, theatre staff and recovery-room nurses want to use the drug. The Chief Executive asks the Director of Surgery to provide the management committee with a summary of the evidence of the product *vis-à-vis* what is currently being used in the hospital.

The Director of Surgery briefs his team and delegates the task of finding, sorting and summarising the evidence to the Senior House Officer (SHO). The SHO works with the information pharmacist, who has experience in systematic reviews. Despite the Chief Executive's arrival and ambition, the management committee is not up to speed with the intricacies of evidence-based care. The SHO and librarian discuss their ideas with the Director of Surgery and decide to present their findings in part to the management committee in a diagram. They use a L'Abbe plot.

You can see from the figure that:

- three reports support A over B (reports 3, 6 and 7)
- two reports suggest equivalence (reports 2 and 4)
- two reports support B over A (reports 1 and 5).

The main strengths of L'Abbe plots are as follows.

- They pictorially summarise the balance of the evidence.
- They can be used to simplify complex issues.
- They allow mixing of different types of reports.
- They indicate which reports favour what intervention.
- They indicate how many reports are used in the analysis.

The main weaknesses of L'Abbe plots are as follows.

- They do not indicate what types of reports are in the picture (e.g. report 1 may be a randomised controlled trial, report 2 may be a systematic review, report 3 may be a case–control study, report 4 may be a meta-analysis, and so on).
- They do not indicate how the reports were identified, sifted or summarised.
- They do not indicate how much better one intervention is over another.
- They can only deal with two options (A or B).

In addition to the L'Abbe plot, the SHO should tell the committee about its caveats. As with any diagrammatic representation, there is debate about its merits and about what it can and cannot reveal. See **Data-display formats; Due process; Hierarchies of the evidence; Meta-analysis; Systematic review; Transparency; Ways of presenting results**.

Label

A label is a short phrase that identifies, for example, a product's strength, dose, administration, contraindications, side-effects, precautions and intended use. The label is usually attached to the product's packaging. See **Medicines Control Agency; Off label; Open label; Open label trial**.

○ Conroy S, Choonara I, Impicciatore P *et al.* on behalf of the European Network for Drug Investigation in Children (2000) Survey of unlicensed and off-label drug use in children's wards in European countries. *BMJ*. **320**: 79–82.

Lag

A lag is something that occurs after a particular period of time. *See* **Induction period; Latent period; Lead; Period effects; Washout period**.

Lakatosian's hard-core, protective belt

Lakatosian's hard-core, protective belt is the set of metaphysical beliefs unifying adherents to a research programme. The hard-core beliefs are not testable. Around the hard core there is claimed to exist a 'protective belt' of theories that are testable. *See* **Bayesian analysis; Duhem's irrefutability theory; Falsificationism; Lakatosian research programme**.

Lakatosian research programme

A Lakatosian research programme is a collection of interconnected theories from a Lakatosian hard core. A progressive Lakatosian research programme captures all facts anticipated by another research programme and provides new facts. A degenerating Lakatosian research programme does not capture all of the facts anticipated by another research programme, nor does it provide new facts. *See* **Duhem's irrefutability theory; Falsificationism; Hypothesis testing; Lakatosian's hard-core, protective belt**.

Last observation carried forward

Last observation carried forward is a method of analysis in which we take the last observation of the patient and carry those data forward to the end of the study. So, for example, if the trial lasts 12 weeks but some patients withdraw early, the last data we have on them, say at 8 weeks, are carried forward and analysed as if those data applied at 12 weeks. The validity of these techniques has yet to be established in each particular study. *See* **Adjusting for baseline; Analysis by administered treatment; Analysis by assigned treatment; Intention-to-treat analysis; Lost; Missing values; Statistical tests diagram; Statistical tests: ten ways to cheat with statistical tests**.

Latent period

The latent period is the particular period during which a disease develops but remains undetected in a person, tissue or culture. It is sometimes loosely called the induction period. *See* **Induction period; Lag**.

Latin square

The Latin square is a useful concept that provides a way to examine the effects of different interventions in different groups. For example, you could compare different hormone replacement therapy treatments in different age groups in different practices. Table 31 gives an example of four primary care groups, four HRT interventions A, B, C and D, and four patient age groups.

Table 31 A Latin square of HRT in four PCGs and four patient age groups

| Patient age group (years) | PCG | | | |
	1	2	3	4
35–44	A	B	C	D
	1	2	3	4
45–54	D	A	B	C
	5	6	7	8
55–64	C	D	A	B
	9	10	11	12
≥65	B	C	D	A
	13	14	15	16

The above example used a 4×4 Latin square of different HRT products. Any size of Latin square can be used, the commonest being 2×2.

Latin squares are often used when a large number of products are being tested in different groups of people in different places. There is no reason why the 'interventions' under study could not be different styles of management, different care packages, different technologies, different strengths, dosages, regimens, and so on.

One attraction of the Latin square system is that each of the four interventions is used in each primary care group and in each patient age group. As shown in Table 31 above, each intervention appears once in each row (PCG group) and once in each column (age group).

Another attraction is that the Latin square system can be considered to be generally efficient. What does this mean? In the HRT experiment above the table produces results from only 16 cells or classes. If you used another system and wanted to look at the effect of four HRT interventions on four different age groups of patients in four different PCGs, this would involve a need for $4 \times 4 \times 4 = 64$ classes. Thus a Latin square system could run with a smaller number of patients in the trial. This is important in terms of patient recruitment, trial feasibility, trial management, trial cost and trial analysis. *See* **Clinical trial; Cluster randomisation; Cross-over trial; Parallel trial.**

Leading question

A leading question is phrased in such a way that it leads the respondent to think that a certain answer is required. Responders are usually reluctant to contradict the questionnaire.

Examples that have been seen recently include the following:

- (to the patient) 'Do you agree that the hospital doctor is the best person to help you?'
- (to the caregiver) 'You don't have difficulty in recruiting patients into the trial, do you?'
- (to the potential purchaser) 'This is a brand new procedure, it incorporates the latest advanced technology, it is easy to use and highly recommended. Would you like to try it in your clinic free of charge for six months?'

See **Acquiescence response; Types of question.**

Licence

A licence is an official permit to own or do something.
     To obtain the licence may require:

- a willingness to have laboratories and manufacturing facilities inspected
- special application (e.g. submitting evidence)
- acceptance of official market rules and regulations.

In terms of UK medicines, the licencing authorities can grant licences for:

- conducting clinical trials (clinical trial certificates or CTCs)
- being exempt from certain aspects of a full clinical trial regulation (clinical trial exemption certificate CTC-X)
- manufacturing (a manufacturer's licence)
- wholesaling (a wholesale dealer's licence)
- product licences (a product licence).

For example, all medicines for human consumption need to have a product licence before they can be put on the market.
     Having a product licence does not necessarily:

- compel the licence holder to market the product
- confer any intellectual property rights on the licence holder
- mean that no further serious research should be conducted on the product
- mean that people will buy the product in the quantities expected
- mean that people will pay the price that the licence holder wants.

See **Food and Drug Administration; Medicines Control Agency; Phases of clinical trials; Research governance in the NHS.**

Likelihood
Likelihood generally means 'being possible'. *See* **Likelihood ratio.**

○ Hill G, Forbes W, Kazak J and MacNeill I (2000) Likelihood and clinical trials. *J Clin Epidemiol.* **53**: 223–7.

Likelihood ratio
The likelihood ratio is a measure that compares the likelihood of a result in one group of patients with that in another group of patients.

In a clinical trial, patients may be assigned to a new care regimen or what is called 'usual care'. Table 32 shows some indicative results.

Table 32 Likelihood ratio

	Event occurs	Event does not occur	Total
New care	a (100)	b (200)	a + b = 300
Usual care	c (300)	d (400)	c + d = 700
Total	a + c = 400	b + d = 600	a + b + c + d = 1000

+LR is the likelihood of an event or a positive result. It expresses how likely we are to find a positive test result in a patient with the disease compared with the likelihood of finding a positive test result in a patient without the disease. Using the symbols in Table 32:

$$+LR = (a/a + c)/(b/b + d)$$

Using the values in Table 32 as an example:

$$+LR = (a/a + c)/(b/b + d)$$
$$= (100/400)/(200/600)$$
$$= 0.75$$

This suggests that patients in new care are less likely to experience the event (e.g. a heart attack), or test positive than those in the usual care regimen.

How does one interpret +LR generally?

• If +LR > 1, this means that the new care group is more likely to experience the event.

• If +LR = 1, this means that the groups are equally likely to experience the event.

- If +LR < 1, this means that the new care group is less likely to experience the event than the usual care group.

−LR is the likelihood of no event or a negative result. It expresses how likely we are to find a negative test result in a patient with the disease compared with the likelihood of finding a negative test result in a patient without the disease. Using the symbols in Table 32:

$$-LR = (c/a + c)/(d/b + d)$$

Using the values in Table 32 as an example:

$$
\begin{aligned}
-LR &= (c/a + c)/(d/b + d) \\
&= (300/400)/(400/600) \\
&= 1.125
\end{aligned}
$$

This suggests that patients in new care are more likely to test negative or not to experience the event (e.g. not have a heart attack) than those in the usual care regimen.

How does one interpret −LR generally?

- If −LR > 1, this means that the new care group is more likely to test negative than the usual care group.

- If −LR = 1, this means that the groups are equally likely to test negative.

- If −LR < 1, this means that the new care group is less likely to test negative than the usual care group.

Likelihood ratios have also been used to express how likely it is that a particular test result will be found in patients.

Likelihood ratios are argued to be:

- unaffected by changes in the prevalence of disease

- usable when the test results are grouped into more than two categories

- convertible into a post-test probability by knowledge of the pre-test probability and likelihood ratio.

See **Absolute risk; Absolute risk reduction; Incidence; Odds; Odds ratio; Relative risk; Relative risk reduction**.

○ Pereira-Maxwell F (1998) *A–Z of Medical Statistics: a companion for critical appraisal*. Edward Arnold, London.

Loaded question

A loaded question is one that is phrased in such a way that it suggests an outcome. For example, if you agree and go ahead with something, things will get better, or if you do not agree and get involved, things will get worse.

Here is an example found in an invitation to patients to take part in a clinical trial:

(to patients at a chest clinic) Does your chest pain cause you severe discomfort and anxiety? Are you registered at this clinic, male, aged between 45 and 60 years? Would you like to enter a trial of a new product that aims to reduce your discomfort and anxiety?

The loaded aspect is that the patient is seduced into believing that if they get involved in the trial the drug will reduce their discomfort and anxiety. This raises questions about the research, the primary question, the null hypothesis, patient selection, volunteer bias, patient expectations, the type of trial, how the trial obtained ethics committee approval, and who is monitoring the recruitment. *See* **Equivalence trial; Leading question**.

Local research ethics committee

Guidance was issued by the Department of Health during 1991 requiring each of the then district health authorities to establish by February 1992 a Local Research Ethics Committee (LREC). LRECs are neither a management arm of the health authority nor a sub-committee of any other committee.

The general purpose of a LREC is:

- to maintain ethical standards of practice in research, and to ensure that guidelines issued by relevant bodies are adhered to
- to protect subjects of research from harm
- to preserve the subject's rights
- to provide reassurance to the public that these aims are being done.

LRECs have been consulted on the ethical issues of a proposed research project where it involves:

- NHS patients, including those under contracts with private sector providers
- foetal material and IVF involving NHS patients
- the recently dead, in NHS premises
- access to the records of past or present NHS patients
- use of, or potential access to, NHS premises or facilities.

Audits and clinical governance investigations are two types of analysis that have not usually been sent to LRECs for consideration. This does not mean that these types of analyses could not be improved by independent ratification by such a committee.

From experience, if there is any doubt about the suitability of a study for ethical review then the researcher should actively seek the advice of the chairman of the committee well in advance of commencing the study.

Any investigator who bypasses or ignores the recommendations of a properly authorised ethics committee does, in fact, create a potentially serious situation. They create for themselves a situation that could make him or her vulnerable to professional disciplinary or even legal proceedings. In addition to this, if their study is flawed they will be wasting patients', administrators' and their colleagues' time. Developments in research governance in the NHS mean that NHS organisations must be aware of what research is being undertaken in their organisation.

LRECs submit an Annual Report to the health authority. These include details such as the number of meetings held and a list of the proposals considered (including whether they were approved, approved after amendment, rejected or withdrawn). Copies of the report are sent to other NHS parties and are made available for public inspection.

A typical LREC may include the following members:

- two lay persons (one acting as chairman or vice-chairman)

- two general practitioners

- one from the nursing profession

- three medical practitioners from the local NHS hospital(s)

- a medical practitioner from the community (non-general practice)

- a pharmacist.

The membership should be representative of both sexes and cover a wide experience. Members do not, and should not, act in a representative capacity. Appointments are usually for an initial period of three years. Some LRECs have excellent induction programmes for new members.

While the members should cover a wide experience, LRECs may seek the advice of specialist referees or co-opt members to the committee so as to cover any aspect (e.g. professional, scientific or ethical) of a research proposal which lies beyond the expertise of the existing members. Investigators are asked to attend the meeting where their application is being discussed. This is especially true where there is a complicated or controversial proposal.

More details of LRECs, individual LREC contact information, how LRECs are fitting in with the research governance programmes and other information can be found on the Central Office for Research Ethics Committees' (COREC) website at http://www.corec.org.uk.

See **Caldicott Guardians; Consent; Ethical issues; European Union Directive on clinical trials of medicinal products for humans; Research ethics committee: possible progress report form; Research governance: baseline assessment; Research governance implementation plan; Research governance in the NHS.**

○ Ah-See KW, MacKenzie J, Thakker NS and Maran AG (1998) Local research ethics committee approval for a national study in Scotland. *J Royal Coll Surg Edin.* **43**: 303–5.

○ Alberti GM (1995) Local research ethics committees. *BMJ.* **311**: 639–41.

○ Busby A and Dolk H (1998) Local research ethics committees' approval in a national population study. *J Royal Coll Phys Lond.* **32**: 142–5.

○ Lux AL, Edwards SW and Osborne JP (2000) Responses of local research ethics committees to a study with approval from a multicentre research ethics committee. *BMJ.* **320**: 1182–3.

○ NHS Executive (1997) *Ethics Committee Review of Multicentre Research: establishment of multicentre research ethics committees.* HSG(97)23. NHS Executive, Leeds.

○ NHS Executive (1998) *Guidance Points to Local Research Ethics Committees.* NHS Executive, Leeds.

○ MREC Central Office (2000) *Revised MREC Paperwork.* NHS Executive South Thames, London.

○ Tulley J, Ninis N, Booy R and Viner R (2000) The new system of review by multicentre research ethics committees: prospective study. *BMJ.* **320**: 1179–82.

○ While AE (1995) Ethics committees: impediments to research or guardians of ethical standards? *BMJ.* **311**: 661.

Long term

In clinical trials, the long term is a period of at least one year.

Two quite different areas to consider are that the long term could relate to:

- the length of treatment
- the period of follow-up study.

The intervention may be given over a long period of time (e.g. in osteoarthritis trials), or the analysis may be over a long period of time. Some trials (e.g. involving surgery) have very short periods of intervention and longer periods of follow-up.

When you come across the expression 'long term' in a clinical trial, start by asking the following questions.

- What was long term (i.e. intervention or follow-up)?
- How long was it?
- How long would patients be on the intervention or followed up in clinical practice?

See **Long-term analysis.**

Long-term analysis

A long-term analysis is a study of patients in a clinical trial, where the patients have been in the trial for at least a year. It is important to be aware that the patients may not have received the intervention for the whole year. For example, they may have received 16 weeks of treatment and 2 weeks of washout, but are now being followed up over 2 years. *See* **Compliance**; **Long term**.

○ Hartigan C, Rainville J, Sobel JB and Hipona M (2000) Long-term exercise adherence after intensive rehabilitation for chronic low back pain. *Med Sci Sports Exerc.* **32**: 551–7.

Longitudinal study

A study that follows patients over a period of time. *See* **Accountability**; **Cohort**; **Comparing research methods**; **Experimental study**; **Observational study**; **Prospective analysis**; **Research questions and research methods**.

Lost

Information that was recorded in a clinical trial but which is now missing is described as lost. It is not the same as information that was not recorded. *See* **Audit**; **Lost in follow-up**; **Missing values**; **Protocol**.

Lost in follow-up

Lost in follow-up refers to patients or data that are not recorded in the records of the clinical trial when you try to follow up the patient (e.g. after their previous visit to the clinic). They are sometimes just described as 'lost'. *See* **Accountability**; **Audit**; **CONSORT**; **Dropout**; **Fate of clinical research**; **Intention-to-treat analysis**; **Interim analysis**; **Last observation carried forward**; **Long-term analysis**; **Lost**; **Number needed to treat**; **Stopping rules**.

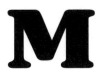

M

Mask

To mask means to cover, disguise, conceal or hide. Various aspects of a clinical trial can be masked. A mask is another term for concealment or blinding. Masks must be lifted in some circumstances (e.g. if there are concerns about side-effects or mortality rates).

Examples include the following:

- masking the system of allocating patients to arms of the trial
- masking the specific intervention from the patient
- masking the specific intervention a patient receives from the doctor
- not allowing the data analysts to know which patients received which intervention in the trial.

Masking reduces the opportunities for bias in the clinical trial. For example, patients may respond differently if they find out what intervention they have (e.g. if they believe that 'new' means 'better'). *See* **Bias; Blind; Blinding; Concealment; Data dredging; Data-monitoring committee; Interim analysis; Stopping rules; Transparency.**

Matched pair

A matched pair occurs when two individuals in a clinical trial share similar characteristics except for the intervention that they received. Factors that have been matched have included age, gender, ethnicity, initial health status and prognosis. Analysis is performed on other factors (e.g. intervention, compliance, outcomes). *See* **Baseline; Baseline balance; Matching; Matching cases and controls; Paired design; Statistical test diagram; Subgroup analysis.**

Matching

This involves selecting a group that has some similar characteristics. Examples include matching on the following characteristics:

- age
- gender

- disease history

- disease state at the start of the trial

- health state at the start of the trial

- lifestyle issues (e.g. smoking status)

- clinic

- ethnicity.

See **Controls; Matched pair; Matching cases and controls**.

Matching cases and controls

This involves selecting groups of patients who have similar characteristics but receive different interventions. The 'cases' receive the new regimen, whereas the 'controls' do not receive the new regimen (e.g. they may receive a placebo or the current standard care). The idea is to try to tease out the specific effects of factors on which they are not matched (e.g. the different interventions).

Patients may be matched on various dimensions. *See* **Baseline; Matched pair; Matching**.

Medical Devices Agency

The Medical Devices Agency is an organisation in the UK that assesses the safety and performance of medical devices. Unlike medicines, medical devices do not as yet need to receive official licences before they can go on the market. This means that most medical devices do not yet have to undergo rigorous clinical trials before they can go on the market. Some medical devices are in fact being subjected to pre-market clinical trials as the makers seek to offer more robust information about the merits of their product. *See* **Medicines Control Agency**.

Medical Research Council Guidelines for Good Practice in Clinical Trials

This is a set of guidelines from the UK's Medical Research Council (MRC) purporting good practice in clinical trials.

As the MRC is a major funder of clinical trials in the UK, it needs to be assured that those who conduct research which it has funded agree to and adhere to guidelines that safeguard study participants and ensure that the data which are collected are of high quality. This needs to be done without destroying the essential element of trust that underpins all research funding, or adding a cumbersome layer of bureaucracy that may stifle legitimate research activity.

The MRC Guidelines are based on the principles laid down by the ICH Harmonisation Tripartite Guidelines for Good Clinical Practice agreed in May 1996.

These principles are as follows.

1 Clinical trials should be conducted in accordance with the ethical principles that have their origin in the Declaration of Helsinki and are consistent with good clinical practice and the applicable regulatory requirements.

2 Before a trial is initiated, foreseeable risks and inconveniences should be weighed against the anticipated benefits for the individual trial's participants and society. A trial should be initiated and continued only if the benefits justify the risks.

3 The rights, safety and well-being of the trial participants are the most important consideration, and they should prevail over the interests of science and society.

4 The available non-clinical and clinical information on an investigational product should be adequate to support the proposed trial.

5 Clinical trials should be scientifically sound and described in a clear detailed protocol.

6 A trial should be conducted in compliance with the protocol that has received prior ethical committee favourable opinion.

7 The medical care given to and the medical decisions made on behalf of participants should always be the responsibility of a qualified physician or, when appropriate, a qualified dentist.

8 Each individual involved in conducting a trial should be qualified by education, training and experience to perform his or her respective task(s).

9 Freely given informed consent should be obtained from every participant prior to clinical trial participation.

10 All clinical trial information should be recorded, handled and stored in a way that allows its accurate reporting, interpretation and verification.

11 The confidentiality of records that could identify participants should be protected, respecting the privacy and confidentiality rules in accordance with the applicable regulatory requirement(s).

12 Investigational procedures should be manufactured, handled and stored in accordance with good manufacturing practice (GMP). They should be used in accordance with the approved protocol.

13 Systems with procedures that ensure the quality of every aspect of the trial should be implemented.

Do not just skip through these principles. They are not only being used to support high standards in trials, but they are also now being used as a checklist by some people who want to find a weakness or raise a question about a clinical trial. If someone finds out that your trial violates one of the principles, then your work and the patients' and your host institutions' goodwill will be seriously damaged. Maintaining high standards is important in terms of medical research, professional reputation, funding, patient care and the law.

If you are not involved in a clinical trial you can always question those who are by asking them to prove that they are adhering to the principles. What else can you do with the principles? Contact a colleague in your trust, board or region who is involved in an MRC clinical trial (see the National Research Register for details) and ask them to show how well they are following the MRC principles. Then go to a trial sponsored by another party and see what principles they have to follow, and what principles they are in fact following. In both exercises, ask the principal investigators of the trials for proof.

As a third exercise, suppose you want to get involved in a clinical trial. Use each of the principles and turn them into questions. For example, principle 10 could be turned into the following question: 'How is the trial information to be gathered, collated, audited and stored?'

The MRC Guidelines include details on the following:

- the host institution

- the principal investigator

- independent trial supervision

- the trial steering committee

- trial management

- investigational products

- randomisation procedures

- medical care of trial participants

- respect for trial participants and informed consent

- protocol compliance

- safety reporting

- data handling and record keeping

- quality assurance and audit

- progress of the trial

- consideration of new information

- dissemination and implementation of trial results

- complaints procedures and compensation for individuals

- communication with local and multicentre research ethics committees

- peer review of scientific, ethical and management arrangements

- documentation

- MRC proforma application form

- MRC trial steering and data-monitoring committees

- key documentation.

See **Audit; Benchmarking; Declaration of Helsinki; International Conference on Harmonisation; Local research ethics committee; Meta-analysis; Multicentre research ethics committee; Peer review; Protocol; Research governance in the NHS; Systematic review.**

○ Department of Health (1996) *The Protection and Use of Patient Information.* Department of Health, London.

○ Medical Research Council (1998) *Guidelines for Good Practice in Clinical Trials.* Medical Research Council, London.

Medical subject headings (MeSH)

Medical subject headings (MeSH) are terms used in some information databases to index the articles in the database. When you search for information in the database, it may be best if you look for and then use the particular relevant terms in the index. Unfortunately, two databases may not use the same MeSH terms. *See* **Cochrane Collaboration; Critical appraisal; Evidence-based medicine; Meta-analysis; National Research Register; Systematic review.**

Medicines Control Agency

The Medicines Control Agency is an organisation in the UK that assesses the safety, efficacy and quality of medicines prior to a market-licensing decision being made. The Medicines Control Agency also covers post-licensing issues relating to pharmacovigilance, licence variation, 5-yearly renewals of marketing authorisations, reclassification of the legal status of a licence, product information, advertising and promotion control (including advertising medicines on the Internet), and the inspection of manufacturing and laboratory facilities.

The Committee on Safety of Medicines (CSM) advises the Medicines Control Agency on questions relating to the safety, efficacy and quality of the product under consideration. On the basis of the evidence and advice, the licensing authority then makes a decision as to whether and on what terms the product should be licensed on the UK market.

The Medicines Control Agency also acts as a rapporteur for products seeking a European licence (i.e. permission to go on all EU member states' markets). *See* **Accountability; Committee on Safety of Medicines; Food and Drugs Administration; Licence; Medical Devices Agency; Transparency.**

Mega-trial

A mega-trial is a clinical trial which:

- generally involves a large number of patients
- includes various clinics *and*
- is of a simple design.

How 'large' a mega-trial has to be remains the subject of debate. Mega-trials could:

- maximise the number of patients under trial
- enrol a large number of patients very quickly
- improve the co-ordination of trial centre staff
- provide results sooner than other types of trials
- make the results more acceptable to a wider audience.

The main problems associated with mega-trials include, for instance:

- relatively high cost
- problems of practicality
- problems of management
- difficulties in recruiting suitable numbers of physicians
- variations in local clinical practice
- variations in ethical committee requirements
- problems in simplifying the care protocol
- the problem of what to include as the comparator intervention.

See **Clinical trial; Definitive clinical trial; Generalisability of trial results; Meta-analysis; Systematic review**.

○ Barer D (1999) Simple mega-trials are not sufficient. *BMJ*. **318**: 1138.

○ Davey Smith G and Egger M (1998) Meta-analysis: unresolved issues and future developments. *BMJ*. **316**: 221–5.

○ Ioannidis JP, Capapelleri JC and Lau J (1998) Issues in comparisons between meta-analysis and large trials. *JAMA*. **279**: 1089–93.

○ le Lorier G, Gregoire G, Benhaddad A, Lapierre J and Derderian F (1997) Discrepancies between meta-analysis and subsequent large-scale randomisation, controlled trials. *NEJM*. **337**: 536–42.

○ Lubsen J and Tijssen JGP (1989) Large trials with simple protocols: indications and contraindications. *Control Clin Trials*. **10**: 151–60S.

○ Peto R and Baigent C (1998) Trials: the next 50 years. Large-scale randomised evidence of moderate benefits. *BMJ*. **317**: 1170–1.

Meta-analysis

Meta-analysis is a method of synthesising the data from more than one study, in order to produce a summary statistic.

Despite what some people say and others seem to think, the basic ideas behind meta-analysis are certainly not new. Astronomers combined the estimates made by different observers as early as 1722, using sophisticated mathematics to attach weights of importance to different people's measures and thus obtain summary measures. In the 1930s, Cochrane combined estimates in agricultural experiments to produce summary data.

The aims of meta-analysis are to:

• use summary statistics to identify the direction and strength of the evidence

• synthesise the available data

• establish where agreement and disagreement exist

• show where gaps in the evidence exist.

Listed below are some points to consider with regard to meta-analysis.

• How were the trials identified?

• Are the trials independent of each other?

• Is there any common ground in terms of settings, investigators or sponsorship?

• How do the individual trials match up in terms of method, entry, exclusion, duration, setting, blinding, treatment, control group, objectives, outcome measures and results?

• Where did the data come from?

• How were the data generated?

• How were the data compiled?

• What data were not included?

• What periods of time do the trials relate to?

• Which trials had independent trial-monitoring committees attached to them?

• Have the meta-analysts themselves been involved in the trials?

• Have the meta-analysts honestly and openly stated their financial and professional interests in the work?

• How sensitive are the results to adding or removing one piece of data?

In some cases very little will be known about the particular topic. If that is the case, then you must be able to state that no meta-analysis was performed because there was no evidence to put together. However, apart from very basic, fundamental clinical trials, there are very few cases where no evidence exists on the topic being studied. So if someone says 'No meta-analysis was possible/required/done', ask them why not.

If one considers that some types of studies are better than others (e.g. some consider randomised controlled trials to be superior to case–control studies), then one can weigh the results more heavily for these studies in the meta-analysis. In other cases, only specific types of studies have been used in a meta-analysis (e.g. published, double-blind, randomised, placebo-controlled trials). *See* **Evidence-based medicine; Fixed-effects model; Heterogeneity; L'Abbe plot; Peto method; Pooled analysis; Random-effects model; Systematic review; Triangulation**.

○ Ballier JC III (1997) The promise and problems of meta-analysis. *NEJM*. **337**: 559–60.

○ Capapelleri JC, Ioannidis JPA, Schmid CH *et al*. (1996) Large trials vs. meta-analysis of smaller trials: how do their results compare? *JAMA*. **276**: 1332–8.

○ Davey Smith G and Egger M (1998) Meta-analysis: unresolved issues and future developments. *BMJ*. **316**: 221–5.

○ Dersimonian R (1996) Meta-analysis in the design and monitoring of clinical trials. *Stat Med*. **15**: 1237–48.

○ Egger M, Davey Smith G and Phillips A (1997) Meta-analysis: principles and procedures. *BMJ*. **315**: 1533–7.

○ le Lorier G, Gregoire G, Benhaddad A, Lapierre J and Derderian F (1997) Discrepancies between meta-analysis and subsequent large-scale randomisation, controlled trials. *NEJM*. **337**: 536–42.

○ Lindbaek M and Hjortdahl P (1999) How do two meta-analyses of similar data reach opposite conclusions? *BMJ*. **318**: 873–4.

Missing values

Missing values are pieces of information in a clinical trial that have not been recorded even though they should have been.

They may seriously impair the validity of the clinical trial and raise questions for research management and research ethics.

There are various ways to deal with missing values, each of which has its own strengths and weaknesses.

- Analyse only the available data.

- Previous estimates of the data can be used to estimate the missing data (e.g. carrying the last observation forward, or using the worst available observation).

- Estimate the missing value by interpolation.

- Estimate the missing value by extrapolation.

- Impute a value by more complex advanced statistical techniques.

See **Audit; Accountability; Available case analysis; Data cleaning; Data-monitoring committee; Lost; Lost to follow-up; Protocol; Statistical tests: ten ways to cheat with statistical tests.**

○ European Agency for the Evaluation of Medicinal Products (1999) *Concept paper on the development of a Committee for Proprietary Medical Products (CPMP) position paper on biostatistical/methodological issues arising from recent CPMP discussions on licensing applications: missing data.* EMEA, London.

○ Lachin JM (1999) Worst rank score analysis with informatively missing observations in clinical trials. *Control Clin Trials.* **20**: 408–22.

Morality

Morality is the subjective belief about what is right or wrong, or good or bad. *See* **Ethical issues.**

Morbidity

Morbidity is a term used to reflect a state of health, not death. *See* **Composite endpoint; Endpoint; Health; Mortality; Multiple endpoints; Outcomes pyramid; Primary outcome; Quality of life; Surrogate endpoint.**

Mortality

Mortality is a term used to signify death. *See* **Endpoint; Health; Morbidity.**

Multicentre research ethics committee

A new system for obtaining ethical approval for multicentre research was announced in the 1997 Health Service Guidelines document HSG(97)23. In order to facilitate the process of ethical review of multicentre research, Multicentre Research Ethics Committees (MRECs) were established in 1997 to complement the work of existing Local Research Ethics Committees (LRECs).

The MREC system is an attempt to solve various problems of multilocation research. These include:

- a diversity of local ethical requirements and systems

- a multiplicity of applications

- delayed time to receive decisions

- variations in decisions

- duplication of effort

- lack of co-ordination.

It was hoped that the MREC system would facilitate useful research, raise the standards, and dilute the problems outlined above.

In addition, the general purpose of a MREC is:

- to maintain ethical standards of practice in research, and to ensure that guidelines issued by relevant bodies are adhered to
- to protect subjects of research from harm
- to preserve the subject's rights
- to provide reassurance to the public that these aims are being adhered to.

For the new system, multicentre research is defined as that which is carried out within five or more LRECs' geographical boundaries. All such research must be considered by a MREC.

The MREC application should be made by a single named 'principal researcher' to the NHS region within which they are based. Interestingly, the decision of the MREC will then apply to all regions in England. Reciprocal arrangements are in place with similar committees established in Scotland, Wales and Northern Ireland.

Once MREC approval has been obtained the principal researcher will receive a letter of approval which must be sent to any local researchers who are to be involved. The local researchers must then submit the application, together with the MREC approval, to the LREC, for consideration of issues that may affect local acceptability. LRECs will not consider applications for multicentre research without the MREC approval letter.

MRECs in each region are given the responsibility of reviewing research proposals taking place within the boundaries of five or more LRECs. The study need not involve a clinical trial: for example, it could involve a plan for database research, patient interviews, or pharmacy practice observation. Approval by one MREC for the research has national acceptance. However, even with such approval there is no compulsion to conduct the trial on a national scale.

MRECs have been established in accordance with the advice given in HSG(97)23 and MEL(1997)8, and in the context of the guidance given in HSG(91)5 and Circular 1992(GEN)93. As of February 1998, the standing orders for MRECs in the UK NHS are as follows.

The Committee will be responsible for considering multicentre research where the principal researcher is based in [the relevant area] and the research is to be conducted within five or more LRECs' geographical boundaries in the UK.

Membership
The Chairman and Vice-Chairman are appointed by the Chief Medical Officer, and one of these appointments is to be lay. They will serve initially for 2 years and will be reappointed in such a way as to ensure continuity of experience. Members will serve for a period of 3 to 5 years, renewable for one term. The composition of the MREC is set out in Table 33.

The Chairman has the authority, in consultation with the Department of Health and the membership, to approach any member whose conduct is felt to be detrimental to the cohesion and work of the Committee, and to discuss this matter for the benefit of the whole Committee. Ultimately, if this cannot be resolved the member can be asked to resign.

Attendance at meetings

Members should not have deputies. If a member fails to attend three consecutive meetings or less than 50% of the meetings taking place in the year, he/she will be deemed to have resigned.

Legal liability

The Department of Health will indemnify MREC members in respect of any loss which they may incur resulting from any claim made against them arising out of the exercise of their function as a member of the MREC, including their legal costs and any compensation and expenses for which they may be found to be liable, provided that the member notifies the Department of any such claim and assists it in all reasonable ways.

Declaration of interest

If a member of the Committee has a financial or personal interest in a project or with a project sponsor, he/she must inform the Chairman, who will decide whether the interest disqualifies the member from the discussion.

Confidentiality

Members will keep confidential all paperwork and discussions connected with the work of the MREC.

Accountability

The MREC will be accountable to the Secretary of State – in practice this function has been delegated to the Chief Medical Officer. The main formal mechanism for achieving accountability will be an annual report.

Number and frequency of meetings

The MREC will meet as often as is reasonable and consistent with its workload. This will be on a monthly basis initially.

Agenda papers

Agenda papers will be sent to members, wherever possible, at least 2 weeks before the meeting at which they will be discussed.

Dates of meetings

Dates of all meetings will be published for the year ahead to enable researchers to target meeting dates. Researchers should send applications to the MREC administrator 3 weeks before the meeting being targeted.

Attendance at meetings by researchers

Applicants may be asked to attend the MREC meeting at which their project is discussed.

Decisions of the committee

The decisions of the Committee will be reached by full discussion of all of the ethical issues. Wherever possible a consensus will be reached. All decisions will be notified to the researcher in writing within 10 working days of the meeting at which the project was discussed. Reasons for approval or rejection will always be given. Any significant minority view will be noted in the minutes, and the comments may be forwarded to the researcher anonymously if this is thought to be helpful.

The following decisions on an application may be taken:

- *approve*: the application is granted ethical approval without amendment

- *approve subject to amendment*: the application is granted ethical approval subject to relatively minor amendments, and authority is delegated to the Chairman to confirm that the response received from the principal researcher conforms with the Committee's requirements

- *defer*: consideration of the application is deferred to a future meeting pending receipt of substantial amendments, clarification or further information

- *reject*: the application is refused ethical approval as it is intrinsically unethical and not capable of easy amendment

- *transfer*: the application is not appropriate for the particular MREC and will be transferred to a more appropriate one.

General conditions of approval

The MREC will offer ethical approval subject to the following general conditions:

- there is no divergence from the original protocol without first contacting the Committee

- regular updates of the progress of the research and a report of the outcome of the trial are received

- the project is started within 3 years of the date approval is given – extensions can be applied for

- adverse events are notified to the MREC, relevant LRECs and the sponsor using the procedure set out in the MREC guidelines.

MREC cross-referrals

A heavily loaded MREC may, by agreement between the secretariats, pass work to another MREC. Proposals may also be passed to another committee where a MREC has expertise in a specialised area. No MREC can hear appeals against another MREC or LREC. Any differences between a researcher and a MREC must be resolved between themselves. It will be possible to seek referral to another MREC if an outcome cannot be resolved, provided that there is agreement with the initial MREC and researcher. The advice of the second MREC will be final.

Chairman's action

Chairman's action will never be used to decide an initial proposal. It is appropriate for confirming minor amendments in applications approved subject to amendment, where the principal researcher has fulfilled the requirements. It is also appropriate for determining whether amendments to applications already approved are sufficiently substantive to require consideration by the full Committee, or whether they are sufficiently minor to be approved by Chairman's action. Decisions made under Chairman's action should be reported to the next meeting of the Committee.

Quorum

A quorum will consist of half of the members, provided that it includes either the Chairman or Vice-Chairman, at least two lay members and two medically qualified members. The Administrator should ensure that each meeting will be quorate prior to the meeting.

Minutes of meetings

Minutes will be taken of all Committee meetings. These will be confidential but may be sent to the Chief Medical Officer, Chief Scientist and LREC Chairmen on request.

Retention of applications

The Administrator of the MREC will retain copies of all applications received by the Committee for a period of 3 years beyond the conclusion of the research.

Annual report

An Annual Report will be sent to the Secretary of State or his representative. Copies of the Annual Report will also be available to LREC Chairmen and the Department of Health. The Annual Report will be available for public inspection.

Reviewing approved research

The MREC will expect to be advised of any adverse results, failure to complete research or any other information that may be considered of interest to the MREC in the conduct of its work. In addition, the MREC requires an annual progress report and a final report on completion of the project. Pro forma are provided in the Guidelines for this purpose. The researcher is also required to advise the MREC if the research is withdrawn or if difficulties are experienced in recruiting research subjects.

Application fee

An application fee of £1000 per application will be charged for research sponsored by commercial companies.

Figure 34 provides an illustration of a flowchart for a MREC system.

Table 33 below sets out the composition for the MRECs. In practice, variations of composition within agreed parameters are permissible.

In September 1998, the NHS Executive issued points of guidance to LRECs stating that:

- a standing subcommittee of the LREC should be established to consider applications approved by MRECs (quorum shall be two members)

- a meeting of this LREC executive subcommittee should be called within 2 weeks of receipt of an application approved by a MREC

- the decision of the LREC executive subcommittee should be communicated to the researcher within 5 working days. This does not require ratification by the full committee, and if approval is granted, the research work may commence

- rejection of the application by the LREC executive subcommittee can only be for local reasons (see below), and must be accompanied by a full explanation for this decision.

Reasons for LREC rejection could be based on:

- the suitability of the local researcher
- the suitability of the site
- the suitability of the subjects
- the requirement that patient information sheets and consent forms carry local information as required or are produced in a locally appropriate language. No other changes to the information sheets or consent forms can be made.

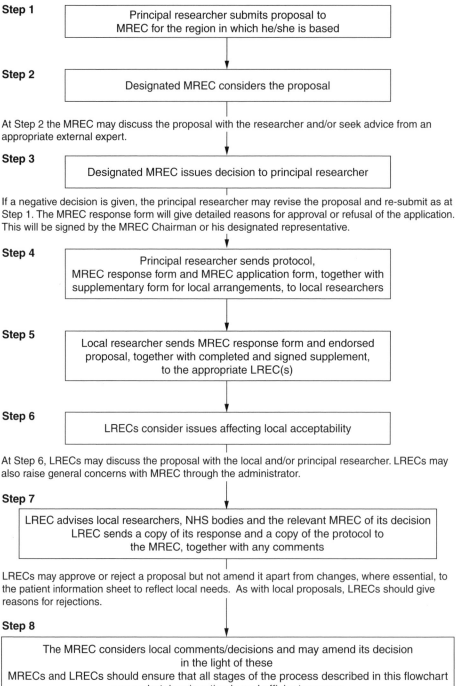

Step 1

> Principal researcher submits proposal to
> MREC for the region in which he/she is based

Step 2

> Designated MREC considers the proposal

At Step 2 the MREC may discuss the proposal with the researcher and/or seek advice from an appropriate external expert.

Step 3

> Designated MREC issues decision to principal researcher

If a negative decision is given, the principal researcher may revise the proposal and re-submit as at Step 1. The MREC response form will give detailed reasons for approval or refusal of the application. This will be signed by the MREC Chairman or his designated representative.

Step 4

> Principal researcher sends protocol,
> MREC response form and MREC application form, together with
> supplementary form for local arrangements, to local researchers

Step 5

> Local researcher sends MREC response form and endorsed
> proposal, together with completed and signed supplement,
> to the appropriate LREC(s)

Step 6

> LRECs consider issues affecting local acceptability

At Step 6, LRECs may discuss the proposal with the local and/or principal researcher. LRECs may also raise general concerns with MREC through the administrator.

Step 7

> LREC advises local researchers, NHS bodies and the relevant MREC of its decision
> LREC sends a copy of its response and a copy of the protocol to
> the MREC, together with any comments

LRECs may approve or reject a proposal but not amend it apart from changes, where essential, to the patient information sheet to reflect local needs. As with local proposals, LRECs should give reasons for rejections.

Step 8

> The MREC considers local comments/decisions and may amend its decision
> in the light of these
> MRECs and LRECs should ensure that all stages of the process described in this flowchart
> are undertaken in a timely and efficient manner

Figure 34 A multicentre research ethics system flowchart (simplified example).

Table 33 MREC membership

Description	Maximum number	Minimum number
General practitioner	2	1
Nurse/midwife	2	1
Professional allied to medicine	1	1
Clinical pharmacologist/pharmacist	2	1
Hospital consultant	4	3
Public health physician/epidemiologist	1	1
Lay person*	6	4
Total	18	12

* a person who is not and never has been:
i) a doctor, dentist, ophthalmic medical practitioner, optician or pharmacist
ii) a registered dispensing optician
iii) a registered nurse, registered midwife or registered health visitor
iv) an officer of, or someone otherwise employed by, any health board, health authority, local health council or community health council.

Exactly what is meant by the term 'suitability' remains unclear. Some studies are reported to have been deemed 'unsuitable' by one LREC but not by another LREC. This divergence in opinion could be for legitimate reasons – further research is required.

One development for MRECs is to use a standard progress report form (*see* Table 34). Such a form is reproduced here to indicate what information the MREC would obtain if these forms were sent out, completed, returned and analysed.

Information from these forms would not only help the trialists to provide an update of the status of the trial, but would provide the approving committee with a valuable insight into the progress of work they have recommended. More generally, that information could be used to help to share real lessons and insight into the fate of research with host institutions, non-trial doctors, trial sponsors generally and, of course, patients and their advocates.

At the time of writing, the MREC system in the UK is very much part of a larger emerging system for ratifying trial applications. As indicated above, there is still some work to do in terms of actually monitoring the approved trials, monitoring the system of approving trials, making the ethics committees' decisions more transparent, and encouraging better public dissemination of the results of trials using NHS patients ratified by NHS ethics committees.

The clinical research ethics committee system in the UK is undergoing another period of reflection, revision and reform. It is doing this under the guise of improvements to research governance in the NHS and in light of the European Union Directive on clinical trials of medicinal products for humans. Exactly what new system will emerge, why, and how well it does, remain to be seen.

See **Benchmarking; Causes of delay and failure to complete a clinical trial; Ethical issues; European Union Directive on clinical trials of medicinal products**

Table 34 A MREC research progress report

1 Name and address of principal researcher.		
2 Short title of study.		
3 Research ethics committee reference number.		
4 Date of research ethics committee approval.		
5 Has the study started? If No, please give reasons.	Yes	No
6 Number of local research sites recruited.	Proposed	Actual
7 Number of subjects/patients recruited into study.	Proposed	Actual
8 Number of subjects/patients completing study.	Proposed	Actual
9 Number of withdrawals because of: (i) lack of efficacy (ii) adverse events (iii) self-withdrawal (iv) non-compliance.		
10 Have there been any serious difficulties in recruiting subjects to the study? If Yes, please give details.	Yes	No
11 Have there been any untoward events? (before you answer this, please refer to our definition in the enclosed booklet *Information for Researchers*) If Yes, have these been notified to the Committee?	Yes Yes	No No
12 If untoward events have not been notified to the Committee, please state why, as notification is a condition of research ethics committee approval.		
13 Have there been any amendments to the study? If Yes, have these been notified to the Committee? If amendments have not been notified to the Committee, please state why, as you know that notification is a condition of the Committee's approval.	Yes Yes	No No
14 Has the study finished? If Yes, please answer questions 15 and 16 below. If No, what is the expected completion date?	Yes	No
15 If the study will not now be completed, please give reason(s).		

16 Results – please include details of outcomes and conclusions (attach a separate page if necessary).
How the findings have been disseminated
• Used for licensing/regulatory purposes
• Presentations
• Publications: – planned
                          – in press
                          – published
	
	Yes
	Yes
	Yes
	Yes
	Yes
		
		No
		No
		No
		No
		No

Please give details below and send copies of publications and presentations as soon as they are available.		
17 Signature of principal investigator.		
18 Print principal investigator's name.		
19 Signature(s) of the Chief Executive(s) of the organisation(s) where the research takes place.		
20 Date of submission of progress report to the Ethics Committee.		

for humans; Fate of research studies; Local research ethics committee; Institutional review board; Multicentre trial; Research governance in the NHS; Research governance implementation plan; Research questions and research methods; Reasons given by the investigator for a study being abandoned or in abeyance; Reasons given by the investigator for a study never being started.

○ Ah-See KW, MacKenzie J, Thakker NS and Maran AG (1998) Local research ethics committee approval for a national study in Scotland. *J Royal Coll Surg Edin.* **43**: 303–5.

○ Alberti KG (1995) Local research ethics committees. *BMJ.* **311**: 639–41.

○ Alberti KG (2000) Multicentre research ethics committees: has the cure been worse than the disease? *BMJ.* **320**: 1157–8.

○ Busby A and Dolk H (1998) Local research ethics committees' approval in a national population study. *J Royal Coll Phy Lon.* **32**: 142–5.

○ Lux AL, Edwards SW and Osborne JP (2000) Responses of local research ethics committees to a study with approval from a multicentre research ethics committee. *BMJ.* **320**: 1182–3.

○ NHS Executive (1997) *Ethics Committee Review of Multicentre Research: establishment of multicentre research ethics committees.* HSG(97)23. NHS Executive, Leeds.

○ NHS Executive (1998) *Guidance Points to Local Research Ethics Committees.* NHS Executive, Leeds.

○ MREC Central Office (2000) *Revised MREC Paperwork.* NHS Executive South Thames, London.

○ Tulley J, Ninis N, Booy R and Viner R (2000) The new system of review by multicentre research ethics committees: prospective study. *BMJ.* **320**: 1179–82.

○ While AE (1995) Ethics committees: impediments to research or guardians of ethical standards? *BMJ.* **311**: 661.

Multicentre trial
A multicentre clinical trial is one that takes place in more than one setting or location. For example:

• Carman and colleagues ran a trial to find out whether vaccination of healthcare workers in 20 long-term elderly-care hospitals lowered mortality and the frequency of virologically proven influenza in the elderly patients

• Shum and colleagues ran a multicentre, randomised, controlled trial to assess the acceptability and safety of a minor illness service led by practice nurses in primary care

• Oderda and colleagues published the results of a multicentre study of the detection of *Helicobacter pylori* in stool specimens by non-invasive antigen enzyme immunoassay in children.

Multicentre trials can be used to:

• recruit the necessary number of patients

• recruit more quickly

- help to obtain a more representative sample of the study population
- encourage co-operation between experts
- familiarise a wide group of health professionals with the new intervention
- improve the generalisability and acceptability of study results in different locations.

Examples of the main problems include the following:

- their relatively high cost
- issues of practicality
- management
- difficulties in recruiting suitable numbers of physicians
- variations in local clinical practice
- variations in ethical committee requirements
- problems in simplifying the care protocol
- the problem of what to include as the comparator intervention.

Some multicentre trials include centres in different countries, while many do not. In one recently published paper, Akkerhuis and colleagues sought to determine the factors that might contribute to geographical variations in patient outcomes and treatment in an international multicentre trial.

Multicentre trials need not be mega-trials, as they could include a relatively small number of patients in different clinics.

In terms of language, you have to be careful as there is a general rule that all international trials are multicentre trials, but not all multicentre trials are international trials. Therefore if someone says that a trial is multicentre, you need to find out whether it is also an international trial. *See* **Advantages of evidence from clinical trials; Bias; Generalisability of trial results; Mega-trial; Multicentre research ethics committee; Trial site**.

○ Akkerhuis KM, Deckers JW, Boersma E *et al.* (2000) Geographic variability in outcomes within an international trial of glycoprotein IIb/IIIA inhibition in patients with acute coronary syndromes. *Eur Heart J.* **21**: 371–81.

○ Carman WF, Elder AG, Wallace LA *et al.* (2000) Effects of influenza vaccination of healthcare workers on mortality of elderly people in long-term care: a randomised controlled trial. *Lancet.* **355**: 93–7.

○ Oderda G, Rapa A, Ronchi B *et al.* (2000) Detection of *Helicobacter pylori* in stool specimens by non-invasive antigen enzyme immunoassay in children: multicentre Italian study. *BMJ.* **320**: 347–8.

○ Shum C, Humphreys A, Wheeler D *et al.* (2000) Nurse management of patients with minor illnesses in general practice: a multicentre randomised controlled trial. *BMJ.* **320**: 1038–43.

Multilevel modelling

Suppose that you come across literature on an international trial, and the trial has various levels of data, for example:

- aggregate data across all centres

- data for each country

- data for each centre

- data for each clinician

- data for each arm of the trial

- data for each patient subgroup

- data for each patient.

Multilevel modelling provides a structure on the basis of which you can review and reflect on the results at different levels. In the model, the assessment will make use of multiple levels of information.

In clinical practice, for example, multilevel modelling can be used to identify and analyse those practices in primary care groups (PCGs) that are quickest to use certain newly launched medicines, with further analysis looking at PCG structure, personnel and PCG characteristics.

A multilevel model will have a hierarchy of parameters, some of which are simplified while others are more complex. Such models can be used to determine relationships and subgroup analysis at different levels.

One strength of multilevel modelling is that it can include non-healthcare issues such as economic status, familial status, geography and other service providers (e.g. social services, patient support groups).

Multilevel modelling opportunities actually exist in clinical practice. For example, you can analyse data reflecting the following:

- one of your patients receiving a certain medication for a particular condition

- all of your patients receiving that medication for that condition

- all of your patients receiving other medication for that condition

- all of the patients in the locality with the condition

- all of the patients in the region with the condition.

Suppose that a recently published trial shows clinical superiority of one product over another. Then multilevel modelling can be used in the PCG, health authority or hospital, and you may see that prescribing of this new product is conditioned by patient characteristics, doctor characteristics, practice characteristics, wider PCG policy systems, national policy and advisory characteristics, and a raft of wider socio-economic characteristics. *See* **Audit; Parsimony principle**.

○ Greenland S (2000) Principles of multilevel modelling. *Int J Epidemiol.* **29**: 158–67.

Multiple causation

Multiple causation occurs when there is more than one reason for an effect.

For example, the recovery rate of a patient undergoing a hip replacement may depend on their pre-operative health status, the success of the operation, the post-operative rehabilitation therapy, family support and the patient's mental attitude. *See* **Causal relationship; Confounding factor; Multiplicative effect; Outcome; Statistical tests: ten ways to cheat with statistical tests**.

Multiple endpoints

Multiple endpoints occur when there is more than one outcome of any particular clinical trial.

For example, in a clinical trial of oxygen administration to patients with chronic obstructive lung disease, the outcomes of interest may include the following:

• pulmonary function

• neuropsychological state

• quality of life

• mortality rate.

See **Composite endpoint; Multiplicative effect; Outcomes pyramid; Primary outcome; Surrogate endpoint**.

○ Ghosh D (2000) Methods for analysis of multiple events in the presence of death. *Control Clin Trials.* **21**: 115–26.

Multiplicative effect

A multiplicative effect is the product of effects from more than one healthcare intervention.

Suppose that three interventions are provided to a patient in a clinical trial:

• T is the kidney transplant

• D is the kidney transplant anti-rejection medication

• E is an appropriate patient education video.

If T results in t, D in d, and E in e, and if the effects are considered to be multiplicative, then the final effect of the three interventions is:

$$t \times d \times e$$

Whenever you come across multiplicative effects, various issues should immediately spring to mind.

- Two negative results will, when multiplied together, yield a positive result. For example:

$$1 \times (-2) \times (-3) = 6 = 1 \times 2 \times 3$$

- Each effect may have different importance (weights) to different people involved in the trial.
- Can a collection of effects really be multiplied together?
- Does the collection make clinical sense?
- Does the collection make practical sense?

See **Additive effect; Composite endpoint; Scales of measurement.**

N

National Institute for Clinical Excellence

The National Institute for Clinical Excellence (NICE) is an authority in the UK NHS that was established in April 1999 to give coherence, authority and prominence to information about the clinical effectiveness and cost-effectiveness of healthcare interventions.

It conducts clinical and economic assessments of products and procedures. It has also started to produce guidelines to aid clinical practice.

NICE is a special health authority, which means that it has unique national or supraregional functions which, it is claimed, cannot be effectively undertaken by certain other types of NHS bodies. NICE brings together work currently undertaken by other professional organisations in receipt of Department of Health funding.

As expected, NICE is developing relationships at local, regional and national levels to help to try to improve the use of resources in the NHS.

The Secretary of State for Health, who is a politician, appoints a small body of executives and non-executives to the NICE Board. NICE is to be held to account by the Secretary of State for Health for its resources, the delivery of its work programme and the guidance that it produces.

In terms of clinical and economic assessment, NICE employs a six-step strategy as described below.

- *Step 1. Identification and examination*: of medicines, devices and procedures that are likely to have a significant impact on the NHS; examining current practice to identify unjustified variations in use, or uncertainty about clinical and cost-effectiveness of healthcare interventions

- *Step 2. Evidence collection*: undertaking research to assess the clinical and cost-effectiveness of health interventions

- *Step 3. Appraisal and guidance*: carefully considering the implications for clinical practice of the evidence on clinical and cost-effectiveness and producing guidance for the NHS

- *Step 4. Dissemination*: of the guidance and supporting audit methodologies

- *Step 5. Implementation*: at a local level, through clinical governance and other approaches

- *Step 6. Monitoring*: the impact and keeping advice under review, taking into account the views of patients and their representatives, and any relevant new research findings.

Visit the NICE website for further details of its evolving programme, staff and decisions to date (www.nice.org). The UK government has said that it will consider developing the role and function of NICE as it gathers momentum and experience. In fact, NICE is undergoing review of its work and impact.

You may (quite rightly) be wondering why NICE is included in this handbook of clinical trials. The simple reason is that NICE will be looking very closely at the clinical evidence surrounding healthcare products, and much of that evidence will stem from clinical trials.

Therefore:

- major purchasing recommendations are going to be made public and will be based more than ever before on a robust review of the clinical evidence

- more people than ever before will be interested in clinical trials

- more people will feel more comfortable and confident about asking NICE-type questions about any product or service

- more people will be asking you very simple questions, such as 'Where is the evidence to support your decision/statement?'.

Those sponsoring or running clinical trials have to realise (and realise quickly) that their research and the results of their research will come under ever closer scrutiny. *See* **Accountability; Due process; Economic analysis and clinical trials; Evidence-based medicine; Research governance in the NHS; Systematic review; Transparency.**

National Research Register

The National Research Register is a database of research projects that are funded or taking place within the National Health Service. It includes a wide variety of studies, gives an impression of the objectives and methods of the studies, and provides the contact details of the lead researcher.

So if you have thought of questions like these, the National Research Register can help you.

- Have you ever wanted to find out what research is taking place in the NHS?

- Is there someone conducting research of interest to your formulary service nearby?

- Are you curious about who is doing what research in the next primary care group area?

- Do you want to call on an expert who is involved in trials of a new drug, but do not know who to call?

- Who paid for a particular piece of research?

- What research projects are about to report?

- Is there any connection between a consultant demanding a new drug be put on the formulary and the sponsors or study participants?

- Who can a doctor talk to about a particular piece of research in practice?

- Can one of your nurses who is keen to learn research find a mentor involved in a clinical trial?

- Do you want to commission some research but are uncertain whether it is already being conducted somewhere else?

- Do you want to get a grasp of what is currently under study?

- Do you want to know when a new study is due to report and who to contact in order to find out when it will actually report?

The National Research Reigister offers the following:

- quick and easy access to a wide range of projects that are taking place or of interest to the NHS

- a keyword search facility to identify relevant material more efficiently

- updates throughout the year

- names and contact information about those leading certain projects.

Project information comes from the following:

- the NHS Health Technology Programme

- the NHS National Priority Programmes in research and development (R&D)

- Scottish and Welsh Office-funded work

- work supported by the NHS R&D Levy within NHS provider units

- the Medical Research Council clinical trials directory

- information about other registers holding R&D-type project information

- the NHS Centre for Reviews and Dissemination database information.

There is scope for the register to give more information on the following:

- whether or not the trials had data-monitoring committees

- issues of blinding in the trials

- the results of completed work

- where the results were published

- who has used the results.

The National Research Register can be found by contacting the NHS Executive in England or on the Internet (www.doh.gov.uk/research/nrr.htm or www.update-software.com). *See* **Accountability; Blinding; Due process; Fate of research studies; Institutional reviews board; Local research ethics committee; Multicentre trial; National Institute for Clinical Excellence; Reasons given by the investigator for a study being abandoned or in abeyance; Reasons given by the investigator for a study never being started; Research governance in the NHS; Research questions and research methods; Transparency; Value-for-money table.**

Natural history studies

Natural history studies are methods of assessing the natural course of events. They can help to improve:

- the understanding of a disease

- the development of a hypothesis

- thinking about possible courses of intervention.

See **Natural response; Non-experimental study; Observational study; Qualitative analysis.**

Natural response

A natural response is a result that is not due to any particular intervention. *See* **Natural history studies.**

Non-experimental study

A non-experimental study is an analysis of an intervention that does not involve an experiment (e.g. analysing current care).

In general, it is not a clinical trial, as clinical trials are by definition experiments. *See* **Clinical trial; Cohort study.**

Non-inferiority trial

A non-inferiority trial is a clinical trial with the primary objective of testing the hypothesis that one regimen is no worse than another. That is the null hypothesis – different regimens are not inferior.

Predefinition of a trial as non-inferiority is necessary for a nujmber of reasons, including the following:

- proper setting of the appropriate hypothesis
- to ensure that the comparator treatments, doses, patient populations and endpoints are appropriate
- the setting up of relevant statistical tests
- to allow proper power calculations to be performed
- to ensure that the non-inferiority criteria are predefined
- to permit appropriate analysis plans to be prespecified in the trial protocol
- to ensure that the quality of the trial matches its objectives.

Some key issues to think about include the following.

- Why is the trial being designed as a non-inferiority trial and not an equivalence trial?
- On what dimensions are the results examined?
- What is the regimen being compared with (is the comparator sensible)?
- What is meant by the term 'non-inferior' (e.g. is there a range of results that would be accepted as showing non-inferiority, or is it a single number)?
- One regimen could turn out to be better than another. What does this imply for the trial statistics and the acceptability of the results?

See **Clinical trial; Data dredging; Data fishing; Equivalence trial; Hypothesis; Primary objective; Statistical test diagram; Superiority trial.**

○ European Agency for the Evaluation of Medicinal Products (1999) *Committee for Proprietary Medical Products (CPMP) points to consider on biostatistical/methodological issues arising from recent CPMP discussions on licensing applications: superiority, non-inferiority, and equivalence.* EMEA, London.

Non-randomised clinical trial

This is a clinical trial where patients are allocated to interventions in ways which do not include randomisation.

For example, they could be allocated by a system based on:

- their date of birth
- the day on which they visit the clinic
- the last digit in their health record number

- the intervention the previous patient went into.

See **Adaptive–adoptive trial; Bernoulli trial; Non-randomised studies; Play-the-winner rule; Random; Randomisation; Randomised controlled trial**.

Non-randomised studies

This is a collection of studies where chance does not have a role to play in allocating patients to regimens.

These have been used, for example, in observational studies and adaptive–adoptive trials.

See **Adaptive–adoptive trial; Case–control study; Cohort study; Non-randomised clinical trial; Observation analysis; Play-the-winner rule; Qualitative analysis; Randomisation**.

Non-response

A non-response in a clinical trial is evidence of absence of a response.

For example, the absence of a patient response may occur for the following reasons:

- because of their sensitivity to the question(s)

- because they interpret the question(s) as being inappropriate or irrelevant

- because they do not actually understand the question

- due to lack of interest, time, payback or conviction about the study

- due to administrative errors

- due to a general failure to reply.

Non-response is not the same as no response.

See **Analysis by assigned treatment; Audit; Closed question; Compliance; Concordance; Dropouts; Intention-to-treat analysis; Leading question; Long-term analysis; Lost; Missing values; Open question; Outcome**.

Null hypothesis

A statement that there is no relationship or difference between the factors under study, or that the answer is 'No', is called the null hypothesis. It usually represents a theory that has been put forward, either because it is believed to be true or as the basis for an argument which has yet to be proven.

Suppose that you believe there is no difference between taking drug X and taking drug Y in terms of outcomes. Then you can write the null hypothesis as follows:

$$H_0 : X = Y \text{ (which is the same as } H_0 : x - y = 0)$$

Or suppose that clinical evidence suggests that the incidence of stroke for a 45 to 50-year-old is a function of five factors, P, Q, R, S and T. Then you can suggest that the null hypothesis is a particular function of these:

$$H_0 : Z = F (p,q,r,s,t)$$

For instance, you may have reason to believe that the formula is:

$$Z = 2p + 3q - 4r \times s^2 \times e^t$$

Do not worry about the details of that particular formula (it is only included here to illustrate how complicated some null hypotheses can become mathematically).

Just remember that in general the null hypothesis is either:

- that there is no difference between X and Y *or*

- that Z is the particular function of the factors under study.

As an example, recent studies have derived their null hypothesis from the following questions.

- In patients with suspected acute pulmonary embolism, what is the diagnostic accuracy of dual-section helical computed tomography?

- In patients with minor head injury, can using a clinical decision rule of seven clinical criteria identify those patients who do not need computed tomography?

- In women with breast cancer in remission, does the level of satisfaction with health service delivery differ when follow-up is undertaken in a primary care setting rather than in a specialist-care hospital outreach setting?

- In women with heavy menstrual bleeding, is transcervical resection of the endometrium better than medical management for relieving menstrual symptoms in the long term?

- In postmenopausal women receiving tamoxifen for breast cancer, does clonidine reduce hot flushes?

- In patients who need long-term oral anticoagulation treatment, is self-management as effective as specialist anticoagulation clinic management?

- In patients with severe congestive heart failure caused by systolic left ventricular dysfunction, does spironolactone combined with usual care reduce all-cause mortality?

The null hypothesis is the primary building block of the trial. Once the results have been analysed and interpreted, we have the following choice:

- either we do not reject the null hypothesis *or*

- we reject the null hypothesis in favour of the alternative hypothesis.

If we conclude 'do not reject the null hypothesis' this does not, curiously, mean that it is true! It only suggests that there is insufficient evidence against the null hypothesis and in favour of the alternative hypothesis.

If we conclude that 'we reject the null hypothesis in favour of the alternative hypothesis', this at best only suggests that the alternative hypothesis may be true.

It has been argued that we should never:

- reject the alternative hypothesis *or*

- accept the alternative hypothesis.

In certain types of trials the null hypothesis is not as outlined above. For example, in an equivalence trial the null hypothesis is that the treatments are not equivalent. *See* **Alternative hypothesis; Equivalence trial; Non-inferiority trial; Primary objective; Research question; Superiority trial; Systematic review.**

○ Luft HS (2000) Identifying and assessing the null hypothesis. *Health Serv Res.* **34**: 1265–71.

Number needed to harm

The number needed to harm (NNH) is the number of patients who must be treated in order for one of them to have an adverse event. For instance, you may have to treat 1000 patients with medication for rheumatoid arthritis before one of them develops drug-related ulcers.

NNH can be calculated as the inverse of the absolute risk increase (ARI).

Thus if ARI = 0.02, then NNH = 1/(0.02) = 50. *See* **Absolute risk increase; Confidence interval; Number needed to treat.**

Number needed to treat

The number needed to treat is the number of patients who must be treated in order to achieve a result (e.g. to avoid one patient having a clinical event). It can, with care, be regarded as a measure of treatment effectiveness. For example, 30 patients may need to be treated with one particular medicine in order to avoid one of them having a myocardial infarction.

Recent examples of NNTs include studies on the following:

- stroke

- myocardial infarction

- falls in the elderly

- leg ulcers

- smoking cessation

- childhood obesity

- avoidance of institutionalisation in patients with Alzheimer's dementia
- prevention of suicide among young males
- epilepsy
- Parkinson's disease
- abstinence from alcohol intake in detoxified alcoholics.

The number needed to treat (NNT) can be calculated in three ways, as described below.

1 NNT is the reciprocal of the absolute risk reduction (ARR): $NNT = 1/ARR$. Suppose that a primary care practice nurse is given responsibility for delivering a new myocardial infarction management programme with the purpose of reducing mortality in the group's population. Suppose that after 1 year the ARR = 0.106. Then the NNT is 9.4 (1/0.106). Rounding up to the nearest integer, 10 patients will have to be treated in the programme in order to avoid one having a myocardial infarction.

2 The second method depends on knowing the patient expected event rate (sometimes called the control event rate) and the odds. Suppose that you are interested in preventative care. Then the NNT can be calculated from Table 35 below.

   Table 35 has 8 rows on the control event rate (CER) and 9 columns on the odds ratios. It is possible to choose data that are relevant to local practice to determine the NNT.

   Suppose that your primary care group is interested in the prevention of ulcerative colitis. After a study of the practice records you find that the primary care group control event rate is 0.3 and the odds ratio is 0.7. Reading along row 0.3 and down column 0.7, you will find the number 14. This suggests that the primary care group needs to treat 14 patients with the intervention in order to avoid one patient having ulcerative colitis.

Table 35 NNT calculator

Control event rate	Odds ratio								
	0.50	0.55	0.60	0.65	0.70	0.75	0.80	0.85	0.90
0.05	41	46	52	59	69	83	104	139	209
0.1	21	24	27	31	36	43	54	73	110
0.2	11	13	14	17	20	24	30	40	61
0.3	8	9	10	12	14	18	22	30	46
0.4	7	8	9	10	12	15	19	26	40
0.5	6	7	8	9	11	14	18	25	38
0.7	6	7	9	10	13	16	20	28	44
0.9	12	15	18	22	27	34	46	64	101

3 A third way to calculate the numbers needed to treat is by reference to Figure 35 below.

Consider the following example. A doctor, dietitian, exercise counsellor, smoking adviser and chest physician run a programme to reduce mortality in patients with heart disease. Suppose that the programme has a patient expected event rate (PEER) of 2. The PEER reflects the susceptibility of the patients to the event. Suppose that the preventative intervention has an associated relative risk reduction (RRR) of 20.

Now plot these points 2 and 20 on the PEER and RRR scales, respectively, draw a line between the two points, and extend the line to the NNT scale. The extended line crosses the NNT scale at a value of 250. In Figure 35, this suggests that 250 patients need to be treated in the programme in order to avoid one death from heart disease.

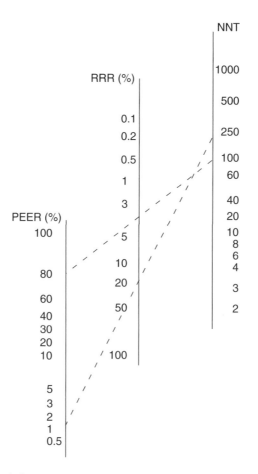

Figure 35 Numbers needed to treat.

If the PEER is 80 and RRR is 4 then, using the same technique as described above, 100 patients have to be treated in order to avoid one patient dying from heart disease. You can use other combinations of PEERs and RRRs to obtain other results that are pertinent to your local circumstances.

NNTs can be made more patient specific. You can convert the NNT to patient-specific NNT (PSNNT).

The calculation is that PSNNT = NNT/(f), where f is the patient type factor.

On the second example of a heart disease programme the NNT was 250. Now if $f = 0.5$ then:

$$\text{PSNNT} = \frac{250}{0.5} = 500.$$

How can you interpret the values of f?

- If f lies between 0 and 1, the healthcare professional believes that their patient cohort is less susceptible to the event.

- If f is equal to 1, this means that the healthcare professional believes that there is no discernible difference between their patients and the other evidence.

- If f exceeds 1, this means that the health professional believes that their patients are more susceptible to the event.

Finally, NNTs can, with caution, be enveloped inside confidence intervals showing, to a degree of certainty (usually 95%), the range of patients that need to be treated in order to achieve a result. Indeed, it has been argued that they should always be enclosed in confidence intervals.

Suppose, after studying the details in the primary care group, that the 95% confidence interval for heart disease mortality in males aged 45-60 years with no prior myocardial infacrction is ± 40. Recall that the NNT above was 250. Now on the basis of these results one would be 95% confident that treating between 210 (250–40) and 290 (250+40) patients in the primary care group would avoid one dying of heart disease.

The increasing use of NNT is welcome in some respects, but caution is required for at least four reasons.

1 They may not be better understood than other measures.

2 The methods of presenting the results of trials influence healthcare decisions.

3 They may differ if we are looking at prevention, therapeutic procedures or palliative care.

4 The numbers needed to treat are sensitive to factors that change the baseline risk, such as the outcome considered, patients' characteristics, secular trends in incidence and case fatality, data analysis and the clinical setting.

See **Absolute risk reduction; Bayesian analysis; Confidence interval; Data-display formats; Number needed to harm; Odds ratio; Patient expected event rate; Relative risk reduction; Systematic review; Value-for-money table.**

○ Altman DG (1998) Confidence intervals for the number needed to treat. *BMJ*. **317**: 1309–12.

○ Cates C (1999) Pooling numbers needed to treat may not be reliable. *BMJ*. **318**: 1764.

○ de Craen AJM, Vickers AJ, Tijssen JGP and Kleijnen J (1998) Number needed to treat and placebo-controlled trials. *Lancet*. **351**: 310.

○ Lesaffre E and Pledger G (1999) A note on number needed to treat. *Control Clin Trials*. **20**: 439–47.

○ Smeeth L, Haines A and Ebrahim S (1999) Numbers needed to treat derived from meta-analysis – sometimes informative, usually misleading. *BMJ*. **318**: 1548–51.

Number-of-1 trial

This is a clinical trial that seeks to establish the efficacy of an intervention in a specific patient (sometimes called an N-of-1 trial or individual patient trial). *See* **Clinical trial; Individual patient trial; Mega-trial.**

Observational study

An observational study is a method of assessment that is used by a researcher who, at best, identifies, observes, records, classifies and analyses relevant information in a study without interfering with the course of events. *See* **Case–control study; Clinical trial; Cohort study; Hierarchy of evidence**.

- ○ Black A (1996) Why we need observational studies to evaluate the effectiveness of health care. *BMJ*. **312**: 1215–18.

- ○ Bowling A (1997) Unstructured and structured observational studies. In: *Research Methods in Health: investigating health and health services*. Open University Press, Buckingham.

- ○ Ioannidis JPA, Haidich AB and Lau J (2001) Any casualties in the clash of randomised and observational evidence? *BMJ*. **322**: 879–80.

Observer

An observer is someone who watches and may record developments and impressions in a particular clinical trial or other study. *See* **Blinding; Data-monitoring committee; Participant**.

Obsolescence

Obsolescence occurs when a product, service or idea becomes outdated or superseded.

For example:

- laboratory equipment becomes outdated or obsolete due to technical improvements
- clinical trials may show that new medication may be clinically superior to older medication
- new ways of developing clinical trial protocols may be superior to older methods
- new materials may be superior to older materials in hip replacements
- new methods of disseminating the evidence from a clinical trial may be superior to older methods.

See **Data-display formats; Product life cycle; Value-for-money table**.

Odds

Quite often in practice you will be interested in how frequently an event occurs in one group compared with how often it does not occur. This means that you have an interest in the odds of the event.

Suppose that a clinical trial looked at the number of strokes occurring in high-risk patients under different regimens, namely a new regimen of care and what we shall call the 'usual PCG-led care' regimen. The results are shown in Table 36.

Table 36 Odds

	Stroke occurs	Stroke does not occur
New care	a (100)	b (200)
Usual care	c (120)	d (180)

Using the data shown in Table 36 as an example, the odds of a stroke occurring under the new care regimen are as follows:

$$\text{odds}_{\text{new care}} = \frac{a}{b} = \frac{100}{200} = 0.5$$

The odds of a stroke occurring in the usual PCG care group are as follows:

$$\text{odds}_{\text{usual PCG care}} = \frac{c}{d} = \frac{120}{180} = 0.67$$

From this you can see that the odds of stroke are lower in the new care regimen than in to the usual PCG regimen.

In general, the lower the odds the better. *See* **Absolute risk; Absolute risk reduction; Likelihood; Odds ratio; Relative risk; Relative risk reduction; Sensitivity; Specificity**.

Odds ratio

The odds ratio is a measure of treatment effectiveness. It is the ratio of two odds.

Odds ratios have become widely used in clinical studies. Suppose that a pharmaceutical company, the primary care group, the hospital and your local social services get together to design and deliver a new regimen for patients at high risk of stroke. They are not sure whether the new programme is better than the existing services, so they obtain approval and some funding to run a clinical trial comparing the existing regimen with the new regimen.

Eligible and consenting patients are randomly assigned to either the new regimen or usual care. After 6 months the data-monitoring committee presents the results shown in Table 37.

In the new care regimen, 100 high-risk patients had a stroke and 200 did not. In the usual care regimen, 120 high-risk patients had a stroke and 180 did not.

Table 37 Odds ratio

	Stroke occurs	Stroke does not occur
New care	a (100)	b (200)
Usual care	c (120)	d (180)

Referring to Table 37, the odds ratio (OR) can be written as follows:

$$OR = \frac{a/b}{c/d}$$

Using the data from Table 35, then:

$$OR = \frac{100/200}{120/180} = 0.75$$

How do you interpret the OR results? In general:

- if OR = 1, the odds of the event are the same in both groups (i.e. the odds are equivalent)
- if OR < 1, the odds of the event are lower in the new care group than in the usual care group
- if OR > 1, the odds of the event are higher in the new care group than in the usual care group.

Thus in the example above, the odds ratio was 0.75. This means that the risk of stroke is lower in the new care regimen than in usual care. *See* **Absolute risk; Absolute risk reduction; Baseline; Matched pairs; Number needed to treat; Odds; Odds reduction; Relative risk; Relative risk reduction.**

○ Bland JM and Altman DG (2000) The odds ratio. *BMJ*. **320**: 1468.

○ Sackett DL, Deeks JJ and Altman DG (1996) Down with odds ratios! *Evidence-Based Med*. **Sep–Oct**: 164–6.

Odds reduction

The odds reduction is the complement of the odds ratio (OR). Mathematically it is simple to determine. The formula is as follows:

$$\text{odds reduction} = 1 - \text{odds ratio}$$

In the example above the odds ratio was 0.75. So:

$$\text{odds reduction} = 1 - 0.75 = 0.25$$

The odds reduction is comparable to the relative risk reduction. In terms of interpretation, in many cases the larger the odds reduction the better. Care has to be taken in interpretation when the odds reduction value falls below zero. Its exact meaning depends on the question being addressed in the study. *See* **Odds; Odds ratio; Relative risk reduction**.

Off-label use

Off-label use refers to the prescribing and use of a medicine for conditions that are not specified on the label (Summary of Product Characteristics, SPC). *See* **Licence; Medicines Control Agency**.

○ Conroy S, Choonara I, Impicciatore P *et al.* (2000) Survey of unlicensed and off-label drug use in paediatric wards in European countries. *BMJ.* **320**: 79–82.

One-tailed test

If you were interested in knowing the probability that a trial result is greater (or less) than some particular value, then you would apply a one-tailed test.

For example, a test of whether the average improvement in diastolic blood pressure for the group of patients exceeds 10% is a one-tailed test. Generally, the context of the problem will determine whether a one-tailed or two-tailed test is performed. Statistical testing is a complex topic, and our best advice is to develop a good rapport with a qualified statistician. *See* **Acceptance area; Outcome; Questions to ask before getting involved in a clinical trial; Research questions and research methods; Statistical test diagram; Two-tailed test**.

Open-label trial

A fully open-label trial is a clinical trial in which the patient, clinicians, administrators and data assessors know what intervention the patient is receiving.

Open-label trials are conducted in order to establish additional data on the following characteristics of what is under trial:

• safety

- efficacy

- quality

- compliance issues.

For example:

- Taylor and colleagues conducted an open-label randomised multicentre trial comparing tacrolimus and cyclosporine immunosuppressive regimens in cardiac transplantation.

Open-label studies may also be conducted when it is difficult, impractical or impossible to blind the interventions.

Open-label trials are sometimes called open clinical trials. *See* **Bias; Blind; Clinical trial; Label; Post-marketing surveillance; Unblinded**.

○ Taylor DO, Barr ML, Radovancevic B *et al.* (1999) A randomised multicentre comparison of tacrolimus and cyclosporine immunosuppressive regimens in cardiac transplantation. *J Heart Lung Transplant*. **18**: 336–45.

Open question

An open question in a clinical trial is one that does not have a pre-set list of answers. Open questions are used in situations where possible replies to the question are unknown, too complex or too numerous to pre-code. They are also used to help to determine a person's awareness, reasoning, articulation and values. In some cases open questions have been used in pilot studies to help to refine research areas for subsequent clinical trials.

Examples of open questions include the following:

- (to the patient) 'What are the qualities about your current GP which you appreciate?'

- (to the doctor) 'What three things about the trial protocol did you like the most?'

- (to the data-monitoring committee) 'From your experience, what key messages would you offer to those planning a phase-three, double-blind, placebo-controlled, multicentre, parallel clinical trial in primary care?'

- (to the retiring ethics committee member) 'Looking back on your work with this ethics committee, what are your most memorable experiences?'

- (to the trial sponsor) 'In the light of past experience and reality, how are you actually going to ensure appropriate and rapid recruitment into this trial?'.

The advantages of open questions are as follows.

- They may provide a better motivation to answer the questions.
- They can encourage spontaneity.
- They do not superimpose answers or expectations.
- They can elicit a wide variety of responses.
- They can lead to the development of measurement scales.
- They can lead to new areas of research or understanding.
- They need to be of good design.

The disadvantages of open questions are as follows.

- They can be time-consuming to categorise.
- they can be difficult to analyse.
- they may have a lower response rate.

See **Closed question**; **Leading question**.

○ Bowling A (1997) *Research Methods in Health: investigating health and health services.* Open University Press, Buckingham.

Open sequential trial

When there is no limit to the number of patients who are recruited into a sequential trial, then it is called an open sequential trial. *See* **Closed sequential trial**; **Interim analysis**; **Sequential trial**; **Stopping rules**.

Order

This is a particular sequence of events. The order may or may not matter in terms of outcomes achieved. *See* **Order effects**.

Order effects

Order effects are effects in a clinical trial that are either:

- influenced by the order of the interventions *or*
- occur in a particular sequence.

For example, in a study of parenterally fed patients, Ang and colleagues found that the order of euglycaemic hyperinsulinaemic clamping influenced the effects of insulin.

Order effects are sometimes also called period effects. *See* **Order; Outcome**.

○ Ang B, Wade A, Halliday D and Powell-Tuck J (2000) Insulin reduces leucine oxidation and improves net leucine retention in parenterally fed humans. *Nutrition*. **16**: 221–5.

Outcome

An outcome is a result.

Helleberg and colleagues conducted a trial study of laparoscopic versus open appendectomy in patients with suspected acute appendicitis. Their outcome measures were as follows:

• subjective full recovery from pain

• functional status

• incidence of major and minor complications

• duration of sick leave.

See **Clinical versus statistical significance; Composite outcome; Endpoint; Health; Health gain; Outcome measures; Outcomes pyramid; Primary outcome; Surrogate endpoint**.

○ Helleberg A, Rudberg C, Kullman E *et al*. (1999) Prospective randomized multicentre study of laparoscopic versus open appendectomy. *Br J Surg*. **86**: 48–53.

Outcome measures

When you use an instrument to measure outcomes or change, that instrument should have some desirable properties.

The following checklist can be used to help to determine how many desirable properties any particular instrument possesses.

1 Is it appropriate for the issues being studied?

2 Is it valid (i.e. does it measure what it claims to measure)?

3 Is it responsive (i.e. can it detect change)?

4 Is it reliable?

5 Is it precise?

6 Can the results be translated into meaningful terms?

7 Is it practicable to administer?

8 Is it acceptable to the patient?

Outcomes pyramid

The outcomes pyramid is a conceptual device in the shape of a two-dimensional pyramid. On the base of the pyramid are six elements of health status, higher up the pyramid are health profiles, and at the top of the pyramid are health indices. Figure 36 shows an example.

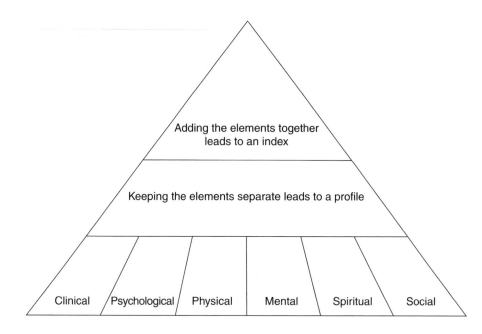

Figure 36 Outcomes pyramid.

In a clinical trial, keeping the base elements separate leads to a health *profile*, whereas adding the base elements together leads to a health *index*. It may be argued that reading along the base of the pyramid from left to right, the elements become more subjective, whereas reading from right to left, the elements become less subjective or more scientific.

When you see results from a clinical study (e.g. a trial), you can refer to the outcomes pyramid and ask the following questions.

- What elements were measured in the trial?

- What elements were missed?

- Are the results reported in the format of a profile or index?

- How do these outcomes compare with outcomes from other trials?

- How do these outcomes compare with results from clinical practice?

See **Baseline**; **Health**; **Outcome**; **Outcome measures**; **Primary outcome**; **Surrogate endpoint**.

Outlier

An outlier is a result that appears to deviate markedly from other results in the clinical trial.

For example, when measuring systolic blood pressure we may obtain values of 126 mmHg, 129 mmHg, 134 mmHg, 121 mmHg, 181 mmHg, 130 mmHg, and 132 mmHg. The 181 mmHg result can be regarded as an outlier. It may arise from a measurement or recording error, or it may be a genuine reading. *See* **Censoring**; **Data cleaning**; **Data dredging**; **Statistical tests: ten ways to cheat with statistical tests**; **Truncated data**.

P

Paired design

A paired design in a clinical trial occurs when patients are put into pairs, and then one member of the pair is allocated to the experimental regimen, while the other is allocated to the control group. The pairs may be matched on the basis of, for example, prognostic variables, age, gender, medical status or lifestyle status.

Pairing may in practice be tedious for the trialists and frustrating for the patient as they wait to have a match before they can enter the trial. *See* **Baseline**; **Matched pairs**.

Paradigm

A paradigm is a set of ideas about an issue.

The concept was popularised by Kuhn from the early 1960s. Kuhn regards 'normal science' (i.e. problem-solving activity in the context of an orthodox theoretical framework) as the rule, and 'revolutionary science' (i.e. the overthrow of one framework by another as a consequence of repeated refutations and mounting anomalies) as the exception in the history of science.

For Kuhn, the history of science is marked by long periods during which a status quo was preserved, interrupted on occasion by discontinuous jumps from one paradigm to another with no conceptual bridge between them. Thus scientific revolutions are sharp breaks from the general status quo. You could argue that evidence-based medicine is an example of 'revolutionary science'.

The term 'paradigm' remains undefined. Indeed it has been pointed out that Kuhn had over 20 definitions of the term in his first book. Over time the term has been recoined as 'disciplinary matrix' (*disciplinary* because it refers to the common possession of practitioners of a particular discipline, and *matrix* because it is composed of orders, layers and links of elements, each requiring further specification).

Mark Blaug's book, which is rather difficult to find now but worth the effort, is an excellent and palatable script that should be read if you are looking for a deeper and wider analysis of paradigms and research methodology. *See* **Analytic perspective**; **Bayesian analysis**; **Duhem's irrefutability theory**; **Falsificationism**; **Lakatosian research programme**; **Paradigm shift**; **Systematic review**.

○ Blaug M (1980) *The Methodology of Economics*. Cambridge Surveys on Economic Literature. Cambridge University Press, Cambridge.

Paradigm shift

A paradigm shift occurs when a set of ideas (a disciplinary matrix in modern terminology) is changed in the light of new evidence, debate or understanding.

Recent paradigm shifts include the following:

- the enterprise and philosophy of evidence-based medicine

- Bayesian analysis.

See **Bayesian analysis; Evidence-based medicine; National Institute for Clinical Excellence; Paradigm**.

Paradox of voting

This is the situation whereby in a system of majority voting, individual preferences cannot be fully reflected by community preferences. If Mrs Green votes in order of priority for drug programmes A, B and C, Mr Brown votes for B, C and A, and Ms Red votes for C, A and B, then any majority voting system cannot reflect all of these individuals' preferences. *See* **Analytic perspective**.

Parallel trial

A parallel trial is a type of clinical trial in which two or more groups of patients are studied concurrently but never change group.

It is the commonest form of clinical trial.

The advantages of this type of trial are as follows.

- Baseline data are needed for each patient.

- Clinician equipoise is needed before the patient is entered into the trial.

- Patients do not cross over to other arms of the trial.

- It can be used to determine causality.

- It can be used to determine the relative merits of each regimen.

- It can be used to dilute bias.

The disadvantages of parallel trials are as follows:

- the need to have comparable patients at the start of the trial

- the time to recruit

- the cost involved in case finding and case enrolment

- the cost involved in setting up and monitoring protocol compliance

- some patients will always leave or try to cross over.

Figure 37 gives an example of a three-arm parallel trial.

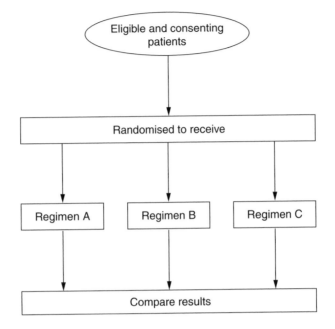

Figure 37 A parallel clinical trial with randomisation.

Parallel trials are sometimes called parallel-group trials, as the groups in each arm are followed up over time. *See* **Adaptive–adoptive trial; Balaam's design; Clinical trial; Consent; Cross-over trial; Equipoise; Preference trial; Sequential trial.**

Parsimony principle

The parsimony principle is the idea that if various clinical models or trials provide similar results, then the one with the fewest parameters or assumptions is to be preferred. *See* **Generalisability; Mega-trial; Principal component analysis; Systematic review; Transitivity.**

Participants

Participants are individuals (either healthy volunteers or patients) who are subject to a regimen in a clinical trial.

They may receive any of the following:

- the new product under examination
- what is termed 'usual care'

- a placebo

- another regimen.

Participants may:

- not necessarily be ill (e.g. healthy volunteers in phase 1 or 2 clinical trials)

- not necessarily fully reflect the type of patients who would receive the intervention in clinical practice.

See **Advantages of evidence from clinical trials; Consent. Equipoise; Phase 1 clinical trial; Phase 2 clinical trial; Phases of a clinical trial; Problems with regard to putting evidence into practice; Questions to ask before getting involved in a clinical trial; Subject.**

Patient information sheet and consent forms

Various guides exist to help in the formation and use of patient information sheets and consent forms. The following notes of guidance are available in the NHS.

Some notes of guidance for researchers

First, potential recruits to your research study must be given sufficient information to allow them to decide whether or not they want to take part. An information sheet should contain information under the headings given below, where appropriate, and in the order specified. It should be written in simple, non-technical terms and be easily understood by a lay person. Use short words, sentences and paragraphs. The 'readability' of any text can be roughly estimated by the application of standard formulae. Checks on readability are provided in most word-processing packages.

Use headed paper of the hospital/institution where the research is being carried out. If you are a local researcher the patient information sheet should be printed on local hospital/surgery paper, with local contact names and telephone numbers. Unheaded paper is not acceptable.

1 Study title

Is the title self-explanatory to a lay person? If not, a simplified title should be included.

2 Invitation paragraph

This should explain that the patient is being asked to take part in a research study. The following may be a suitable example:

> You are being invited to take part in a research study. Before you decide it is important for you to understand why the research is being done and what it

will involve. Please take time to read the following information carefully and discuss it with friends, relatives and your GP if you wish. Ask us if there is anything that is not clear or if you would like more information. Take time to decide whether or not you wish to take part. Consumers for Ethics in Research (CERES) publish a leaflet entitled *Medical Research and You*. This leaflet gives more information about medical research and looks at some questions you may want to ask. A copy may be obtained from CERES, PO Box 1365, London, N16 0BW. Thank you for reading this.

3 What is the purpose of the study?
The background and aim of the study should be given here. Also mention the duration of the study.

4 Why have I been chosen?
You should explain how the patient was chosen and how many other patients will be studied.

5 Do I have to take part?
You should explain that taking part in the research is entirely voluntary. You could use the following paragraph:

It is up to you to decide whether or not to take part. If you do decide to take part you will be given this information sheet to keep and be asked to sign a consent form. If you decide to take part you are still free to withdraw at any time and without giving a reason. This will not affect the standard of care you receive.

6 What will happen to me if I take part?
You should say how long the patient will be involved in the research, how long the research will last (if this is different), how often they will need to visit a clinic (if this is appropriate), and how long these visits will be. You should explain if the patient will need to visit the GP (or clinic) more often than for his/her usual treatment, and if travel expenses are available. What exactly will happen, e.g. blood tests, X-rays, interviews, etc? Whenever possible you should draw a simple flowchart or plan indicating what will happen at each visit. What are the patient's responsibilities? Set down clearly what you expect of them. You should also set out simply the research methods you intend to use. The following simple definitions may help.

- *Randomised trial*: Sometimes because we do not know which way of treating patients is best, we need to make comparisons. People will be put into groups and then compared. The groups are selected by a computer that has no information about the individual, i.e. by chance. Patients in each group then receive a different treatment and these are compared. You should tell the patients what chance they have of getting the study drug/treatment, e.g. a one in four chance.

- *Blind trial*: In a blind trial you will not know which treatment group you are in. If the trial is a double-blind trial, neither you nor your doctor will know which treatment group you are in (although, if your doctor needs to find out he/she can do so).

- *Cross-over trial*: In a cross-over trial the groups each receive the different treatments in turn. There may be a break between treatments so that the first drugs are cleared from your body before you start the new treatment.

- *Placebo*: A placebo is a dummy treatment, such as a pill that looks like the real thing but is not. It contains no active ingredient.

7 What do I have to do?

Are there any lifestyle restrictions? You should tell the patient if there are any dietary restrictions. Can the patient drive, drink, take part in sport? Can the patient continue to take his/her regular medication? Should the patient refrain from giving blood? What happens if the patient becomes pregnant? Explain (if appropriate) that the patient should take the medication regularly.

8 What is the drug or procedure that is being tested?

You should include a short description of the drug, device, surgery or procedure and give the stage of development. You should also state the dosage of the drug and method of administration. Patients entered into drug trials could be given a card (similar to a credit card) with details of the trial they are in. They should be asked to carry it at all times.

9 What are the alternatives for diagnosis or treatment?

For therapeutic research the patient should be told what other treatments are available.

10 What are the side-effects of taking part?

For any new drug or procedure you should explain to the patients the possible side-effects. If they suffer these or any other symptoms, they should report them next time you meet. You should also give them a contact name and number to phone if they become in any way concerned.

The known side-effects should be listed in terms the patient will clearly understand (e.g. 'damage to the heart' rather than 'cardiotoxicity', 'abnormalities of liver tests' rather than 'raised liver enzymes'). For any relatively new drug it should be explained that there may be unknown side-effects.

11 What are the possible disadvantages and risks of taking part?

For studies where there could be harm to an unborn child if the patient were pregnant or became pregnant during the study, the following (or similar) could be said:

> It is possible that if the treatment is given to a pregnant woman it will harm the unborn child. Pregnant women must not therefore take part in this study, neither should women who plan to become pregnant during the study. Women who are at risk of pregnancy may be asked to have a pregnancy test before taking part, to exclude the possibility of pregnancy. Women who could become pregnant must use an effective contraceptive during the course of this study. Any woman who finds that she has become pregnant while taking part in the study should immediately tell her research doctor.

Use the pregnancy statement carefully. In certain circumstances (e.g. terminal illness) it would be inappropriate and insensitive to raise the issue of pregnancy. There should also be an appropriate warning and advice for men if the treatment could damage sperm, which might lead to a risk of a damaged foetus.

If future insurance status, e.g. for life insurance or private medical insurance, could be affected by taking part this should be stated (if, for example, high blood pressure is detected). If the patient has private medical insurance you should ask him/her to check with the company before agreeing to take part in the trial, to ensure that their participation will not affect their medical insurance.

You should state what happens if you find a condition of which the patient was unaware. Is it treatable? What are you going to do with this information? What might be uncovered, e.g. high blood pressure, HIV status?

12 What are the possible benefits of taking part?

Where there is no intended clinical benefit to the patient from taking part in the trial, this should be stated clearly. It is important not to exaggerate the possible benefits to the patient during the course of the study, e.g. by saying they will be given extra attention, as this could be seen as coercive. It would be reasonable to say something similar to:

> Through this trial we hope to be able to identify and better understand the merits of the products under investigation. However, this cannot be guaranteed. The information we get from this study may help us to treat future patients with [name of condition] better.

In contrast, an invitation to join a research study in November 2001 in England included the following text:

> We are looking for healthy volunteers aged 5–16 years to help us with research, which will lead to improvements in the management (surgical treatment and physiotherapy) in children who have cerebral palsy ...

13 What if new information becomes available?

If additional information becomes available during the course of the research, you will need to tell the patient about this. You could use the following:

> Sometimes during the course of a research project, new information becomes available about the treatment/drug that is being studied. If this happens, your research doctor will tell you about it and discuss with you whether you want to continue in the study. If you decide to continue in the study, you will be asked to sign an updated consent form. Also, on receiving new information your research doctor might consider it to be in your best interests to withdraw you from the study. He/she will explain the reasons and arrange for your care to continue.

14 What happens when the research study stops?

If the treatment will not be available after the research finishes this should be explained to the patient. You should also explain to them what treatment will be available instead. Occasionally, the company sponsoring the research may stop it. If this is the case the reasons and implications should be explained to the patient.

15 What if something goes wrong?

You should inform patients how complaints will be handled and what redress may be available. Is there a procedure in place? You will need to distinguish between complaints from patients about their treatment by members of staff (doctors, nurses, etc.), and something serious happening during or following their participation in the trial, i.e. a reportable serious adverse event.

Where there are no Association of the British Pharmaceutical Industry (ABPI) or other no-fault compensation arrangements, and the study carries risk of physical or significant psychological harm, the following (or similar) should be said:

> If you are harmed by taking part in this research project, there are no special compensation arrangements. If you are harmed due to someone's negligence, then you may have grounds for a legal action but you may have to pay to pursue the case. Regardless of this, if you wish to complain about any aspect of the way you have been approached or treated during the course of this study, the normal National Health Service complaints mechanisms are available to you.

Where there are ABPI or other no-fault compensation arrangements, the following (or similar) could be included:

> Compensation for any injury caused by taking part in this study will be in accordance with the guidelines of the Association of the British Pharmaceutical Industry (ABPI). Broadly speaking, the ABPI guidelines recommend that 'the sponsor', without legal commitment, should compensate you without you having to prove that it is at fault. This applies in cases where it is likely that

such injury results from giving any new drug or any other procedure carried out in accordance with the protocol for the study. 'The sponsor' will not compensate you where such injury results from any procedure carried out which is not in accordance with the protocol for the study. Your right at law to claim compensation for injury where you can prove negligence is not affected. Copies of these guidelines are available on request.

16 Will my taking part in this study be kept confidential?

You will need to obtain the patient's permission to allow restricted access to their medical records and to the information collected about them during the course of the study. You should explain that all information collected about them will be kept strictly confidential. A suggested form of words for drug company sponsored research is:

> If you consent to take part in the research, any of your medical records may be inspected by the company sponsoring (and/or the company organising) the research for purposes of analysing the results. They may also be looked at by people from the company and from regulatory authorities to check that the study is being carried out correctly. Your name, however, will not be disclosed outside the hospital/GP surgery

or for other research:

> All information that is collected about you during the course of the research will be kept strictly confidential. Any information about you which leaves the hospital/surgery will have your name and address removed so that you cannot be recognised from it.

You should explain that for studies not being conducted by a GP, the patient's own GP will be notified of their participation in the trial. This could include other medical practitioners not involved in the research who may be treating the patient. You should seek the patient's agreement to this. In some instances, agreement from the patient that their GP can be informed is a precondition of entering the trial.

17 What will happen to the results of the research study?

You should be able to tell the patients what will happen to the results of the research. When are the results likely to be published? Where can they obtain a copy of the published results? Will they be told which arm of the study they were in? You might add that they will not be identified in any report/publication.

18 Who is organising and funding the research?

The answer should include the organisation or company sponsoring or funding the research (e.g. Medical Research Council, pharmaceutical company, charity or academic institution). The patient should be told whether the doctor conducting the research is being paid for including and looking after the patient in the study. This means payment other than that to cover necessary expenses such as laboratory tests arranged locally by the researcher, or the costs of a research nurse. You should say:

> The sponsors of this study will pay [name of hospital department or research fund] for including you in this study

or

> Your doctor will be paid for including you in this study.

19 Who has reviewed the study?

You should give the name of the research ethics committee(s) that reviewed the study (you do not, however, have to list the members of the committee).

20 Contact for further information

You should give the patient a contact point for further information. This can be your name or that of another doctor/nurse involved in the study.

Whilst various guides do exist to help researchers in the formation and use of patient information sheets and consent forms, the notes above provide a useful starting point. Nevertheless, you should be aware that local practice, ethics committee requirements, organisational requirements, professional rules and obligations, and legal requirements can often indicate other issues to be considered in the particular formation and use of patient information sheets and consent forms. *See* **Advantages of evidence from clinical trials; Caldicott Guardians; Clinical trial; Fate of clinical research; Multicentre trial; Patient preferences; Patient preferences in clinical trials; Placebo; Placebo effect; Qualitative research; Questions to ask before getting involved in a clinical trial; Random; Reasons given by the investigator for a study being abandoned or in abeyance; Research governance in the NHS; Types of questions.**

Patient preferences

Patients may have an inclination, penchant or preference for one product, service or scheme over another. This is known as a patient preference.

For instance:

- Meredith and colleagues reported on a survey of cancer patients' views of their information needs

- Moffett and colleagues reported on a randomised controlled trial of a progressive exercise programme compared with usual primary care management in a community setting for patients with low back pain. The patients' preferences for the type of management were elicited independently of randomisation

- Protheroe and colleagues investigated the impact of patients' preferences on the treatment of atrial fibrillation

- Silvestri and colleagues reported on a study of preferences for chemotherapy in patients with advanced non-small-cell lung cancer.

The advantage of patient preferences is that they may improve compliance, but the drawback is that the basis of their preferences may be questioned. In a clinical trial we do not know whether one regime is better than another – hence the experiment – so where do patients derive their preferences from in these cases? *See* **Patient preferences in clinical trials; Qualitative analysis**.

○ Meredith C, Symonds P, Webster L *et al.* (1996) Information needs of cancer patients in west Scotland: cross-sectional survey of patients' views. *BMJ.* **313**: 724–6.

○ Moffett JK, Bell-Syer S, Jackson D *et al.* (1999) Randomised controlled trial of exercise for low back pain: clinical outcomes, costs and preferences. *BMJ.* **319**: 279–83.

○ Protheroe J, Fahey T, Montgomery AA and Peters TJ (2000) The impact of patients' preferences on the treatment of atrial fibrillation: observational study of patient-based decision analysis. *BMJ.* **320**: 1380–4.

○ Silvestri G, Pritchard R and Welch G (1998) Preferences for chemotherapy in patients with advanced non-small-cell lung cancer: descriptive study based on scripted interviews. *BMJ.* **317**: 771–5.

Patient preferences in clinical trials

In some clinical trials, patients are allowed to state their preference for:

- a particular course of treatment

- whether or not they are to be randomised.

Recent examples include the following.

- Chilvers and colleagues reported on a randomised trial with patient preference arms consisting of antidepressant drugs and generic counselling for treatment of major depression in primary care. In this trial the patients were either randomised to counselling or antidepressant drugs, or if they had a preference they were allowed to go into their preference arm (e.g. counselling). Patients were followed up at 8 weeks and 12 months.

- Ward and colleagues reported on a randomised controlled trial of non-directive counselling, cognitive-behaviour therapy and usual general practitioner care for patients with depression.

There is a series of letters in the *British Medical Journal* following on from these articles. These letters are certainly worth looking at in order to gain a wider and deeper understanding of the trials and their relevance.

The actual foundation of patients' preferences has yet to be fully examined.

In general, there are three main types of preference trials:

- the comprehensive cohort design
- the Wennberg design
- the Zelen design.

See **Comprehensive cohort design; Declaration of Helsinki; Equipoise; Patient preferences; Preference trial; Wennberg design; Zelen consent design.**

○ Ashcroft R (2000) Giving medicine a fair trial. *BMJ.* **320**: 1686.

○ Brewin CR and Bradley C (1989) Patient preferences and randomised clinical trials. *BMJ.* **299**: 684–5.

○ Chilvers C, Dewey M, Fielding K *et al.* (2001) Antidepressant drugs and generic counselling for treatment of major depression in primary care: randomised trial with patient preference arms. *BMJ.* **322**: 772–5.

○ Lambert MF and Wood J (2000) Incorporating patient preferences into randomized trials. *J Clin Epidemiol.* **53**: 163–6.

○ MacPharson K, Britton AR and Wennberg JA (1997) Are randomized controlled trials controlled? Patient preferences and unblind trials? *Lancet.* **90**: 652–6.

○ Silverman WA and Altman DG (1996) Patients' preferences and randomised trials. *Lancet.* **347**: 171–4.

○ Torgerson DJ, Klaber-Moffett J and Russell IT (1996) Patient preferences in randomised trials: threat or opportunity? *J Health Serv Res Policy.* **1**: 194–7.

○ van der Windt DAWM, Koes BW, van Aarst M *et al.* (2000) Practical aspects of conducting a pragmatic randomised trial in primary care: patient recruitment and outcome assessment. *Br J Gen Pract.* **50**: 371–4.

○ Ward E, King M, Lloyd M *et al.* (2000) Randomised controlled trial of non-directive counselling, cognitive-behaviour therapy, and usual general practitioner care for patients with depressions. I. Clinical effectiveness. *BMJ.* **321**: 1383–8.

Patient's expected event rate

The patient's expected event rate (PEER) reflects the susceptibility of the patient to the event (e.g. breast cancer). *See* **Bayesian analysis; Number needed to treat.**

Patients' register

This is a list of the relevant patient details logged by the trial investigator and assessed by the data-monitoring committee. *See* **Audit; Baseline characteristics; Blind; Data-monitoring committee; Protocol.**

Peer review

Whatever profession you are currently in, there will always be others in that same profession. When some of these people review what you say, do or write, this is peer review.

Peer review may or may not:

- be systematic
- be representative
- be constructive
- have an ulterior motive
- include a lot of subjectivity.

See **Accountability; Due process; Peer reviewers' checklist (*BMJ* recommended); Research governance in the NHS; William's agreement measure**.

○ Godlee F and Jefferson T (1999) *Peer Review in Health Sciences*. BMJ Books, London.

Peer reviewers' checklist (*BMJ* recommended)

The *BMJ* produces guidelines for peer reviewers (i.e. those who review their colleagues' work). Although other peer review checklists do exist, the *BMJ* checklist offers a good point for opening the discussion and debates about what should and should not be included in such a checklist. More fundamentally it helps to highlight the issue of the need for such a checklist.

General guidance

The *BMJ* writes to the reviewer to say that the manuscript is a confidential document, and states that the reviewer should not discuss it even with the author. The *BMJ* now has a system of open peer review. This means that you, as a reviewer, will be asked to sign your report on any paper for consideration for publication in the *BMJ* that the journal sends to you. It does not mean that authors should contact you directly (we will continue to ask them to direct any queries through us). Openness also means that we ask reviewers and authors to declare any competing interest that might relate to the papers considered by the *BMJ*.

As a *BMJ* reviewer you will be advising the editors who make the final decision (aided by an editorial 'hanging committee' for some papers). The *BMJ* will advise you of their decision, and will pass on your signed report to the author, so they advise you not to make any comments that you do not wish the author to see. Even if the *BMJ* does not accept a paper, they consider it useful to pass on constructive comments that might help the author to improve it. Please give detailed comments (with references whenever possible) that will help both the editor(s) to make a decision on the paper and the authors to improve it.

For all papers, the following questions need to be addressed.

1 Is the paper important?

2 Will the paper add enough to existing knowledge?

3 Does the paper read well and make sense?

For research papers, you need to comment on the points listed in Table 38 below.

Table 38 Peer reviewers' checklist (*BMJ* recommended)

1 *Originality* – Does the work add enough to what is already in the published literature? If so, what does it add? If not, please cite relevant references.

2 *Importance of the work to general readers* – Does this work matter to clinicians, patients, teachers or policymakers? Is a general journal the right place for it?

3 *Scientific reliability*

4 *Research question* – Is it clearly defined and appropriately answered?

5 *Overall design of study* – Is it adequate?

6 *Participants studied* – Are they adequately described and their conditions defined?

7 *Methods* – Are they adequately described? For randomised trials: CONSORT style? Are they ethical?

8 *Results* – Do they answer the research question? Are they credible? Are they well presented?

9 *Interpretation and conclusions* – Are they warranted by and sufficiently derived from/focused on the data? Is the message clear?

10 *References* – Are they up to date and relevant? Are there any glaring omissions?

11 *Abstract/summary/key messages/This Week in BMJ* – Do they reflect accurately what the paper says?

12 *Not all of these points will be relevant for non-research papers.* Please use your discretion about the above list when reporting on other types of paper.

See **Accountability; Peer review; Statisticians' checklist (*BMJ* recommended); Transparency**.

Period effects
Another term for order effects. *See* **Order effects**.

Peto's method
Peto's method is a statistical method of combining odds ratios in a meta-analysis. It has been used in clinical trials where sample sizes of the groups tended to be quite similar. However, Peto's method can lead to biased results if the odds ratio is close to 1. *See* **Mega-trial; Meta-analysis; Odds ratios**.

○ Pereira-Maxwell F (1998) *A–Z of Medical Statistics: a companion for critical appraisal*. Edward Arnold, London.

○ Petrie A and Sabin C (2000) *Medical Statistics at a Glance*. Blackwell Science, Oxford.

Pharmacodynamics

Pharmacodynamics is the study of the relationships between the dose of the drug and its effect. *See* **Dose-ranging trial; Pharmacokinetics; Phase 1 clinical trial; Phase 2 clinical trial; Titration.**

Pharmacokinetics

Pharmacokinetics is the study of the absorption, distribution and elimination properties of a drug and its metabolites. It is often seen in the early phase of clinical trials. *See* **Pharmacodynamics; Phase 1 clinical trial; Phase 2 clinical trial; Washout period**.

○ Muirhead GJ, Harness J, Holt PR, Oliver S and Anziano RJ (2000) Ziprasidone and the pharmacokinetics of a combined oral contraceptive. *Br J Clin Pharmacol*. **49 (Supplement 1)**: 49–56S.

Phase I clinical trial

When a product is first studied in healthy humans, it is called a phase 1 clinical trial. The primary objective of a phase 1 clinical trial is usually to determine the product's:

- safety
- safe dose range
- clinical pharmacology (e.g. pharmacokinetics, pharmacodynamics).

Phase 1 clinical trials:

- usually involve 10–80 healthy volunteers
- may or may not involve a placebo
- may or may not involve randomisation.

If the results are promising, the product would be put into a phase 2 clinical trial for further analysis. *See* **Causes of delay and failure to complete a clinical trial; Clinical trial; Fate of clinical research; Phase 2 clinical trial; Phase 3 clinical trial; Phase 4 clinical trial; Phases of clinical trials; Primary question; Randomisation; Randomised controlled trial; Reasons given by the investigator for a study being abandoned or in abeyance; Reasons given by the investigator for a study never being started.**

Phase 2 clinical trial

A product that successfully comes through a phase 1 clinical trial may be put into a phase 2 clinical trial.

The primary objectives of a phase 2 clinical trial are as follows:

- to determine the product's efficacy

- to further determine its safety, at different doses and frequencies of administration

- to confirm the product's pharmacokinetic and pharmacodynamic properties.

Phase 2 clinical trials:

- usually involve 100–300 patients who have the disease of interest. Sometimes there is a mix of healthy volunteers and patients

- generally benefit from identification of the ratio of healthy volunteers to patients

- may or may not involve a placebo

- may or may not involve randomisation.

If the results of phase 2 are promising, further analysis would be performed under a phase 3 clinical trial. *See* **Causes of delay and failure to complete a clinical trial; Clinical trial; Control group; Fate of clinical research; Phase 1 clinical trial; Phase 3 clinical trial; Phase 4 clinical trial; Phases of clinical trials; Primary question; Randomisation; Randomised controlled trial; Reasons given by the investigator for a study being abandoned or in abeyance; Reasons given by the investigator for a study never being started.**

○ Pectasides D, Cunnigham D, Roth AD *et al.* (2000) Chemotherapy with cisplatin, epirubicin and docetaxel in transitional cell urothelial cancer: phase II trial. *Eur J Cancer.* **36**: 74–9.

Phase 3 clinical trial

A product that successfully comes through a phase 2 trial may be put into a phase 3 clinical trial.

The primary objective of a phase 3 clinical trial is usually to determine and collect more evidence of the product's:

- safety and efficacy

- side-effects

- risks and benefits, by providing information that will enable an assessment of these.

Most phase 3 clinical trials:

- involve a placebo
- involve randomising the patients to different regimens in the trial
- involve 100–3000 patients who have the disease of interest
- last between 1 week and 1 year.

There is no regulatory requirement in phase 3 trials to test the experimental intervention with current best practice. This is because:

- we rarely find a consensus on what current best practice is supposed to be
- many practices may not be following 'current best practice'
- there is often more than one alternative in current practice.

If the results are promising, the company behind the product would use the trial and other information in its application to bring the product on to the market. Thus the information from phase 3 trials provides part of the foundation for the licensing application.

Phase 3 trials can be stopped because of their success or because of their apparent lack of success. A recent example is GlaxoSmithkline's development of tranilist for the prevention of restenosis following percutaneous coronary intervention. Over 11 500 patients were enrolled and randomised to one of two treatment doses of tranilist or placebo, given over 3 months. The endpoints were a reduction in major adverse cardiac events due to restenosis (i.e. death, myocardial infarction, and the need for revascularisation). In July 2001, GlaxoSmithkline announced that it was abandoning the PRESTO development (Prevention of REStenosis with Tranilist and its Outcomes) as it had failed to meet the efficacy endpoints. The trial data and analysis were due to be presented at the American Heart Association meeting in November 2001.

This does not automatically mean that no other work will be done on the product, and indeed it is currently on the Japanese market for a range of indications, including asthma, dermal allergies and keloids. *See* **Causes of delay and failure to complete a clinical trial; Clinical trial; Control group; Fate of clinical research; Medicines Control Agency; Phase 1 clinical trial; Phase 2 clinical trial; Phase 4 clinical trial; Phases of clinical trials; Primary question; Randomisation; Randomised controlled trial; Reasons given by the investigator for a study being abandoned or in abeyance; Reasons given by the investigator for a study never being started.**

Phase 4 clinical trial

A phase 4 clinical trial is an investigation of the attributes of a product that is on the market.

By describing it as phase 4, we are assuming that the product in question has successfully undergone the first three phases of clinical trials (*see* above).

The objectives of a phase 4 clinical trial can include establishing the merits of the product in practice and increasing practitioners' knowledge of the product.

Phase 4 clinical trials:

- involve from around 20 to 20 000 patients

- can generally run from 1 day to 5 or more years

- do not usually, if ever, involve a placebo

- may or may not involve randomisation.

Phase 4 clinical trials are sometimes called post-marketing studies. Although a phase 4 clinical trial is indeed a post-marketing study, not all post-marketing studies are phase 4 clinical trials. *See* **Causes of delay and failure to complete a clinical trial; Clinical trial; Control group; Fate of clinical research; Local research ethics committee; Medicines Control Agency; Multicentre research ethics committee; Phase 1 clinical trial; Phase 2 clinical trial; Phase 3 clinical trial; Phases of clinical trials; Post-marketing study; Primary question; Randomisation; Randomised controlled trial; Reasons given by the investigator for a study being abandoned or in abeyance; Reasons given by the investigator for a study never being started; Research governance in the NHS.**

Phases of clinical trials

Products that are subject to clinical trials generally go through particular phases of study. From basic research, biological testing and screening in the preclinical period, the product would go through phase 1, 2, 3 and maybe 4 trials (*see* above). Figure 38 gives an indication of how knowledge of a product changes throughout different phases of the trials.

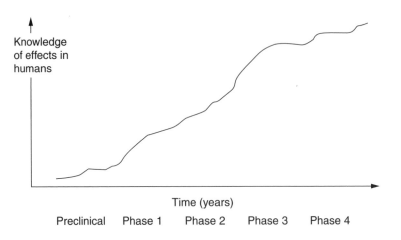

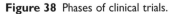

Figure 38 Phases of clinical trials.

While Figure 38 does indeed show a growing amount of knowledge of the effects of the product under study in humans, the line may be different in particular cases. The figure is a concept, for illustration only. It may not reflect knowledge of a particular product, and many products in development do not get past phase 2 trials. Furthermore, knowledge evaporates over time, so there is a possibility of broken lines. The diagram does not necessarily relate to any one individual's knowledge. It could relate to groups of individuals (e.g. those following the clinical trial all the way through the series of phases).

The key message of the figure is that each phase should provide more knowledge than existed before. *See* **Medicines Control Agency**; **Phase 1 clinical trial**; **Phase 2 clinical trial**; **Phase 3 clinical trial**; **Phase 4 clinical trial**; **Post-marketing surveillance**.

Pilot trial

A pilot trial is a relatively small-scale clinical trial designed to establish the following:

- the possible number of patients that could be recruited

- the issues involved in finding and recruiting patients

- the issues involved in finding and recruiting healthcare professionals (e.g. doctors, consultants, nurses or midwives)

- the feasibility of gathering data

- the practicalities involved with questionnaire design and administration

- protocol adherence

- key clinical outcomes to look for

- the primary research question.

See **Clinical trial**; **Feasibility trial**; **Hypothesis**; **Mega-trial**.

○ Ross-McGill H, Hewison J, Hirst J *et al*. (1999) Antenatal home blood pressure monitoring: a pilot randomised controlled trial. *Br J Obstet Gynacol.* **107**: 217–21.

Pitfalls of interviewing

Many of us are involved in interviewing every week.

- When we interact with a patient we ask some questions in order to gain a better understanding of their impressions and condition. They interview us in order to gain a better appreciation of what we think, what we advise, and what options are available to them.

- When we are presented with the results of clinical trials, we can ask the presenter a series of questions and they should be able to answer them.

- When we are thinking of getting involved in a clinical trial, we usually interviewed (and we should be surprised if the lead researcher does not interview us).

- When we are considering recruiting a patient to a clinical trial they will be interviewed, and they should be encouraged to (in effect) interview us.

- In assessing the experiences and outcomes of clinical trials, interviews often help to reveal important information.

Interviewing has many pitfalls, and although there is no comprehensive evidence showing how common certain pitfalls are, a list of possible ones would be helpful when designing an interview schedule, conducting an interview and interpreting results from an interview. Table 39 presents a list of 20 pitfalls that may be encountered in interviewing.

Table 39 Twenty pitfalls of interviewing

1 Not making clear the purpose of the interview.
2 Not making clear what the answers will be used for and how this will help the interviewee.
3 Interruptions from outside (e.g. telephone, visitors).
4 Competing distractions (e.g. others in the room, children).
5 Stage fright in interviewer.
6 Stage fright in interviewee.
7 Jumping from one subject to another.
8 Lack of logical flow in questions.
9 Asking the interviewee embarrassing or awkward questions.
10 Asking leading or loaded questions.
11 Asking imprecise questions.
12 Asking questions that are open to questioning.
13 Asking complex questions.
14 Teaching (e.g. giving interviewee medical advice).
15 Counselling (e.g. summarising responses too early).
16 Presenting one's own perspective and thus potentially biasing the interviewee.
17 Superficial interviews.
18 Ethical issues – what do you do if you receive specific allegations, contradictory information or secret information?
19 Deviating from the main objectives of the interview.
20 Translating from the interviewee's story and reinterpreting it in your own words.

See **Qualitative analysis; Types of questions.**

○ Field PA and Morse JM (1989) *Nursing Research: the application of qualitative approaches*. Chapman and Hall, London.

○ Pope C and Mays M (eds) (2000) *Qualitative Research in Health Care*. BMJ Books, London.

Placebo

A placebo is a product that is indistinguishable from a medicine in terms of packaging, taste, smell, texture, form, colour and size. The only difference between the placebo and the medicine is that the placebo does not contain the active pharmacological ingredient.

Some people regard placebos as deceitful. A more enlightened interpretation is that placebos can:

- highlight the importance of good care and psychological aspects of healthcare intervention

- provide a benchmark against which to gauge an intervention.

There has been, and will continue to be, considerable debate about the use of placebos in clinical trials. *See* **Active control; Benchmarking; Control group; Ethical issues; Hawthorne effect; Hello–goodbye effect; Multicentre research ethics committees; Placebo-controlled trial; Placebo effect; Research governance in the NHS.**

○ Balar JC III (2001) The powerful placebo and the wizard of Oz. *NEJM.* **344**: 1630–2.

○ Hrobjartsson A and Gotzsche PC (2001) Is the placebo powerless? An analysis of clinical trials comparing placebo to no treatment. *NEJM.* **344**: 1594–602.

○ Rothman KJ (1996) Placebo mania. *BMJ.* **313**: 3–4.

○ Vickers AJ and de Craen AJ (2000) Why use placebos in clinical trials? A narrative review of the methodological literature. *J Clin Epidemiol.* **53**: 157–61.

○ Welton AJ, Vickers MR, Cooper JA, Meade TW and Marteau TM (1999) Is recruitment more difficult with a placebo arm in a randomised controlled trial? *BMJ.* **318**: 1114–17.

Placebo-controlled trial

A placebo-controlled trial is a clinical trial in which the control group receives a placebo. The key objective of a placebo-controlled trial is usually to help to determine whether changes in the experimental group can be attributed to the experimental substance received. *See* **Baseline; Benchmarking; Clinical trial; Control group; Placebo; Placebo effect; Randomised controlled trial.**

Placebo effect

Suppose that a new medicine is to be tested for its safety, quality and efficacy in patients. Then patients may be allocated to one of two groups. Group 1 receives the medicine of interest, while Group 2 receives the placebo. Measured results from Group 2's consumption of the placebo are called placebo effects.

Hrobjartsson and Gotzsche have reported on a systematic analysis of clinical trials in which patients were randomly assigned to either placebo or no treatment. They reported on 114 trials and found little evidence that placebos had powerful clinical effects. However, they did not report fully on the possibility of non-clinical effects. *See* **Hawthorne effect; Placebo**.

○ Balar JC III (2001) The powerful placebo and the wizard of Oz. *NEJM.* **344**: 1630–2.

○ Collier J (1995) Confusion over the use of placebos in clinical trials. *BMJ.* **311**: 821–2.

○ Hrobjartsson A and Gotzsche PC (2001) Is the placebo powerless? An analysis of clinical trials comparing placebo to no treatment. *NEJM.* **344**: 1594–602.

○ Rothman KJ (1996) Placebo mania. *BMJ.* **313**: 3–4 (There is a series of papers following this article, *see BMJ* dated 19 October 1996).

○ Vickers AJ and de Craen AJ (2000) Why use placebos in clinical trials? A narrative review of the methodological literature. *J Clin Epidemiol.* **53**: 157–61.

○ Welton AJ, Vickers MR, Cooper JA, Meade TW and Marteau TM (1999) Is recruitment more difficult with a placebo arm in a randomised controlled trial? *BMJ.* **318**: 1114–17.

Play-the-winner rule

The play-the-winner rule occurs in a clinical trial when allocation of the next patient depends on how well the last patient fared in the trial. In general it is part of the adaptive–adoptive family of trials.

You need to be able to see the outcome from the previous patient before the next patient goes into the trial. If their outcome is favourable, the next patient who goes into the trial receives the same intervention that they received. If the previous patient's outcome was not successful, the next patient goes into another regimen in the trial. Generally the method is used to maximise the number of successful patients, but it depends heavily on identifying outcomes relatively quickly and accurately. *See* **Adaptive–adoptive trial; Bernoulli trial; Clinical significance; Outcomes pyramid; Primary outcome; Statistical significance; Surrogate endpoint**.

Pooled analysis

A pooled analysis is an assessment of a collection of evidence. It may or may not:

• be systematic

• state where one looked for the information

• reveal how the information was selected

• show how it was pooled

• be reproducible.

You should compare this with the entries for systematic review and meta-analysis. *See* **Bias; Due process; Evidence-based medicine; L'Abbe plot; Meta-analysis; Peer review; Systematic review; Transparency**.

○ Cates C (1999) Pooling numbers needed to treat may not be reliable. *BMJ.* **318**: 1764.

Post hoc

Post hoc generally means after the event. *See* **Bayesian analysis**; **Data dredging**; **Data fishing**.

Post-marketing surveillance

Post-marketing surveillance is the study of a product in the marketplace.

By law, the holder of a product licence (usually the drug company) has a statutory obligation to maintain a record of reports (of which they are aware) of adverse effects in one or more human beings or animals associated with the use of any medicinal product to which the licence relates. These records must also be available for inspection by anyone who is authorised to ask to inspect them. However, they are not required by law or regulation to reveal and make available for inspection to a wider audience their methods, results, analyses or implications.

Product licences for medicines for human consumption are only valid for a particular period, generally 5 years. The licence holder has to submit evidence to support the continuation of that licence. This information, which would include post-marketing data, could also be useful, if it were made available, to a wider audience such as market analysts, companies, patients, healthcare practitioners, healthcare managers and funders.

At best, post-marketing surveillance can contribute to the better understanding of product safety, efficacy, compliance and administration, it can help to determine new uses of existing drugs, and it can help to identify issues for particular subgroups of patients. At worst it can be used as a mask for promoting the product. *See* **Clinical trial**; **Observational study**; **Phase 4 clinical trial**; **Research governance in the NHS**; **Transparency**; **Yellow card scheme**.

○ Rathman W, Haastert B, Delling B *et al.* (1998) Postmarketing surveillance of adverse drug reactions: a correlation study approach using multiple data sources. *Pharmaco-Epidemiol Drug Safety.* 7: 51–7.

Post-randomisation consent

Post-randomisation consent occurs when a patient agrees to the treatment option after they have been randomly assigned to it (sometimes loosely called deferred consent). It has recently been argued to be an unethical, immoral, unprofessional and probably illegal practice. *See* **Comprehensive cohort design**; **Consent**; **Deferred consent**; **Ethical issues**; **Preference trial**; **Pre-randomisation consent**; **Research governance in the NHS**; **Wennberg's design**; **Zelen consent design**.

Post-test odds

The post-test odds (PTO) are the odds that the patient has the target disorder after the diagnostic test has been carried out.

Mathematically the PTO is written and can be calculated as follows:

$$\text{PTO} = \text{pre-test odds} \times \text{likelihood ratio of a positive test result}$$

So, if the pre-test odds for a patient are 0.8 and the likelihood ratio is 0.2, then the PTO of the patient having the condition of interest are:

$$\text{PTO} = 0.8 \times 0.2 = 0.16$$

In this case, the lower the PTO the better. PTO are sometimes called 'posterior odds'. *See* **Odds; Post-test probability; Pre-test odds; Pre-test probability.**

- Katz DL (2001) *Clinical Epidemiology and Evidence Based Medicine.* Sage Publications, London.
- Pereira-Maxwell F (1998) *A–Z of Medical Statistics: a companion for critical appraisal.* Arnold Publishing, London.
- Petrie A and Sabin C (2001) *Medical Statistics at a Glance.* Blackwell Science, Oxford.

Post-test probability

The post-test probability (PTP) is the proportion of patients with that particular test result who have the condition of interest.

The PTP is related to the post-test odds as follows:

$$\text{PTP} = \frac{\text{post-test odds}}{1 + \text{post-test odds}}$$

So, if the post-test odds are 0.16, then the PTP is:

$$\text{PTP} = \frac{0.16}{1 + 0.16} = 0.138$$

Generally, the lower the PTP the better. PTP is sometimes called 'posterior probability'. *See* **Post-test odds; Pre-test odds; Pre-test probability.**

- Katz DL (2001) *Clinical Epidemiology and Evidence Based Medicine.* Sage Publications, London.
- Pereira-Maxwell F (1998) *A–Z of Medical Statistics: a companion for critical appraisal.* Arnold Publishing, London.
- Petrie A and Sabin C (2001) *Medical Statistics at a Glance.* Blackwell Science, Oxford.

Power

A clinical trial has sufficient power if it can reliably detect a statistically significant difference if one actually exists. It is generally taken to be the probability of finding a difference in a study to be statistically significant when the difference actually exists. *See* **Power calculation; Power of a test; Protocol.**

Power calculation

When setting up a clinical trial, you could specify in advance that you are looking to see whether a particular statistically significant difference between regimens exists. A power calculation is a measure of how likely it is that the clinical trial will produce a statistically significant result if that difference is indeed found to exist.

There are tables and diagrams available in most good-quality statistical books that show you how to do the power calculation in practice. *See* **Power; Power of a test; Sample size; Statistical significance; Statistical test diagram; Statistical tests: ten ways to cheat with statistical tests; Superiority trial**.

Power of a test

Suppose you are looking at the merits of different cholesterol-lowering drugs. You can set up a clinical trial with the standard null hypothesis that there is no significant difference between cholesterol regimens after 48 weeks on specific predefined outcomes.

The power of a test is the probability that a null hypothesis will be rejected if it is in fact false. In this example, it is the probability of rejecting the hypothesis that there is no difference between cholesterol-lowering regimens in favour of the alternative hypothesis. More generally, it is the power to make a correct decision (it is sometimes just called power).

You can set up a simple calculation for power (P) where:

$$P = 1 - \text{probability of a type 2 error}$$

The maximum value of P is 1 and the minimum value of P is 0. In general, the higher the power the better – P closer to 1 is preferable to P closer to 0. This means that you want the probability of a type 2 error to be as small as possible. *See* **Hypothesis test decisions; Null hypothesis; Power; Research governance in the NHS; Type 2 error**.

Pragmatic trial

This is another term for efficiency trial.

For example:

- Morrison and colleagues from Aberdeen and Glasgow, Scotland, reported on a pragmatic cluster randomised controlled trial to evaluate guidelines for the management of infertility across the primary care–secondary care interface (*see* the letters published on the *BMJ* website (www.bmj.com) by Dr Rashidian and Professor Freemantle for a discussion of the methods, results, analysis and implications of the paper by Morrison and colleagues)

- Williams and colleagues used a pragmatic randomised trial to evaluate whether follow-up of patients with inflammatory bowel disease is better through open access than through routine booked appointments.

See **Clinical trial; Efficiency trial.**

○ Charlton BG (1994) Understanding randomised controlled trials: explanatory or pragmatic? *Fam Pract.* **11**: 243–4.

○ Freemantle N (2001) Methodological weakness and poor reporting undermine author's conclusions. *BMJ.* **323**: 808.

○ Morrison J, Carroll L, Twaddle S *et al.* (2001) Pragmatic randomised controlled trial to evaluate guidelines for the management of infertility across the primary care–secondary care interface. *BMJ.* **322**: 1282–4.

○ Roland M and Torgerson DJ (1998) Understanding controlled trials: what are pragmatic trials? *BMJ.* **316**: 285.

○ van der Windt DAWM, Koes BW, van Aarst M, Heemskerk MAMB and Bouter LM (2000) Practical aspects of conducting a pragmatic randomised trial in primary care: patient recruitment and outcome assessment. *Br J Gen Pract.* **50**: 371–4.

○ Williams JG, Cheung WY, Russel IT *et al.* (2000) Open-access follow-up for inflammatory bowel disease. *BMJ.* **320**: 544–8.

Preference group

In a trial, a preference group is a collection of patients who are allowed to express a preference of some kind. For example:

• whether or not they will be randomised

• which regimen they will go into.

See **Assent; Comprehensive cohort design; Consent; Preference trial; Wennberg design; Zelen consent design.**

Preference trial

A preference trial is a clinical trial in which patients' preferences are taken into account.

Thus in a trial of regimen A versus regimen B we may have four groups, namely those randomised to A (RA), those with a preference for A (PA), those randomised to B (RB) and those with a preference for B (PB). How that trial is then analysed remains the subject of debate. For instance, it has been argued that we can compare the two randomised groups RA and RB as in a standard trial, but how do we compare those whose preferences were for A and B, namely groups PA and PB? Some have argued that the preference groups should be assessed as if they were in 'observational studies'. Others have suggested that if patients have a strong preference it would be unethical to enter them into the trial in the first place, so they should not be included.

Then we need to address the question of comparing the two randomised groups (RA and RB) with those who activated their preference (PA and PB). Can it be done? If so, would it be meaningful?

Trials involving patient preferences have an impact on the overall sample size that is required to run appropriate statistical tests. Some estimate that a trial with preferences requires at least two to three times the number of patients in a standard trial with no preferences.

There is also a series of preference trials in which some of the doctors have a preference as to which regimen they work with in the trial.

The methods, ethics, statistics and practicalities of preference trials are currently subject to reconsideration. Some attempts have been made to identify patient preferences initially, and then to randomise the patients regardless of their preferences. This method may show whether those who received their preference differ from those who received the same regimen but had expressed no preference, or indeed had expressed a preference for something else in the trial!

To date there have been no published systematic reviews of preference trials *per se*, nor are there any published systematic reviews comparing trials where preferences had a role to play with trials where preferences had no role. See **Baseline**; **Completer**; **Comprehensive cohort design**; **Confounding factor**; **Consent**; **Cross-over rate**; **Dropout**; **Outcomes pyramid**; **Patient preferences**; **Preference group**; **Wennberg's design**; **Zelen consent design**.

○ Awad MA, Shapiro SH, Lund JP and Feine JS (2000) Determinants of patients' treatment preferences in a clinical trial. *Commun Dental Oral Epidemiol.* **2**: 119–25.

○ Lambert MF and Wood J (2000) Incorporating patient preferences into randomised trials. *J Clin Epidemiol.* **53**: 163–6.

○ McPharson EK (1996) Patients' preferences and randomised trials. *Lancet.* **347**: 1119.

○ McPherson K, Britton AR and Wennberg JE (1997) Are randomized controlled trials controlled? Patient preferences and unblind trials. *J R Soc Med.* **90**: 652–6.

○ Torgerson DJ, Klaber-Moffett J and Russell IT (1996) Patient preferences in randomised trials: threat or opportunity. *J Health Serv Res Policy.* **1**: 194–7.

○ Torgerson D and Sibbald B (1998) Understanding controlled trials: what is a patient preference trial? *BMJ.* **316**: 360 (There is also a series of letters following this article; see *BMJ.* **317**: 78).

○ Ward E, King M, Lloyd M *et al.* (2000) Randomised controlled trial of non-directive counselling, cognitive-behaviour therapy, and usual general practitioner care for patients with depression. I. Clinical effectiveness. *BMJ.* **321**: 1383–8.

Prerandomisation consent

Prerandomisation consent occurs when a patient agrees to be randomly allocated to any one of a variety of alternative regimens in the clinical trial before they are actually randomly assigned to a regimen. It is a common feature of most clinical trials.

In Figure 39, you start out with a pool of patients who are eligible to enter the trial. Some agree to be randomised (group B), and are then randomly allocated to a regimen in the trial.

Notice that some patients did not want to be randomised (group D). What happens to them depends on further particulars of the trial. In some trials the group D members are allowed to choose which arm of the trial they will enter. This is useful in so far as it gives another set of comparisons for the trial – comparing the results from those who were randomised with those who were not randomised. In other cases the

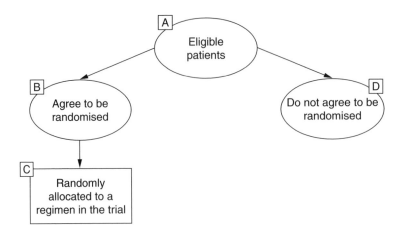

Figure 39 Prerandomisation consent.

group D members are only discussed in passing during the writing up of the trial. *See* **Belmont report; Consent; CONSORT; Declaration of Helsinki; European Union Directive on clinical trials of medicinal products for humans; Post-randomisation consent.**

Pre-test odds

The pre-test odds (Pre-TO) are the odds that the patient has the condition of interest, e.g. a disease, before the diagnostic test is carried out.

The Pre-TO is calculated as follows:

$$\text{Pre-TO} = \frac{\text{pre-test probability}}{1 - \text{pre-test probability}}$$

If the pre-test probability is 0.15, then the Pre-TO are:

$$\text{Pre-TO} = \frac{0.15}{1 - 0.15} = \frac{0.15}{0.85} = 0.176$$

Generally, the lower the Pre-TO the better. Pre-TO are sometimes called 'prior odds'. *See* **Bayesian analysis; Odds; Post-test odds; Post-test probability; Pre-test probability.**

○ Katz DL (2001) *Clinical Epidemiology and Evidence Based Medicine.* Sage Publications, London.

○ Pereira-Maxwell F (1998) *A–Z of Medical Statistics: a companion for critical appraisal.* Arnold Publishing, London.

○ Petrie A and Sabin C (2001) *Medical Statistics at a Glance.* Blackwell Science, Oxford.

Pre-test probability

The pre-test probability (Pre-TP) is the proportion of patients with the particular diagnostic test result who have the condition or disease of interest.

Table 40 Pre-test probability

		Condition present	Condition absent
	Positive	A	B
Test result			
	Negative	C	D

Suppose you are interested in the Pre-TP of a patient having the condition of interest. Using Table 40 you can write the Pre-TP of the patient having the condition as follows:

$$\text{Pre-TP}_{\text{with condition}} = \frac{A + C}{A + B + C + D}$$

For example, if A = 0.14, B = 0.65, C = 0.01 and D = 0.2, then the Pre-TP of the patient having the condition of interest is:

$$\text{Pre-TP}_{\text{with condition}} = \frac{0.14 + 0.01}{0.14 + 0.65 + 0.01 + 0.2} = \frac{0.15}{1} = 0.15, \text{ or } 15\%$$

A curious question that has not been fully answered is this: where do the initial data come from to set up the table that helps establish a pre-test probability? Generally, the lower the Pre-TP the better. Pre-TP is sometimes called 'prior probability'. *See* **Bayesian analysis; Post-test odds; Pre-test odds.**

○ Katz DL (2001) *Clinical Epidemiology and Evidence Based Medicine.* Sage Publications, London.

○ Pereira-Maxwell F (1998) *A–Z of Medical Statistics: a companion for critical appraisal.* Arnold Publishing, London.

○ Petrie A and Sabin C (2001) *Medical Statistics at a Glance.* Blackwell Science, Oxford.

Prevalence

The prevalence is a measure of the proportion of people with a particular characteristic in a given area in a given period of time.

The prevalence (Prev) is usually calculated as follows:

$$\text{Prev} = \frac{\text{Number of cases present in the population in the time period}}{\text{Number of individuals exposed to the risk in that time period}} \times 1000$$

For example:

- the prevalence of women in your region with relapsing remitting multiple sclerosis

- the prevalence of people in the city over 60 years of age with Alzheimer's dementia

- the prevalence of teenagers in your town who use cocaine

- the prevalence of chlamydia in students at your local college

- the prevalence of residents with incontinence in an elderly respite home.

A recently published example includes an investigation of the prevalence of neurological disorders in a prospective community-based study in the UK. *See* **Incidence**.

○ MacDonald BK, Coekerell OC, Sander JW and Shorvon SD (2000) The incidence and lifetime prevalence of neurological disorders in a prospective community-based study in the UK. *Brain.* **123**: 665–76.

Prevention trial

This is a clinical trial that studies the preventative issues relating to disease, disability or death.

Recently published examples involving prevention include the following:

- a randomised trial of in-home disability prevention in community-dwelling older people at low and high risk for nursing home admission

- a randomised trial comparing sibrafiban with aspirin for prevention of cardio-vascular events after acute coronary syndromes.

See **Clinical trial; Outcomes pyramid; Surrogate outcomes**.

○ Bouchet C, Guillemin F, Paul-Dauphin A and Briancon S (2000) Selection of quality-of-life measures for a prevention trial. A psychometric analysis. *Control Clin Trials.* **21**: 30–43.

○ Stuck AE, Minder CE, Peter-Wuest I *et al.* (2000) A randomized trial of in-home prevention for disability prevention in community-dwelling older people at low and high risk for nursing home admission. *Arch Intern Med.* **160**: 977–86.

○ The Symphony Investigators (2000) Comparison of sibrafiban with aspirin for prevention of cardio-vascular events after acute coronary syndromes: a randomised trial. *Lancet.* **355**: 337–45.

Primary outcome

Every clinical trial will have at least one outcome of interest. The primary outcome is the outcome of prime importance in the particular clinical trial. *See* **Analytic perspective; Meta-analysis; Outcome; Outcomes pyramid; Primary question; Surrogate endpoint; Systematic review**.

Primary question

The primary question is the basic question to be addressed in the clinical trial.
   The primary question in a clinical trial should:

- be important

- be carefully selected

- be clearly stated

- have a reasonable chance of being answered.

If the primary question of any trial is difficult to detect, do not take part in the trial, and be cautious about accepting its results. *See* **Clinical trial; Primary outcome; Questions to ask before getting involved in a clinical trial; Research governance in the NHS.**

○ Ewart R (1999) The UKPDS – what was the question? *Lancet.* **353**: 1882.

Principal investigator

The principal investigator in a clinical trial is the person who is identified as being the lead in the trial.
   The principal investigator will normally:

- be the lead applicant in an application for trial research funds

- have significant experience of clinical trials

- have significant knowledge of the subject under trial

- have expert project management skills

- have excellent people management skills.

See **Clinical trial steering committee; Data-monitoring committee; Multicentre research ethics committee; Participant; Research governance in the NHS; Sponsor.**

PROBE

PROBE is an acronym for pragmatic, randomised open blinded entry. It is a term that has increasingly been used in the literature. In effect it seeks to capture the wide family of trials that are pragmatic, randomised and open, but with a blinded or masked system of allocating patients (blind entry). *See* **Blind; Efficiency trial; Masking; Open-label trial; Pragmatic trial; Randomisation.**

Problems with regard to putting evidence into practice

Table 41 lists 10 real-life problems that have occurred, and continue to occur, with regard to attempts to put the evidence from research into clinical practice.

Table 41 Problems associated with putting evidence into practice

1 Limited time for decision making.
2 Lack of political power in locality.
3 Lack of resources and skills for policy analysis and evaluation.
4 Lack of consensus.
5 Evidence found is not fully relevant to the case in hand.
6 Evidence is only part of the basis of any decision.
7 Inability to release resources from current spend.
8 Information overload.
9 Concern about ethical implications of change.
10 Concern about legal implications.

As a small but important learning exercise, get some colleagues together for an hour on the first Tuesday, say, of next month. Your collective task is to consider the evidence on treatments for rheumatoid arthritis in women over 60 years of age. You should bring two sets of evidence to the meeting:

- the evidence from the published literature

- the evidence on how such patients are currently treated in your practice.

Then use Table 41 to consider the following:

- the actual or potential problems involved in putting that evidence into practice

- whether the trial designers considered any such problems when they designed or wrote up the trial

- how important each problem is to getting that evidence into your practice

- the best way to overcome identified problems.

Any one of the problems in Table 41 could reduce the use of the product in clinical practice. Taken together, the list of problems may weigh heavily against putting any evidence from any trial into practice. Of course this is so, and some trials even with robust and clinically important results have failed to make headway in terms of affecting practice – because of the problems involved in putting evidence into practice.

The real significance of the problems identified in Table 41 is that once you have identified the specific problems with regard to putting evidence into practice, you are in a much better position to design appropriate solutions.

Remember that not all of the problems in the table are of equal importance, and the list is not necessarily comprehensive. Your ongoing task will be to find out what the important problems are and to deal with them. *See* **Advantages of using evidence from clinical trials; Disadvantages of using evidence from clinical trials; Evidence-based medicine; National Institute for Clinical Excellence**.

○ Earl-Slater A (1999) Advantages and disadvantages of evidence from clinical trials. *Evidence-based Healthcare.* **3**: 53–4.

○ Earl-Slater A (2001) Barriers to applying clinical trial evidence in practice. *Br J Clin Gov.* **6**: 279–82.

○ Freeman AC and Sweeney K (2001) Why general practitioners do not implement evidence: qualitative study. *BMJ.* **323**: 1100–2 (and see the letters in the *BMJ* (2002) **324**: 674 by de Lusignan, Wells and Singleton).

○ Lilford RJ, Pauker SG, Braunholtz DA and Chard J (1998) Getting research findings into practice: decision analysis and implementation of research findings. *BMJ.* **317**: 405–9.

○ Rosser WM (1999) Application of evidence from randomised controlled trials to general practice. *Lancet.* **353**: 661–4.

Product life cycle

The product life cycle is the notion that all heathcare goods and services follow a cycle in life, from product conception, through birth, growth and maturity to demise.

The length of the product life cycle depends on the following:

- demand for the product

- scientific knowledge and understanding

- the product's therapeutic and technical gains over substitute products

- the time it takes for alternatives to come on to the market

- the relative quality and practicality of the alternatives

- finance

- tastes

- clinical, management and personal fashion.

Products in clinical trials are generally at an early stage of their life, and they will then follow a life cycle. Once a product has been used on the market it may be entered into new clinical trials to establish new indications or uses. Figure 40 provides an illustration of this.

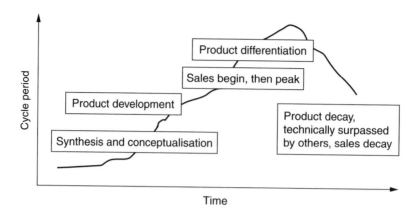

Figure 40 Product cycle.

Prognosis

Prognosis is a forecast of the future status of the health of a patient. *See* **Surrogate endpoints**.

Prospective study

A prospective study is one in which the subjects are followed up over a future period of time. All clinical trials are prospective studies. *See* **Clinical trial; Longitudinal study; Retrospective study; Subject.**

Protocol

A protocol is a detailed plan outlining the content and conduct of a particular clinical trial.

It generally includes the following:

- the primary and secondary objectives of the trial
- the rationale
- the design of the study
- entry and exclusion criteria
- statistical issues (e.g. what tests will be conducted)
- where the trial will take place
- details of the trial investigators
- data collection and monitoring
- how long the trial will last for any one patient

- rules concerning interim analysis

- stopping rules

- protocol violation management issues.

Protocols in clinical trials require ethics committee approval. It has been argued that a trial is more feasible and will be more generalisable if participating practices (trial centres and caregiver staff) are involved in protocol development. All protocols should have escape routes so that in some cases they need not be followed to the letter. *See* **Algorithm**; **Care path**; **Clinical pathway**; **Data-monitoring committee**; **Entry criteria**; **Exclusion criteria**; **Institutional review board**; **Interim analysis**; **Primary objective**; **Protocol: audit of research applications**; **Protocol amendment**; **Research governance in the NHS**; **Stopping rules**.

○ Medical Research Council (MRC) (1998) *MRC Guidelines for Good Clinical Practice in Clinical Trials.* Medical Research Council, London.

○ Wise P and Drury M (1996) Pharmaceutical trials in general practice: the first 100 protocols. An audit by the clinical research ethics committee of the Royal College of General Practitioners. *BMJ.* **313**: 1245–8.

Protocol amendment

Any change to the protocol of the clinical trial is called a protocol amendment. A protocol amendment may need prior approval from the ethics committee. In general, protocol amendments should be agreed with the clinical trial steering committee and the ethics approval board, and be notified to the trial sponsor.

All clinical trial protocol amendments should be set out in writing, stating the following:

- the reasons for the amendment

- the amendment

- who decided on the amendment and how they reached their decision

- who is responsible for making the amendment

- how the amendment will be managed in the trial

- the statistical, clinical, practical and patient implications of the amendment.

See **Protocol**; **Protocol: audit of research applications**.

Protocol: audit of research applications

We do not very often get to see the results of audits of research ethics committees' decisions, and there are few studies showing the fate of research applications.

Peter Wise and Michael Drury, then vice chairman and chairman, respectively, of the Clinical Research Ethics Committee of the Royal College of General Practitioners, reported on an audit of 100 general practice-based, multicentre research projects submitted to the ethics committee of the UK's Royal College of General Practitioners by pharmaceutical companies or their agents. The applications were made between 1984 and 1989. The authors analysed protocols for their stated objectives, study design and outcomes. They reviewed the Royal College's committee minutes and correspondence in relation to amendment and approval of studies. They also made an assessment of the final reports submitted at the conclusion of the studies.

In total, 46 studies were double-blind controlled trials, and nine were single blind, 22 studies were placebo controlled, 38 studies had an open design or were post-marketing surveillance studies, and curiously seven studies did not appear to require clinical endpoints for interpretation.

A total of 82 applications were eventually approved, and 45 protocols required amendment and resubmission, with an average of 1.5 amendment items per protocol. The reasons for amendment are listed in Table 42.

Table 42 Reasons for requesting amendment of submitted protocols

Reasons for requesting amendment of submitted protocols: 66 amendment items in 45 protocols	Number of studies
Safety aspect or inappropriate drug dose	18
Remuneration considerations	14
Logistics or cost of pathology	9
Inadequate information sheet	8
Statistical clarification or modification	4
Imprecise diagnostic criteria	4
Age limit considerations	3
Pregnancy safety aspects	2
No run-in phase	1
Other	3

The authors found that a common feature of their audit was the shortfall of investigators and trial subjects. They also suggest that greater regard for patient welfare is required in terms of information provision and suspension of existing therapy.

With a follow-up of at least six years, Wise and Drury found that of the 82 studies that had been approved, 71 studies had been completed.

Table 43 provides an insight into the fate of the studies that had started.

See **Accountability; Audit; Causes of delay and failure to complete a clinical trial; Due process; Fate of research studies; Open-label trial; Post-marketing surveillance; Reasons given by the investigator for a study being abandoned or in abeyance; Reasons given by the investigator for a study never being started; Research governance in the NHS; Transparency.**

○ Altman DG (1994) The scandal of poor medical research. *BMJ.* **308**: 283–4.

○ Thomas P (2000) The research needs of primary care: trials must be relevant to patients. *BMJ.* **321**: 2–3.

Table 43 Fate of studies that had started

Detail	Number of studies
How many studies were actually started?	74
After 6 years, how many had been completed?	71
Of those that were completed, for how many could we find out what happened to them?	68
What happened to these completed studies?	
How many were used in licensing applications?	31
How many were published in books or journals?	19
How many were presented at scientific meetings?	11
How many were neither promulgated in any way nor used for licensing or registration purposes?	21*
Were open and post-marketing studies less likely to be published or presented?	Yes. These studies represented 30% of completed projects, but only 15% of the publications or presentations

*The numbers do not add up to 68, as some studies were disseminated in more than one way.

○ Tognini G, Alli C, Avanzini F et al. (1991) Randomised clinical trials in general practice: lessons from a failure. *BMJ*. **303**: 969–71.

○ Ward E, King M, Lloyd M et al. (1999) Conducting randomised trials in general practice: methodological and practical issues. *Br J Gen Pract*. **49**: 919–22.

○ Wilson S, Delaney BC, Roalfe A et al. (2000) Randomised controlled trials in primary care: case study. *BMJ*. **321**: 24–7.

○ Wise P and Drury M (1996) Pharmaceutical trials in general practice: the first 100 protocols. An audit by the clinical research ethics committee of the Royal College of General Practitioners. *BMJ*. **313**: 1245–8.

Pseudorandom allocation

This is the term used to describe methods of allocating patients to regimens in the trial that are not considered to be true methods of randomisation.

For example, patients may be allocated according to:

• the order in which they present themselves

• their medical record numbers

• their date of birth

• calendar dates (e.g. day of the month, month of the year)

• their age.

This is also sometimes called quasi-randomisation. *See* **Bias**; **Quasi-randomisation**; **Random allocation**; **Sampling strategies**.

Purposive sampling

Purposive sampling is a non-random method of sampling a group of study subjects by handpicking cases of particular interest. It has been used in pilot studies to help to develop questionnaires, and to generate hypotheses for further study. It may be used for practical reasons. Figure 41 provides an illustration of purposive sampling. *See* **Capture–recapture sampling; Case finding; Sampling strategies; Two-stage sampling.**

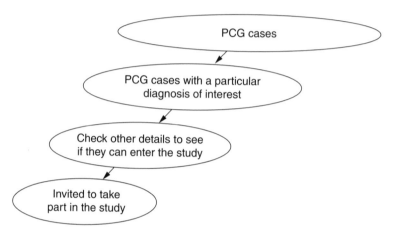

Figure 41 Purposive sampling.

P-value

The *P*-value is the probability that a result occurred by chance. Suppose that the clinical trial data analysts find a *P*-value of 5%. This means there is a 5% probability that the results could have occurred by chance. Alternatively, we can say that there is a 95% probability that the results have not occurred by chance. *See* **Confidence interval; Equivalence trial; Hypothesis; Non-inferiority trial; Power; Sample size; Statistically significant; Superiority trial.**

Quadruple-blind trial

A quadruple-blind trial is one in which all four parties are blind to what the patient received.

These four parties are:

- the patient

- the clinician-caregiver

- the outcome assessors

- the statisticians.

For example:

- Baldwin and colleagues reported on a randomised placebo-controlled trial with a 12-week follow-up of paroxetine in social phobia/social anxiety disorder. They called this a double-blind trial, but it has been reported in *Evidence-Based Medicine* (2000; **5**: 86; www.evidence-basedmedicine.com) as having all four parties (patients, clinicians, outcome assessors and statisticians) blind

- Salazar-Lindo and colleagues reported on a randomised placebo-controlled trial of racecadotril in the treatment of acute watery diarrhoea in children. The patients, the clinicians, the outcome assessors and the statisticians were blinded.

As with any trial, important points to check in terms of blinding are exactly who is blind, why and how. *See* **Blind**; **Double-blind trial**; **Single-blind trial**; **Triple-blind trial**; **Unblinded trial**.

○ Baldwin D, Bobes J, Stein DJ *et al.* on behalf of the Paroxetine Study Group (1999) Paroxetine in social phobia/social anxiety disorder. Randomised double-blind placebo-controlled study. *Br J Psychiatry.* **175**: 120–6.

○ Salazar-Lindo E, Santisteban-Ponce J, Chea-Woo E and Gutierrez M (2000) Racecadotril in the treatment of acute watery diarrhea in children. *NEJM.* **343**: 463–7.

Qualitative analysis

Qualitative analysis seeks to find out a person's opinions, beliefs, feelings, knowledge and articulation about a given topic. It seeks to make sense of or interpret phenomena in terms of the meanings that people attach to them.

For example:

- Benson and Britten reported on a qualitative study of cancer patients' views about disclosure of information to their family, their family's influence on the information given to them, and their preferences with regard to doctors' behaviour if they and their family disagreed

- Britten and colleagues reported on a qualitative study of misunderstanding between patients and doctors associated with prescribing decisions in general practice

- Salmon and colleagues reported on a qualitative study of verbatim records of interviews in which patients recounted doctors' explanations for their symptoms of somatisation disorder

- Silvestri and colleagues reported on a descriptive study based on scripted interviews of patients with advanced non-small-cell lung cancer, with regard to their preferences for chemotherapy

- Tod and colleagues reported on a qualitative study of barriers to uptake of services for coronary heart disease.

Good qualitative analysis:

- starts with a well-specified question

- uses appropriate methods which are systematic, explicit and reproducible

- uses appropriate settings and subjects, with explicit reasons for the choice

- has conclusions that follow from the analysis.

You can turn the criteria for good qualitative analysis into questions. For example, 'Was the question well specified? Does the setting seem appropriate to you? Do the conclusions follow from the analysis?'

Examples of qualitative research include the following:

- documentary analysis

- passive observation (watching and recording behaviour)

- more active observation of participants

- in-depth interviews

- focus groups, delphi techniques.

Qualitative analysis:

- may help to define preliminary questions or routes of enquiry that can be addressed by quantitative studies
- is sometimes added to the quantitative and scientific aspects of a clinical trial
- sometimes leads to new trials being set up.

See **Action research; Compliance; Pitfalls in interviewing; Qualitative research checklist (*BMJ*'s version); Quantitative analysis; Research questions and research methods; Types of questions.**

○ Barbour RS (2001) Checklists for improving rigour in qualitative research: a case of the tail wagging the dog? *BMJ.* **322**: 1115–17.

○ Benson J and Britten N (1996) Respecting the autonomy of cancer patients when talking with their families: qualitative analysis of semi-structured interviews with patients. *BMJ.* **313**: 729–31.

○ Britten N, Jones J, Murphy E and Stacy R (1995) Qualitative research methods in general practice and primary care. *Fam Pract.* **12**: 104–14.

○ Britten N, Stevenson FA, Barry CA *et al.* (2000) Misunderstandings in prescribing decisions in general practice: qualitative study. *BMJ.* **320**: 484–8.

○ Devers KJ (1999) How will we know 'good' qualitative research when we see it? *Health Serv Res.* **34**: 1153–88.

○ Giacomini MK (2001) The rocky road: qualitative research as evidence. *Evidence-Based Med.* **6**: 4–6.

○ Gillies A (2002) *Using Research in Primary Care: a workbook for health professionals.* Radcliffe Medical Press, Oxford.

○ Greenhalgh T and Taylor R (1997) Papers that go beyond numbers (qualitative research). *BMJ.* **350**: 740–3.

○ Howitt A and Armstrong D (1999) Implementing evidence-based medicine in general practice: audit and qualitative study of anti-thrombotic treatment for atrial fibrillation. *BMJ.* **318**: 1324–7.

○ Murphy E, Dingwall R, Greatbatch D *et al.* (1998) Qualitative research methods in health technology assessment – a review of the literature. *Health Technol Assess.* **2**: 1–272.

○ Pope C and Mays N (1995) Reaching the parts that other methods cannot reach: an introduction to qualitative methods in health and health services research. *BMJ.* **311**: 42–5.

○ Pope C and Mays N (eds) (2000) *Qualitative Research in Health Care.* BMJ Books, London.

○ Salmon P, Peters S and Stanley I (1999) Patients' perceptions of medical explanations for somatisation disorders: qualitative analysis. *BMJ.* **318**: 372–6.

○ Silvestri G, Pritchard R and Welch G (1998) Preferences for chemotherapy in patients with advanced non-small-cell lung cancer: descriptive study based on scripted interviews. *BMJ.* **317**: 771–5.

○ Strauss A and Corbin J (1998) *Basics of Qualitative Research* (2e). Sage Publications, London.

○ Tod AM, Read C, Lacey A and Abbot J (2001) Barriers to uptake of services for coronary heart disease: qualitative study. *BMJ.* **323**: 214.

Qualitative research checklist (BMJ's version)

The *British Medical Journal (BMJ)* produces a checklist for qualitative research. Whilst other checklists do exist, the *BMJ* checklist offers a good starting point for opening up discussion and debates about what should and should not be included in such a checklist. More fundamentally, it helps to highlight the need for such a checklist. It is reproduced in Table 44.

Table 44 Qualitative research checklist (*BMJ's* version)

1 Was the research question clearly defined?
2 Overall, did the researcher make explicit in the account the theoretical framework and methods used at every stage of the research?
3 Was the context clearly described?
4 Was the sampling strategy clearly described and justified?
5 Was the sampling strategy theoretically comprehensive, to ensure the generalisability of the conceptual analysis (e.g. diverse range of individuals and settings)?
6 How was the fieldwork undertaken? Was it described in detail?
7 Could the evidence (e.g. fieldwork notes, interview transcripts, recordings, documentary analysis) be inspected independently by others? If relevant, could the process of transcription be independently inspected?
8 Were the procedures for data analysis clearly described and theoretically justified? Did they relate to the original research questions? How were themes and concepts identified from the data?
9 Was the analysis repeated by more than one researcher to ensure reliability?
10 Did the investigator make use of quantitative evidence to test qualitative conclusions where appropriate?
11 Did the investigator give evidence of seeking out observations that might have contradicted or modified the analysis?
12 Was enough of the original evidence presented systematically in the written account to satisfy the sceptical reader of the relationship between the interpretation and the evidence (e.g. were quotations numbered and sources given)?

See **Qualitative analysis.**

○ Barbour RS (2001) Checklists for improving rigour in qualitative research: a case of the tail wagging the dog? *BMJ.* **322**: 1115–17.

Quality of life

Quality of life is the state of well-being of a person. There is no universally accepted definition of quality of life, what factors determine it or how to measure it accurately. Elements of quality of life that need to be measured include clinical, psychological, physical, mental, spiritual and social aspects. There are many instruments which are used to gauge these elements of quality of life (see, for example, the individual books by Bowling and Staquet and colleagues).

Quality of life has importance in terms of choice of the primary and secondary questions for the trial, the primary and secondary measures used, and the interpretation of the results, among other things.

Some of the factors that determine quality of life include employment, the environment, family welfare, healthcare, education, sanitation, housing, income, perceptions, prospects, public health, recreation, feelings of safety and security, spiritual beliefs and practices, food consumption, and transport. It is therefore obvious that healthcare may only have a limited role in changing or maintaining a person's quality of life.

One definition of quality of life is as follows:

> an individual's perception of their position in life in the context of the culture and value systems in which they live and in relation to their goals, expectations, standards and concerns. It is a broad-ranging concept affected in a complex way by the person's physical health, psychological state, level of independence, social relationships, and their relationships to salient features of their environment.

Another definition of quality of life is in relation to the degree to which a person achieves their life goals. More controversially, Shaw argued that quality of life related to one's endowment and the effort made on one's behalf by family and society.

Many attempts continue to be made to establish the impact of healthcare on quality of life. These measurement instruments are a reduced form of measuring quality of life. Reduced-form measurement is useful if the excluded factors either play an unimportant role or are insignificant with regard to the person's quality of life. The reduced form measures can, at best, be seen as important parts of the wider picture.

If the measure of quality of life has more than one component, then are all of the components of the same weight or of equal value? The answer to this depends on the person to whom the factors are important. For example, climbing stairs may not be as important to someone as being able to wash, dress or feed him- or herself.

For instance, Belardinelli and colleagues looked at the effects of long-term moderate exercise training on functional capacity, clinical outcome and quality of life in patients with chronic heart failure. See **Analytic perspective; Generalisability of trial results; Health; Outcome; Outcomes pyramid; Primary question; Surrogate outcome**.

○ Belardinelli R, Georgiou D, Cianci G and Purcaro A (1999) Randomized controlled trial of long-term moderate exercise training in chronic heart failure. Effects on functional capacity, quality of life and clinical outcome. *Circulation*. **99**: 1173–82.

○ Bouchet C, Guillemin F, Paul-Dauphin A and Briancon S (2000) Selection of quality-of-life measures for a prevention trial. A psychometric analysis. *Control Clin Trials*. **21**: 30–43.

○ Bowling A (1995) *Measuring Disease*. Open University Press, Buckingham.

○ Bowling A (1995) *Measuring Health*. Open University Press, Buckingham.

○ Bowling A (1997) *Research Methods in Health: investigating health and health services*. Open University Press, Buckingham.

○ Staquet MJ, Hays RD and Fayers PM (eds) (1998) *Quality of Life Assessment in Clinical Trials. Methods and practice*. Oxford University Press, Oxford.

Quantitative analysis

Studies involving the assessment of data as quantities are called quantitative studies. Some authors consider them to be more robust and scientific than qualitative studies. Most clinical trials are heavily in favour of quantitative studies, but many concerns about putting the trial evidence into practice turn on practical qualitative issues. See **Data types**; **Outcomes pyramid**; **Qualitative analysis**; **Statistical test diagram**; **Statistical tests: ten ways to cheat with statistical tests**.

Quasi-randomisation

Quasi-randomisation is the term used to describe methods of allocating patients that are not truly random.

For example, when allocating patients to regimens in the trial you may have used the following:

- the patient's date of birth

- the day of the week

- the last digit of the patient's medical record number

- the order in which participants arrive at the clinic.

Another term for this is pseudorandomisation. See **Pseudorandomisation**; **Quasi-randomised trial**.

Quasi-randomised trial

This is a clinical trial that uses methods of quasi-randomisation when allocating patients to different regimens. See **Pseudorandomisation**; **Quasi-randomisation**; **Random**.

Questions to ask before getting involved in a clinical trial

Before you get involved in a particular clinical trial, there are various questions that you must ask. Table 45 gives an indication of some of them.

Many of the questions in Table 45 can be used by a variety of people. For example, the questions can be used by the following:

- healthcare professionals to quiz the principal investigator

- healthcare professionals to quiz the trial sponsor

- one healthcare professional to another

- healthcare manager to doctors who are thinking of taking part in the trial in their organisation

Table 45 Questions to ask before getting involved in a clinical trial

1 What is the primary research question?
2 Why is the research being done?
3 What do the researchers want to achieve?
4 What is already known about the intervention(s)?
5 What is already known about the disease?
6 What are the entry and exclusion criteria?
7 What evidence exists to support the entry and exclusion criteria?
8 What type of trial is it?
9 What evidence supports that type of trial?
10 What is the system of recruitment?
11 What is the system of allocation to arms in the trial?
12 What will be done during the trial and for how long?
13 What risks are involved in the trial?
14 What benefits can be expected from the trial?
15 What other treatments are available?
16 If I refuse to enter, will I still get access to the product?
17 How do the possible risks and benefits of the trial compare with current practice?
18 What data will be collected?
19 How will the data be collected?
20 Who will analyse the data?
21 What will be done with the data after the trial has finished?
22 What is the plan for disseminating the study results?
23 Will I see a summary of the results before they are published?
24 Where will the results of the trial be published?
25 Where is the trial site?
26 How often do I have to attend?
27 What do I have to do when I am there?
28 Will I receive any payment?
29 What are my responsibilities during the trial?
30 What happens if things get worse during the trial?
31 Can I talk to anyone about the trial?
32 Can anyone else find out that I am in the trial?
33 What will happen to me after the trial has finished?
34 What will happen if I want to leave the trial early?
35 What will happen if not enough patients are recruited?
36 What will happen if recruitment is slower than expected?
37 What will happen to me if the trial is stopped early?
38 Who is sponsoring the study?
39 Why are they sponsoring the study?
40 Who has reviewed the study?
41 Who has approved the study?
42 Does the trial meet ethical, regulatory and legal requirements?
43 Who is the principal investigator?
44 What skills and experience do the trialists and recruiters actually have?
45 Can I have a copy of the clinical trial protocol?

- healthcare manager to trial sponsor
- ethics review committee to principal investigator
- patients can ask the doctor these questions
- patients can ask the principal investigator these questions.

Although the table is already long and interesting, it is not comprehensive. There will be other questions that you may think of asking.

From experience, you may have been tempted to skip through the above table. If you have, then you have not really done yourself any favours either personally or professionally.

As a short exercise, get a few colleagues together next week for an hour. Make sure that one of them has been involved in a clinical trial. Obtain all of the information on that trial. At your meeting seek to answer every question in Table 45.

Whether you are a patient, a healthy volunteer, the manager of a primary care group, trust or clinic, a member of a review panel, or a healthcare professional, you should not enter into clinical trials lightly, as they are serious scientific experiments. Equally, you should never be afraid to ask questions about a clinical trial. This will show that you are taking the idea of the trial seriously.

It is important to make your own questions count.

The most important thing is that you ask questions and feel comfortable about the answers. It is usually a very good idea to get the answers in writing from the appropriate authority (e.g. the principal investigator).

If you are unhappy or unclear about any of the answers, ask again, and if you are still not sure, discuss this with your colleagues and friends. If you are in any serious doubt, stay out of that particular trial. *See* **Accountability; Advantages of evidence from clinical trials; Declaration of Helsinki; Disadvantages of evidence from clinical trials; Due process; Evidence-based medicine; Institutional review board; International Conference on Harmonisation; Patient information and consent forms; Pitfalls in interviewing; Problems with regard to putting evidence into practice; Randomised controlled trial; Research governance in the NHS; Transparency.**

QUOROM

This is an acronym for quality of reporting of meta-analyses of randomised controlled trials. It is a recently developed system that aims to standardise the reporting of meta-analyses.

The group that developed it consisted of 30 experts, including clinical epidemiologists, statisticians, clinicians, editors and researchers interested in meta-analysis. In conference the group were asked to identify items which they thought should be included in a checklist of standards of reporting meta-analyses. Some of the items were guided by research evidence. After assessing the items and reaching an agreement, the conference produced a checklist (*see* Table 46), and a flow diagram (*see* Figure 42).

Table 46 The QUOROM checklist

Heading	Subheading	Descriptor	Reported (Yes/No)	Page number
Title		Identify the report as a meta-analysis (or systematic review) of randomised controlled trials		
Abstract		*Describe*		
	Objectives	The clinical question explicitly		
	Data sources	The databases (i.e. list) and other information sources		
	Review methods	The selection criteria (i.e. population, intervention, outcome and study design), methods for validity assessment, data abstraction and study characteristics, and quantitative data synthesis, in sufficient detail to permit replication		
	Results	Characteristics of the randomised controlled trials included and excluded; qualitative and quantitative findings (i.e. point estimates and confidence intervals); subgroup analyses		
	Conclusion	The main results		
Introduction		*Describe* The explicit clinical problem, biological rationale for the intervention, and rationale for review		
Methods	Searching	The information sources in detail (e.g. databases, registers, personal files, expert informants, agencies, hand-searching), and any restrictions (years considered, publication status, language of publication)		
	Selection	The inclusion and exclusion criteria (defining population, intervention, principal outcomes and study design)		
	Validity assessment	The criteria and process used (e.g. masked conditions, quality assessment, and their findings)		
	Data abstraction	The process or processes used (e.g. completed independently, in duplicate)		
	Study characteristics	The type of study design, participants' characteristics, details of intervention, outcome definitions and how heterogeneity was assessed		

continued overleaf

Table 46 continued

Heading	Subheading	Descriptor	Reported (Yes/No)	Page number
	Quantitative data synthesis	The principal measures of effect (e.g. relative risk), method of combining results (statistical testing and confidence intervals), handling of missing data, how statistical heterogeneity was assessed, rationale for any a-priori sensitivity and subgroup analyses, and any assessment of publication bias		
Results	Trial flow	Provide a meta-analysis profile summarising trial flow (see Figure 42)		
	Study characteristics	Present descriptive data for each trial (e.g. age, sample size, intervention, dose, duration, follow-up period)		
	Quantitative data synthesis	Report agreement on the selection and validity assessment; present simple summary results (for each treatment group in each trial, for each primary outcome); present data needed to calculate effect sizes and confidence intervals in intention-to-treat analyses; any assessment of publication bias		
Discussion		Summarise key findings; discuss clinical inferences based on internal and external validity; interpret the results in the light of totality of available evidence; describe potential biases in the review process (e.g. publication bias); suggest a future research agenda		

Probably the best way to appreciate the QUOROM checklist is to use it, so get together with a colleague, find one recently published meta-analysis, and together see how well the paper performs against the checklist (i.e. read the paper and fill in the descriptors in column 3).

The second aspect of the QUOROM system is the flow diagram (*see* Figure 42). This is simply a filtering record which shows the number of potentially relevant randomised controlled trials (RCTs) identified and screened right down to the RCTs with usable information.

The QUOROM system is one of a variety of checklists that are used to report meta-analyses. If you use QUOROM, you really should supplement the QUOROM checklist with your own specific questions, such as the following.

• Where did each trial take place?

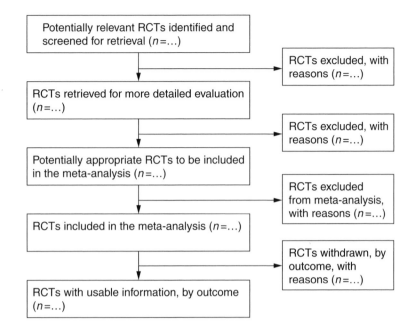

Figure 42 The QUOROM diagram.

- When did each trial take place?

- Who sponsored each trial?

- What links exist between the authors of various trials, the meta-analysts and the trial sponsors?

- Which trials had an independent data-monitoring committee?

- How do the patients in the trials compare with your patients?

- Where were the results of each trial actually published (e.g. in peer-reviewed journals)?

Although the QUOROM system was designed to help to improve the reporting of meta-analysis, it can also be used in the design stage of a new meta-analysis. Like the CONSORT system, the QUOROM system will develop and improve over time, so it is not set in stone. Finally, remember that the QUOROM system is an aid to decision making, not an escape from it. *See* **Clinical trial; CONSORT; Evidence-based medicine; Hierarchy of evidence; Meta-analysis; Primary question; Randomised controlled trial; Systematic review; Transparency.**

○ Moher D, Cook DJ, Eastwood S *et al.* (1999) Improving the quality of reports of meta-analyses of randomised controlled trials: the QUOROM statement. *Lancet.* **354**: 1896–900.

Quota sampling

Quota sampling is the term used to describe methods of sampling from a population up to a certain number (the quota). It is not a randomised procedure.

For example, the quota may be to stop recruiting once 200 patients are in each arm of the study. Quota sampling is sometimes used when randomisation is not possible, ethical or otherwise feasible. More often it is used in market research and in public surveys, being favoured for its general speed and convenience. *See* **Closed sequential trial; Sampling strategies.**

R

Random

The term random means chance.

For instance, a trial could have:

- random selection of patients

- random allocation

- random error in its results.

See **Random allocation; Random effects; Randomisation; Randomised consent design; Randomised controlled trial; Random selection**.

Random allocation

Random allocation means allocating by chance.

Random allocation in a clinical trial is the business of allocating patients to arms of the trial on the basis of chance.

Random allocation does not mean that patients are allocated in a haphazard fashion. The term random allocation means that each patient has a known chance – usually an equal chance – of being assigned to one of the arms of the trial. For example, if we have a trial with two arms, A and B, then each patient may have a 50% chance of being allocated to either A or B.

Reasons for random allocation include the following:

- to compare outcomes when patients only differ in terms of which regimen they entered

- much common statistical theory is based on the principles of random sampling

- to distance the investigator from the method of allocation.

See **Benchmarking; Bias; Equipoise; Play-the-winner rule; Pre-randomised consent; Post-randomised consent; Pseudorandom allocation; Random; Random selection; Randomised consent design; Randomised controlled trial**.

○ Altman DA and Bland JM (1999) Treatment allocation in controlled trials: why randomise? *BMJ*. **318**: 1209.

○ Chalmers I (1999) Why transition from alternation to randomisation in clinical trials was made. *BMJ*. **319**: 1372.

Random-effects models

Used in the context of meta-analysis, a random-effects model can accommodate some aspects of heterogeneity when pooling estimates from different studies.

Suppose we included the study centre as a factor in the analysis. In a random-effects model we would consider those centres in the analysis to be a random selection of all centres that might have taken part in the trials. Therefore, in random-effects models we assume that the meta-analysis results can be applied to all centres that might have taken part.

Consider two sources of variation: you can have variations within a study and you can have variations between the studies in a meta-analysis. In a random-effects model both variations influence the uncertainty of the results (and hence the confidence intervals). As a result of incorporating the extra variation, the confidence intervals of a random-effects model are wider, more conservative, than the confidence intervals from a fixed-effects model.

Tests of heterogeneity are used to help determine the choice of a random- or fixed-effects model. Recent innovations and developments in research methodology have introduced us to two other genres of models: mixed-effects models and Bayesian-effects models.

See **Bayesian analysis; Duhem's irrefutability theory; Error; External validity of clinical trials; Fixed-effects model; Generalisability of trial results; Lakatosian's hard-core, protective belt; Meta-analysis**.

○ Cooper H and Hedges LV (1994) *The Handbook of Research Synthesis*. Russel Sage Foundation, New York.

○ Egger M, Davey Smith G and Phillips AN (1997) Meta-analysis: principles and procedures. *BMJ*. **315**: 1533–7.

○ Fleiss JL (1993) The statistical basis of meta-analysis. *Stat Meth Med Res*. **2**: 121–45.

Random error

Random error is error that has occurred by chance. See **Bias; Confidence interval**.

Random number table

This is a collection of random numbers that are presented in table format. Table 47 shows an example.

The table opposite is only one of many that include random numbers. Therefore when you see a trial reporting that it used a table of random numbers, ask to see the actual table that was used.

Random number tables can be used in a systematic way to:

• identify patients from a list to enter a trial

• allocate patients to different arms of the trial

• sample cases in the trial for data quality-assurance work.

Table 47 Random numbers

29	32	95	99	57	98	08	36	97	08
12	11	80	16	17	01	03	97	59	73
87	58	22	25	55	35	72	79	28	15
02	92	42	87	57	53	53	34	55	75
69	28	63	73	98	45	61	10	43	20
11	95	68	77	86	91	76	11	63	34
06	43	41	02	13	65	23	94	48	88
68	55	98	08	39	59	85	46	66	13
41	01	06	65	10	29	29	91	86	24
46	75	71	76	88	04	42	94	41	42

For instance, if you read the table from the top left-hand corner across the row, the first five cases can be selected as 29, 32, 95, 99 and 57.

If the table is used to allocate patients into arms of the trial, then we could have the even numbers going into arm A and the odd numbers going into arm B. Therefore reading the table from the top left-hand corner down the column, arm A would have patients numbered 12, 02, 06, 68 and 46, and arm B would have patients numbered 29, 87, 69, 11 and 41.

If the data-monitoring committee wanted to select five cases in the trial as part of their quality-control assurance, then they could start anywhere in the table and move along rows and columns to obtain the five numbers.

Note that:

- any number can appear more than once in the table (as at any point in time each number has the same chance of appearing)

- you can read the table in any way (as shown in the above examples)

- pairs of numbers were used, but you could take any relevant combination.

See **Randomisation; Random permuted blocks; Random sample; Random selection.**

Random permuted blocks

These are methods of randomly allocating patients such that at any point in time an equal number of patients have been allocated to each arm of the trial. Random permuted blocks are often used when we want to keep the number of patients in each block equal, or not higher than say differing by 2.

They are sometimes called block randomisation or restricted randomisation.

The size of the block can, if we wish, also be randomised.

See **Block randomisation; Play-the-winner rule; Stratification.**

○ Altman DG and Bland JM (1999) How to randomise. *BMJ.* **319**: 703–4.

Random sample
This is a sample of patients selected by chance. *See* **Random**.

Random selection
Random selection is any method of selecting patients by means of chance. *See* **Random**; **Random allocation**; **Random sample**.

Randomisation
This is the act of selecting or allocating cases by means of chance.
 For example, we could have:

• random selection of individual patients to different arms of the clinical trial

• randomised clusters of patients.

See **Block randomisation**; **Cluster randomisation**; **Random**; **Random allocation**; **Random number table**.

Randomised controlled trial
A randomised controlled trial is a clinical trial in which:

• patients are randomly allocated to different regimens in the trial

• some patients get the regimen of prime interest (e.g. a new drug)

• other patients (the controls) get another regimen (e.g. 'usual care' or placebo).

This design allows the assessment of the relative effectiveness of the different regimens by comparing event rates and outcomes.
 Such a trial could include medicines, surgery, technology, exercise, diet, systems of organisation, grades of staff and educational efforts. There are few limits to what can be included in a randomised controlled trial.
 As an example of a recently published randomised controlled trial plan, Freemantle and colleagues evaluated the effectiveness and efficiency of visits by trained pharmacists in delivering messages to general practitioners. The pharmacists received special training and the messages were derived from four evidence-based clinical practice guidelines.
 Montgomery and colleagues ran a randomised controlled trial to evaluate a computer-based clinical decision support system and risk chart for management of hypertension in primary care. There are many other examples sprinkled throughout the references in this handbook.
 In general, randomised controlled trials are thought to offer the best methods for determining the merits of different regimens. Some argue that they are the

'gold-standard' method of providing information about the relative merits of interventions.

The quality and relevance of any such trial need close attention. *See* **Baseline; Bias; Blinding; Clinical trial; Cochrane Collaboration; Controlled trial; Entry criteria; Equipoise; Exclusion criteria; Gold standard; Hierarchies of the evidence; National Research Register; Phase 1 clinical trial; Phase 2 clinical trial; Phase 3 clinical trial; Phase 4 clinical trial; Random; Randomisation**.

○ Freemantle N, Eccles M, Wood J *et al.* (1999) A randomised trial of evidence-based outreach (EBOR). Rational and design. *Control Clin Trials*. **20**: 479–92.

○ Jadad N (1998) *Randomised Controlled Trials*. BMJ Books, London.

○ Mathews J (2000) *Introduction to Randomized Controlled Clinical Trials*. Edward Arnold, London.

○ Montgomery AA, Fahey T, Peters TJ *et al.* (2000) Evaluation of computer-based clinical decision support systems and risk chart for management of hypertension in primary care. *BMJ*. **320**: 686–90.

○ Pringle M (1995) Randomised controlled trials in general practice. *BMJ*. **311**: 1382.

○ Sacks H, Chalmers T and Smith H (1982) Randomized versus historical controls for clinical trials. *Am J Med*. **72**: 233–40.

○ Sibbald B and Roland M (1998) Why are randomised controlled trials important? *BMJ*. **316**: 201.

Raters

Raters are those who rate the clinical trial in terms of the following:

- protocol adherence
- care paths
- outcomes
- causation.

The term 'raters' is sometimes used as an alternative to 'assessors'. They combine the role of outcome adjudicators, protocol auditors and trial assessors. Try to be clear what they rate and why. *See* **Assessors; Audit; Clinical trial steering committee; Data-monitoring committee; Inter-rater reliability; Participants; Protocol; Research governance in the NHS; Sponsors**.

Reasons given by the investigator for a study being abandoned or in abeyance

Starting a study is one thing, but keeping it going is quite another. Table 48 lists the reasons for 58 studies that were approved by the Central Oxford Research Ethics Committees being abandonded or in abeyance (according to the principal investigator).

These data come from an analysis of 487 studies that were approved by the ethics committee between 1984 and 1987. Although the data are somewhat dated, there is in fact a paucity of contemporary information in the UK about the fate of research.

Table 48 Reasons given by the investigator for a study being abandoned or in abeyance

Main reason	Number of studies (and %)
1 Difficulty in recruiting participants	16 (28%)
2 Technical problems (e.g. unreliable technique, specimens spoiled in transit)	9 (16%)
3 Principal or co-investigator left institution	8 (14%)
4 Withdrawal of funding	6 (10%)
5 Logistical problems (e.g. appropriate equipment not available, associated study abandoned, difficulties with collaborators, closure of research unit)	6 (10%)
6 Adverse effects	5 (9%)
7 Lost interest	1 (2%)
8 Too busy	2 (3%)
9 Null results	5 (9%)
Total	58 (100%)

The reasons cited in Table 48 for suspending or failing to continue an approved study may still be occurring.

- Principal investigators need to attend to these possible issues in the early days of planning the project (e.g. 28% of the reasons cited related to difficulty in recruiting participants).

- Host institutions should determine the fate of research in their institution and the lessons to be learned, and put in place systems to reduce the rates of abandonment and abeyance (e.g. through education, training, monitoring, mentoring, financial support and logistical advice).

- Sponsors of clinical research should take the main reasons and key issues in Table 48 into account when deciding with whom, for what and where to place their funds. They should certainly look into the reasons and implications for withdrawing funding, and provide evidence of this to a wider audience so that lessons can be learned.

- Ethics committees can take the issues listed in Table 48 and cross-examine the research applicants on each reason to see whether they have considered it, how they plan to overcome the potential problem, and what will happen if the study is stopped or put in abeyance.

The main reasons listed in Table 48 are also issues that you as a healthcare professional, approver, sponsor, host institution or patient should consider before getting involved in a study. They are certainly issues that need to be talked through with prospective patients who may enter the study in good faith. *See* **Causes of delay and failure to complete a clinical trial; Fate of research studies; Reasons given by the investigator for a study never being started; Research governance in the NHS.**

○ Altman DG (1994) The scandal of poor medical research. *BMJ.* **308**: 283–4.

○ Easterbrook PJ and Mathews DR (1992) Fate of research studies. *J R Soc Med.* **85**: 71–6.

Reasons given by the investigator for a study never being started

Obtaining ethics committee approval to start a study is one thing, but getting started is quite another. Table 49 lists the reasons cited for 100 studies that were approved by the Central Oxford Research Ethics Committees not being started.

Table 49 Reasons given by the investigator for a study never being started

Main reason	Number of studies (%)
Failure to obtain funding	40 (40%)
Principal or co-investigator left institution	16 (16%)
Logistical problems (e.g. ward closure, limited drug supply, ward staff unwilling to co-operate with protocol, flawed design, publication of identical study)	11 (11%)
Anticipated difficulty in recruiting patients	10 (10%)
Adverse drug effects reported, or drug withdrawn	8 (8%)
Loss of interest	7 (7%)
Too busy	6 (6%)
Technical problems (e.g. flawed assay technique, inadequate laboratory equipment)	2 (2%)
Total	100 (100%)

These data come from an analysis of 487 studies that were approved by the ethics committee between 1984 and 1987. Although the data are somewhat dated, there is in fact a paucity of information in the UK about the fate of research.

The reasons cited in Table 49 for failing to start an approved study may still be occurring.

• Principal investigators need to attend to these possible issues in the early stages of planning the project.

• Host institutions should determine the fate of research in their institution, the lessons to be learned, and put in place systems to reduce the failure rates (e.g. education, training, monitoring, mentoring and financial support).

• Sponsors of clinical research should do all that they can to ameliorate the possible reasons for failing to start (e.g. 60% of the studies that failed to start, failed to start for reasons other than lack of funding).

• Ethics committees should do all that they can to monitor and learn from the fate of research studies which they have approved, and they should learn from other committee experiences.

See **Causes of delay and failure to complete a clinical trial; Fate of research studies; Reasons given by the investigator for a study being abandoned or in abeyance; Research governance in the NHS.**

○ Altman DG (1994) The scandal of poor medical research. *BMJ.* **308**: 283–4.

○ Easterbrook PJ and Mathews DR (1992) Fate of research studies. *J R Soc Med.* **85**: 71–6.

Relative benefit increase

The relative benefit increase (RBI) is a measure of the proportional difference in event rates.

The general formula is as follows:

$$RBI = \frac{\text{experimental event rate} - \text{control event rate}}{\text{control event rate}}$$

Suppose that evidence from a recently published clinical trial shows that a new regimen for dealing with acute myocardial infarction improves the likelihood of certain patients being alive after 30 days, compared with patients on the usual care regimen. Out of 100 patients in the new regimen, 93 individuals are alive at 30 days. Out of 100 patients who received usual care, only 86 individuals are alive at 30 days.

Thus, using the above data we have:

$$RBI = \frac{93/100 - 86/100}{86/100} = \frac{7}{86} = 8.1\%$$

In patients with calcific tendinitis of the shoulder, is pulsed ultrasound therapy clinically effective? This is the question that Ebenbichler and colleagues reported on in their randomised double-blind placebo-controlled trial with a 9-month follow-up. Resolution rates at 9 months after therapy were 42% for ultrasound and 8% for the placebo group. Therefore, calculating the relative benefit increase, we have:

$$RBI = \frac{0.42 - 0.08}{0.08} = 425\%$$

An RBI of 425% looks and sounds very impressive indeed. The RBI measure is to be used when the outcomes in the experimental regimen are better than the outcomes in the control regimen.

However, if we look more closely at the Ebenbichler paper, we find that there was no reported significant difference between the two groups in terms of pain or quality of life at 9 months. Therefore in interpreting the RBI results you may need to think about the rest of the results. In fact, this is true of any trial – it is important to look to see what outcomes they reported and measured, and to examine all of the results. *See* **Absolute benefit increase; Outcomes pyramid; Primary question; Relative risk reduction.**

○ Ebenbichler GR, Erdogmus CB, Resch KL *et al.* (1999) Ultrasound therapy for calcific tendinitis of the shoulder. *NEJM.* **340**: 1533–88.

Relative risk

The relative risk is the ratio of the risk of an event in one regimen compared with the risk of the event in another regimen.

Table 50 provides some data to work with. It relates to high-risk MI patients who were randomised to attend a new chest care clinic or receive their usual cardio-risk care. The risk in question is the risk of a fatal myocardial infarction.

Table 50 Relative risk

	Outcome			
	Fatal heart attack	*No fatal heart attack*	*Total*	*Risk of events*
New chest care clinic	a (100)	b (200)	a + b = 300	X = a/(a + b) = 100/300
Usual cardio-risk care	c (120)	d (180)	c + d = 300	Y = c/(c + d) = 120/300
Total	a + c = 220	b + d = 380	a + b + c + d = 600	

Using the data in Table 50, the relative risk (RR) is calculated as the risk of two events:

$$RR = \frac{a/(a + b)}{c/(c + d)} = \frac{X}{Y}$$

In this case we have:

$$RR = \frac{100/300}{120/300} = 0.83$$

As another example, in a publication of the ISIS-4 trial (Fourth International Study of Infarct Survival collaborative group), of the 29 028 patients who were treated with captopril, 2088 individuals died in the first 35 days. This gives a death rate of 71.9 per 1000 (2088/29 028). Of the 29 022 individuals in the placebo group, 2231 patients died in the first 35 days. This gives a death rate for the placebo group of 76.9 per 1000 (2231/29 022). Thus the relative risk of death in the first 35 days in the captopril group compared with the placebo group is 0.94. The calculation is as follows:

$$RR = \frac{71.9}{76.9} = 0.94$$

In general, how should we interpret the RR results?

- If RR = 1, the risk of the event is the same in both groups.

- If RR < 1, the risk of the event is lower in, say, the new chest clinic or captopril group compared with the usual care or placebo group, respectively.

- If RR > 1, the risk of the event is higher in, say, the new chest clinic or captopril group compared with the usual care or placebo group, respectively.

See **Absolute risk; Absolute risk reduction; Likelihood ratio; Odds; Odds ratio; Relative risk increase; Relative risk reduction; Ways of presenting results.**

Relative risk increase

The relative risk increase (RRI) is a measure of the relative increase in risk of an event in one regimen compared with another. It is used when the risk of the event is found to be greater in the experimental regimen than in the other regimen.

Suppose that a recent study of a new minimally invasive technique shows that 5% of selected patients die, but with standard surgery only 3% die within 1 year.

Using the above data we have:

$$RRI = \frac{5\% - 3\%}{3\%} = 66\%$$

So with these data the new minimally invasive technique has a relative risk increase of 66% compared with the standard surgery. Put this way, it sounds alarming. But is it? Recent examples include the following.

- Small and colleagues reported on a randomised controlled trial with a 6-month follow-up to see whether, in women who give birth by Caesarean section, forceps or vacuum extraction, a debriefing session led by a midwife is more effective than standard care in reducing maternal depression at 6 months postpartum. Their primary outcome measures were maternal depression (a score of 13 or more on the Edinburgh Postnatal Depression Scale, EPDS) and overall maternal health status (from the SF-36 questionnaire). A secondary outcome was satisfaction with care. At 6 months, 14% of those in 'standard care' scored 13 or more on the EPDS scale, whereas 17% of those in the midwife-led debriefing arm of the trial scored 13 or more on the EPDS. Therefore:

$$RRI = \frac{17\% - 14\%}{14\%} = 21\%$$

Look more closely at the paper by Small and colleagues before making any decision about the merits of the midwife-led programme. RRIs alone can only tell us 'something', not everything we need to know.

- Pahor and colleagues reported on a meta-analysis of randomised controlled trials in patients with hypertension. The question to be addressed was whether, in patients with hypertension, calcium antagonists as first-line treatment are superior, equal or inferior to other antihypertensive drugs for reducing major cardiovascular events. For an outcome of myocardial infarction, the weighted event rates were 4.5% for those in the calcium antagonists group and 3.6% for those on other anti-hypertensive agents.

$$RRI = \frac{4.5\% - 3.6\%}{3.6\%} = 25\%$$

However, for an outcome of all-cause mortality, the weighted event rates were 8.3% for those in the calcium antagonists group and 8.1% for those on other antihypertensive agents, giving an RRI of 2.5%. And for an outcome of stroke, the weighted event rates were 4.5% for those in the calcium antagonists group and 5.01% for those on other antihypertensive agents, giving an RRR of 10%.

This is an interesting report because of the way in which data were combined, the baseline risk profile of the patients who were included, and the fact that more research is required because some products in one particular class may be more beneficial to some patients in certain circumstances than other products in the same or other classes of antihypertensives.

In general, therefore, the formula for the relative risk increase (RRI) is as follows:

$$RRI = \frac{\text{experimental event rate} - \text{control event rate}}{\text{control event rate}}$$

See **Absolute risk increase; Relative benefit increase; Relative risk; Relative risk reduction; Statistical significance; Ways of presenting results.**

○ Pahor M, Psaty BM and Alderman MH (2000) Health outcomes associated with calcium antagonists compared with other first-line anti-hypertensive therapies: a meta-analysis of randomised controlled trials. *Lancet.* **356**: 1949–54.

○ Small R, Lumley J, Donohue L *et al.* (2000) Randomised controlled trial of midwife-led debriefing to reduce maternal depression after operative childbirth. *BMJ.* **321**: 1043–7.

Relative risk reduction

By definition, the relative risk reduction (RRR) is a measure of the percentage reduction in risk in the experimental regimen compared with the other regimen. Let us call the other regimen the control. The RRR is written as follows:

$$RRR = \frac{\text{control event rate} - \text{experimental event rate}}{\text{control event rate}}$$

Suppose that a recent audit of your nearest special-care baby unit shows that 9.6% of babies die under standard care. A newly published clinical trial shows that under a different care regimen, only 2.4% of the babies would die. You can then calculate the relative reduction in risk as follows:

$$RRR = \frac{9.6 - 2.4}{9.6} \times 100\% = 75\%$$

This means that the new special-care baby-unit regimen would reduce the risk of death by 75% compared with the usual care regimen.

Fleming and colleagues reported on a randomised controlled trial designed to establish whether brief physician advice reduced alcohol consumption in older adults with potentially excessive drinking habits. At a 12-month follow-up, 31% of the individuals in the brief intervention group experienced episodes of binge drinking, whereas 49% of those in the control group had episodes of binge drinking. Therefore:

$$RRR = \frac{49 - 31}{49} = 37\%$$

The relative risk reduction in the brief intervention group compared with the control group for binge drinking is 37%.

At the 12-month follow-up, 15% of individuals in the brief intervention group experienced episodes of excessive drinking, compared with 34% of those in the control group. Therefore:

$$RRR = \frac{34 - 15}{34} = 56\%$$

The relative risk reduction in the brief intervention group compared with the control group for excessive drinking at the 12-month follow-up is 56%.

The Fleming paper also presents results for excessive and binge drinking in the previous 7 days and the previous 30 days.

Look at the results from a new chest clinic compared with usual cardio-care (see Table 51). The primary outcome of interest is whether or not the patient had a fatal heart attack.

Table 51 Relative risk reduction

	Outcome			
	Fatal myocardial infarction	No fatal myocardial infarction	Total	Risk of events
New chest clinic	a (100)	b (200)	a + b = 300	Y = a/(a + b) = 100/300
Usual cardio-risk care	c (120)	d (180)	c + d = 300	X = c/(c + d) = 120/300
Total	a + c = 220	b + d = 380	a + b + c + d = 600	

Mathematically, the RRR can be written as follows:

$$RRR = 1 - \frac{Y}{X} = \frac{X - Y}{X}$$

Using the data from Table 51 we have:

$$RRR = \frac{120/300 - 100/300}{120/300} = 0.167$$

This means that the new chest clinic lowers the risk of having a fatal heart attack by 16.7% compared with usual cardio-care.

The RRR is a marketing executive's favoured way of presenting results from clinical trials. *See* **Absolute risk; Absolute risk reduction; Incidence; Likelihood ratio; Number needed to treat; Odds; Odds ratio; Relative benefit increase; Relative risk; Relative risk increase; Ways of presenting results.**

○ Fleming MF, Manwell LB and Barry KL (1999) Brief physician advice for alcohol problems in older adults. A randomized community-based trial. *J Fam Pract.* **48**: 378–84.

Research ethics committee: possible progress report form

Giving ethical approval for a research project to begin is one thing, but once given it is certainly not the end of the ethics committee's involvement in the research information process. For what it has approved, each research ethics committee can, and in some countries are required to, ask for an annual progress report from the principal investigator. It is generally considered good business practice for ethics committees to make it known that such reports will be required.

The information in the annual progress report could help form part of the research ethics committee's monitoring and feedback system. It could also provide visible evidence, hopefully available to the general public, of the state of progress of the work the research ethics committee has approved. In some cases, the progress reports have also been successfully used to improve local research governance plans, and in other cases they have been used to help put into place systems to develop research skills and capacities in NHS organisations.

The following provides an example of a possible progress report. Some forms have more questions than the example given here, and some have less. Developments in research governance may begin to standardise these forms. The actual form itself will have more physical space available for the principal investigator to fill in. For reasons of legibility, or the lack of it, it is preferable for the principal investigator to type their answers. One way of aiding that process is to allow the form to be completed electronically, so that an electronic and, for legal reasons, a paper copy can be sent back to the research ethics committee administrator.

Introductory notes in the cover letter

The [name] research ethics committee would like to know how the [named] study has progressed in the last year and whether any difficulties have been experienced. Please complete the questionnaire below and return it to the research ethics committee administrator within 28 days [name/postal address/ email address supplied]. Thank you for your co-operation.

Table 52 Possible research progress report

1 Name and address of principal researcher.		
2 Short title of study.		
3 Research ethics committee reference number.		
4 Date of research ethics committee approval.		
5 Has the study started?	Yes	No
If No, please give reasons.		
6 Number of local research sites recruited.	Proposed	Actual
7 Number of subjects/patients recruited into study.	Proposed	Actual
8 Number of subjects/patients completing study.	Proposed	Actual
9 Number of withdrawals because of:		
(i) lack of efficacy		
(ii) adverse events		
(iii) self-withdrawal		
(iv) non-compliance.		
10 Have there been any serious difficulties in recruiting subjects to the study? Yes		No
If Yes, please give details.		
11 Have there been any untoward events?	Yes	No
(before you answer this, please refer to our definition in the enclosed booklet *Information for Researchers*)		
If Yes, have these been notified to the Committee?	Yes	No
12 If untoward events have not been notified to the Committee, please state why, as notification is a condition of research ethics committee approval.		
13 Have there been any amendments to the study?	Yes	No
If Yes, have these been notified to the Committee?	Yes	No
If amendments have not been notified to the Committee, please state why, as you know that notification is a condition of the Committee's approval.		
14 Has the study finished?	Yes	No
If Yes, please answer questions 15 and 16 below.		
If No, what is the expected completion date?		
15 If the study will not now be completed, please give reason(s).		

continued opposite

Table 52 continued

16	Results – please include details of outcomes and conclusions (attach a separate page if necessary).		

How the findings have been disseminated

	Yes	No
• Used for licensing/regulatory purposes	Yes	No
• Presentations	Yes	No
• Publications: – planned	Yes	No
– in press	Yes	No
– published	Yes	No

Please give details below and send copies of publications and presentations as soon as they are available.

17 Signature of principal investigator.

18 Print principal investigator's name.

19 Signature(s) of the Chief Executive(s) of the organisation(s) where the research takes place.

20 Date of submission of progress report to the Ethics Committee.

See **Audit; Audit cycle; Caldicott Guardians; Causes of delay and failure to complete a clinical trial; Declaration of Helsinki; European Union Directive in clinical trials of medicinal products for humans; Institutional review board; Local research ethics committee; Multicentre research ethics committee; Patient information sheet and consent forms; Reasons given by the investigator for a study being abandoned or in abeyance; Reasons given by the investigator for a study never being started; Research governance in the NHS; Research governance implementation plan; Transparency.**

Research governance: baseline assessment

In March 2001, Lord Hunt outlined the research governance framework for health and social care. In April 2001, Professor Sir John Pattison from the Office of the Director of Research and Development in the Department of Health, outlined a baseline or initial assessment for research-active NHS organisations. Sir John asked the recipients of his letter to take action by 31 May 2001, in making a baseline assessment of compliance with standards set out in the research governance framework for health and social care. Sir John's letter was addressed to Chief Executives of NHS hospitals, primary care trusts, health authorities and special health authorities.

The baseline assessment of compliance with research governance standards is part of the drive to improve quality in the NHS generally, and to provide information upon which a research governance implementation plan would be built.

The baseline assessment cannot be seen solely as a 'policy ploy', as something to do, deal with, be dispatched and dismissed. More accurately, and more generally, baseline assessments can be seen as the first step towards an ongoing and evolving process in improving research and research governance.

The baseline assessment should therefore be seen as something that would:

- provide a candid picture of the state of research governance systems in the NHS
- offer insight into organisations' strengths and weaknesses in research governance
- identify any particular problem areas or areas of success
- assess the extent to which data on research are in place for quality surveillance
- detect links, or the lack of them, with other clinical practice and clinical research activities and obligations
- aid the design and development of underpinning strategies, e.g. information technology, legal compliance, continuing professional development
- enhance knowledge and understanding of integration of quality control.

Sir John's letter, the baseline assessment questionnaire and other related material is available on the Department of Health's website. The responses to the baseline questionnaire were used to help design the research governance implementation plan announced by Sir John in October 2001.

See **Accountability; Audit; Audit cycle; Benchmarking; Research governance implementation plan; Research governance in the NHS; Transparency.**

Research governance implementation plan

In October 2001, Professor Sir John Pattison from the Office of the Director of Research and Development in the Department of Health, sent a letter to various people outlining the DoH's research governance implementation plan. The letter asked the recipients to take action in preparing a local implementation plan to hit the targets. Sir John's letter was addressed to Chief Executives of NHS hospitals, primary care trusts, health authorities and special health authorities.

Earlier, in March 2001, Lord Hunt had sent a letter about the research governance framework for health and social care. In April 2001, Sir John had sent a letter outlining the necessary action needed to make a baseline assessment for research governance compliance. The baseline assessment for research-active organisations in the NHS has since been carried out and analysed. Drawing on the baseline assessment, the research governance implementation plan outlined by Sir John in October 2001 has now been produced.

The health implementation plan sets out targets and milestones for NHS organisations. Table 53 identifies the timescales and milestones. The implementation plan is intended to sustain and develop a research culture in healthcare that promotes excellence, with visible research leadership and expert management to help researchers, clinicians and managers apply standards correctly. As Sir John correctly states:

We must ensure the systems and agreements that we and our partners rely on are ones that command confidence amongst us and with the public.

Table 53 Research governance implementation plan

By December 2001	All research-active NHS care organisations have access to adequate systems for notification of R&D and for checking ethical approval and informed consent.
In 2002	DoH draws the requirements of research governance to the attention of all research-active independent practitioners after consulting the relevant professional bodies and Royal Colleges.
During 2002	DoH works with primary care trusts to develop protocols for the role of host for shared research governance and management services.
By March 2002	DoH arranges for a baseline assessment of the way it complies with the responsibilities of research sponsor and establishes an internal implementation plan.
From April 2002	A funding body makes clear, for each grant it awards for R&D in the NHS, whether it will itself act as research sponsor or whether it expects another organisation to agree to do so.
July 2002	Each research-active NHS care organisation has a local research governance implementation plan.
December 2002	Implementation plan for research governance in social care is published.
March 2003	Research-active NHS care organisations comply with all the requirements in paragraph 3.10.
March 2003	All researchers not employed by the NHS hold a NHS honorary contract that includes research governance procedures and responsibilities if they are to interact with individuals in a way that has a direct bearing on the quality of healthcare.
April 2003	Research-active NHS care organisations report progress.
April 2003	No research with human participants, their organs, tissue or data may begin or continue in the NHS until a research sponsor has confirmed that it accepts responsibility.
By April 2003	There is a national network of primary care trusts ready to act as host for shared research governance and management capacity.
April 2003	The national network of PCTs begins to stand as research sponsor for R&D in health and social care, where it is inappropriate for another organisation to do so.
By March 2004	All primary care practices that lead non-commercial R&D are accredited.
March 2004	All research-active NHS care organisations comply with the research governance framework, unless there are well-documented reasons for a longer timetable.
April 2004	Research-active NHS care organisations report progress.
By May 2004	Member States bring the EU Directive on Good Practice in Clinical Trials into force in domestic law.

An important issue is the first deadline, December 2001. Sir John stated in his October letter that:

> If your NHS organisation does not have access by the end of December 2001 to systems for notification of R&D and for checking ethical approval and informed consent, you should decide whether to suspend R&D in your organisation until you do have access to the systems required.

As seen from Table 53, the implementation plan is ambitious, and will induce changes to the current systems, structures and processes of research governance locally and regionally. The implementation plan also includes particular points where progress reports have to be made. Hopefully, these progress reports will be made available to the wider public in an efficient and timely manner.

The last entry in Table 53 suggests that by May 2004 Member States (of the European Union) bring the EU Directive on Good Clinical Trials into force in domestic law. This is something generally beyond the control of local and regional researchers or research governors. But it is certainly not beyond their interest. Why? Because:

- the Directive is only at the planning stage, in draft form and is not yet fixed in stone

- the Directive only applies to trials involving medicines in humans

- the Directive may change as it moves through the legal and policy making machinery of the European Union

- the Directive has to be ratified by the European Parliament

- the Directive will, in practice, be implemented in different ways in different EU countries – an issue for international multicentre clinical trials

- the Directive will impact on the design, development and delivery of research governance systems, structures and processes.

In general then, the research governance implementation plan is considered to be SMART:

- **S**pecific

- **M**easurable

- **A**ttainable, but challenging

- **R**elevant

- **T**ime oriented.

The plan will enhance accountability, due process and transparency in research and in research governance in the NHS. Hopefully, the quality of research output in terms of publications, conference proceedings, and impact on practice resulting from NHS research will be lifted even higher.

Social care has its own research governance implementation plan.

See **Accountability; Caldicott Guardians; Due process; European Union Directive on clinical trials of medicinal products for humans; Fate of clinical research; Multicentre trial; Institutional review board; Patient preference; Patient preferences in clinical trials; Patient information sheet and consent forms; Research governance: baseline assessment; Research governance in the NHS; Transparency; Volunteer.**

○ Information on the letters and research governance plan is available from the Department of Health's website, http://www.doh.gsi.gov.uk, and Sir John's email contact is john.pattison@doh.gsi.gov.uk.

Research governance in the NHS

Research governance is the system of control of research in an area. For example, it could be the NHS in general, local hospitals, local primary care trusts, community clinics, or private, voluntary or charitable sectors.

By the term 'govern', I mean 'to control with authority'. That authority may, for example, be embedded in law, professional codes of practice, ethical codes of conduct or voluntary codes of conduct. Research governance in general deals with research standards, research systems, rules, expectations, monitoring, auditing, research reporting, ethics and discipline.

Research governance is also affected by issues surrounding data protection acts and good clinical practice (GCP) requirements.

In 2000 the UK Department of Health produced a short document about the management of clinical trials conducted in the NHS.

Essentially the guidance states that NHS trusts, health authorities, general practitioners, primary care groups and primary care trusts should:

- have systems in place to review all ongoing and proposed R&D studies that they fund, intend to fund, or which involve patients in their care

- take action to ensure that good clinical practice standards for clinical trials involving NHS patients are implemented for all relevant research in which they are involved.

The Department of Health guidance also states that:

- all research studies involving patients should have ethics committee approval and clear lines of accountability for ensuring that approved protocols and procedures are adhered to

- those organisations that are involved in the study understand, accept and are equipped to discharge the responsibilities that fall on them

- any NHS organisation or employee with doubts about their ability to meet standards of good practice in the management of trials should seek help from their

Regional Director of Research and Development to ensure that they can continue (or begin) to support this important aspect of the work of the NHS.

See **Accountability; Clinical trial; Data-monitoring committee; Declaration of Helsinki; Due process; Good clinical practice; Host institution; Independent trials steering committee; Local research ethics committee; Medical Research Council Guidelines for Good Practice in Clinical Trials; Multicentre research ethics committee; National Research Register; Principal investigator; Sponsor; Transparency.**

○ Department of Health (2000) *Research Governance in the NHS: guidance on good clinical practice and clinical trials in the NHS.* Department of Health, London.

○ Strobl J, Cave E and Walley T (2000) Data protection legislation: interpretation and barriers to research. *BMJ.* **321**: 890–2.

Research question

Every clinical trial should have one particular research question that it seeks to answer. If the question is not clear, there is a good chance that the rest of the research idea is similarly vague or opaque.

For every clinical trial in which you get involved or on which you base decisions, always ask the following questions.

• What is the primary research question?

• Is it important to you?

• Has it been tackled before?

• Are the methods appropriate?

• Does the study answer the question?

• Do the answers seem plausible?

See **Clinical significance; Primary question; Questions to ask before getting involved in a clinical trial; Research questions and research methods; Statistical significance; Type of question.**

Research questions and research methods

The question that you want to answer will determine the type of methodology that you use to answer it. Table 54 gives an indication of different questions and the types of research methods that may be used.

These are indicative questions that will give you a feel for or flavour of the line of enquiry. In reality, each question would have to be refined and made more specific for you to come up with specific answers to specific questions.

Table 54 Research questions and research methods

General type of research question	Possible research method
Why did this patient develop these complications?	Case study
How many female patients in this hospital developed bedsores during their stay in October 2001?	Case series
What is the nutritional intake of post-surgical patients on recovery wards 9–11 today?	Cross-sectional study
What questions do patients actually ask their doctor before deciding whether or not to enter this clinical trial?	Observational analysis
What are the effects on patients of exposure to a particular risk?	Cohort study
Why do some patients develop a rare type of liver failure whereas others do not?	Case–control study
What is the predicted future demand for this new drug in its first year on the market?	Operations research
What are the merits of care regimen A versus regimen B?	Clinical trial
What is currently known from the published clinical literature about 30-day mortality rates for this type of keyhole surgery on certain types of patients in specific settings?	Systematic review
For specified patients with insomnia, what do the combined clinical trials data show in terms of specific measures of product efficacy?	Meta-analysis

We can design a specific template to help to formulate research questions. The template has four categories as follows:

- patient or problem
- intervention
- comparison treatment
- outcomes.

So, for instance, in patients with heart failure from dilated cardiomyopathy who are in sinus rhythm, would adding anticoagulation with warfarin to standard heart failure therapy, when compared with heart therapy alone, lead to lower mortality or morbidity from thromboembolism? Is this enough to be worth the extra risk of bleeding?

To make matters more complex but more realistic, remember that the same method could be used to answer different questions, and the same question could be answered via different methods. The key is to be able to firm up your question and then justify the method that is or will be used. *See* **Comparing research methods; Hypothesis; Outcomes pyramid; Primary question; Surrogate outcomes; Types of question**.

○ Strobl J, Cave E and Walley T (2000) Data protection legislation: interpretation and barriers to research. *BMJ*. **321**: 890–2.

Retrospective studies

Retrospective studies look back in time – that is, they study events that have already taken place.

For example:

- how quickly a patient was administered thrombolytic treatment after presenting with signs of chest pain in the hospital in the last 12 weeks

- how many patients received thrombolytic therapy en route to the hospital (e.g. in ambulatory care) during the last 12 weeks

- in a 5-year retrospective cohort study of 138 acute-care hospitals, Glasgow and colleagues sought to determine whether higher hospital volume was associated with lower operative mortality and shorter length of stay after hepatic resection

- Reid and colleagues reported on a retrospective cohort study of medically unexplained symptoms in frequent attenders of secondary healthcare.

This information is useful in its own right, and may also feed into the design of a new clinical trial. *See* **Audit; Comparing research methods; Data dredging; Data fishing; Prospective studies; Research questions and research methods**.

○ Glasgow RE, Showstack J, Katz PP *et al.* (1999) The relationship between hospital volume and outcomes of hepatic resection for hepatocellular carcinoma. *Arch Surg*. **134**: 30–5.

○ Reid S, Wessely S, Crayford T and Hotopf M (2001) Medically unexplained symptoms in frequent attenders of secondary health care: retrospective cohort study. *BMJ*. **322**: 767.

Risk–benefit ratio

The risk–benefit ratio is a calculation of the risks of events compared with the benefits. In general, the lower the risk–benefit ratio the better. *See* **Medicines Control Agency; Outcomes pyramid; Risk; Trade-off**.

○ Elwyn G (2000) Explaining risks to patients. *Br J Gen Pract*. **50**: 342–3.

Risk difference

The risk difference is another term for absolute risk reduction. *See* **Absolute risk reduction**.

Risk factor

A risk factor is a factor that affects the probability of an event occurring.

For example:

- Gorelick and colleagues reviewed various risk factors for first stroke (hypertension, coronary artery disease, including blood lipid levels, atrial fibrillation, diabetes mellitus and asymptomatic carotid artery stenosis) and lifestyle factors (e.g. cigarette smoking, alcohol consumption, physical activity and diet)
- in a recently published cohort study by Dixon and colleagues of the Edinburgh Breast Group, an increased risk of breast cancer was seen in women with palpable breast cysts. They found that the risk was greatest during the first year after cyst aspiration and in younger women, but that it did not differ according to cyst type.

See **Association; Causal relationship; Clinical trial; Cohort study; Risk–benefit ratio.**

○ Dixon JM, MacDonald C, Elton RA *et al.* (1999) Risk of breast cancer in women with palpable breast cysts. *Lancet.* **353**: 1742–5.

○ Elwyn G (2000) Explaining risks to patients. *Br J Gen Pract.* **50**: 342–3.

○ Gorelick PB, Sacco RL, Smith DB *et al.* (1999) Prevention of first stroke. A review of guidelines and a multidisciplinary consensus statement from the National Stroke Association. *JAMA.* **281**: 1112–20.

Robust

A test is said to be robust if its *P*-value and power are not appreciably or significantly affected by violations of the assumptions of the test. *See* **Duhem's irrefutability theory; Falsificationism; Hypothesis; Power; *P*-value; Sensitivity analysis.**

Run-in period

The run-in period is the period of time between recruitment into a study and the point just before the intervention starts.

For example, when studying the efficacy of atrovastatin compared with simvastatin in patients with hypercholesterolaemia, Farnier and colleagues used a 6-week run-in period.

A key question concerns when the run-in period actually starts. Is it when the patient agrees to enter the trial, when they start to come off their current treatment, or when they are off their current treatment? Different trials have used different starting points for the run-in period.

The run-in period is sometimes called the lead time. *See* **Baseline; Eligibility; Washout period.**

○ Farnier M, Portal JJ and Maigret P (2000) Efficacy of atrovastatin compared with simvastatin in patients with hypercholesterolemia. *J Cardiovasc Pharmacol Ther.* **5**: 27–32.

Sample size

Sample size is the number of patients in or required for a clinical trial.

When you take part in a clinical trial or look at the evidence stemming from such a trial, you must always be aware that the patients in the trial are not all patients who could receive the treatment. Of course, this may seem rather obvious but, surprisingly, a number of people continue to ignore this fact.

In general, clinical trials involving relatively large sample sizes of patients may be expensive and time-consuming to run, but could be more representative. A small sample size may be too weak to yield significant results even if they exist.

In addition to the importance of sample size, you need to ask questions about the source and nature of the sample. *See* **Baseline; Clinical significance; Disadvantages of evidence from clinical trials; Funnel plot; Generalisability of trial results; Heterogeneity; Mega-trial; Power; Problems with regard to putting clinical trial evidence into practice; Sample size calculation; Sample size determinants; Sampling error; Sampling strategies; Statistical significance.**

○ Moher D, Dulberg CS and Wells GA (1994) Statistical power, sample size and their reporting in randomized controlled trials. *JAMA*. **272**: 122–4.

Sample size calculation

This involves methods of determining how many patients have to be recruited in order to meet the trial objectives. *See* **Closed sequential trial; Primary question; Sample size; Sample size determinants; Sampling error.**

○ Fayers PM, Cushieri A, Fielding J *et al.* (2000) Sample size calculations for clinical trials: the impact of clinician beliefs. *Br J Cancer*. **82**: 213–9.

Sample size determinants

Table 55 shows that there are various factors that predetermine the size of a sample. These factors need to be considered in both the design and analytical stages of any clinical trial.

See **Power; sample; sample size.**

Table 55 Factors that determine the size of a sample

Factor	Comment
Confounding	The more you have to control for confounding factors in the study, the greater the sample size that is required
Error	The more errors there are (e.g. in classification, measurement), the greater the sample size that is required
Frequency of outcome	More frequent outcome requires smaller sample size. It appears that for some methods of analysis, minimum sample size occurs when the frequency of outcome is 50%
Power	Sample size increases as power increases
Strength of association	
Significance level	Sample size decreases as significance level increases
Type of research study	Cross-over trials, in which patients are programmed to switch treatment regimens at specific times, may need smaller samples than other trials (e.g. parallel trials)
Also think about	
The amount of funding necessary for the trial	Greater funding of a trial means that it can use a larger sample size
The number and availability of suitable investigators	What criteria are used to select these investigators?
The number and availability of suitable patients	More patients, or a larger target audience, may mean that a larger sample is required
The ability to recruit investigators and patients	Think about the practicalities and ethics of trial recruitment, retention and compliance

Sampling error

Sampling error is the probability that any particular sample is not fully representative of the population from which it is drawn. *See* **Bias; Confidence interval; Error; Generalisability of trial results; Sample size; Sample size calculation**.

Sampling strategies

Sampling strategies are methods of selecting a sample. Table 56 indicates a variety of sampling strategies, each of which has its own strengths and weaknesses. Each method can affect the type of statistical tests that can subsequently be performed on the data.

See **Power; Questions to ask before getting involved in a clinical trial; Sample size; Sampling error; Scales of measurement; Statistical test diagram; Statistical tests: ten ways to cheat with statistical tests**.

Sampling with replacement

Sampling with replacement involves methods of selecting a sample by choosing a case, replacing it, and then choosing the next case. The main problem is that cases

Table 56 Sampling strategies

1 *Sampling with replacement*
2 *Sampling without replacement*
3 *Probability sampling.* This includes sampling where chance has a role to play in selection.
  For example:
  • simple random sampling (selecting patients at random)
  • cluster sampling (surveying whole clusters of the population)
  • stratified sampling (sampling within groups of the population)
  • systematic sampling (sampling every *n*th case).
4 *Non-probability sampling.* This includes sampling where chance does not have a role to play.
  For example:
  • convenience sampling (sampling those that are most convenient)
  • purposive sampling (hand-picking typical or interesting cases)
  • snowball sampling (building a sample through informants)
  • voluntary sampling (where the sample is self-selected).
5 *Event sampling.* This involves choosing patients according to the particular event. The sample may
  have had the event (e.g. in trials that look at prevention of another myocardial infarction) or the
  sample may be at risk of having the event (e.g. patients at high risk of having a stroke).
6 *Time sampling.* This involves choosing cases according to an aspect of time. For example, the day
  when they last attended hospital, the month when they were first diagnosed with the disease of
  interest, or their date of birth. One study showed that more patients with myocardial infarction
  arrived in hospital on Fridays and Mondays than on any other day of the week. Therefore a trial
  could focus on those patients arriving at hospital on certain days of the week.

may be selected more than once. *See* **Sample size; Sampling strategies; Sampling without replacement; Statistical test diagram.**

Sampling without replacement
Sampling without replacement involves methods of selecting a sample by choosing a case, not replacing it, and then choosing the next case. The main problem is that the pool diminishes each time you extract a sample. *See* **Sample size; Sampling strategies; Sampling with replacement; Statistical test diagram.**

Scales of measurement
Scales of measurement are different types of scales that are used in clinical trials.
  These scales may be used to identify and gauge:

• which patients can enter a trial

• which patients cannot enter a trial

• patient characteristics at the start of the trial

• patient characteristics during the trial

- patient characteristics at the end of the trial

- patient characteristics some time after the trial has stopped (e.g. in follow-up analysis).

Table 57 lists the main types of scale, including their definition and some examples.

Table 57 Scales of measurement

Scale	Meaning and example
Interval	Named because the interval, the difference between two numbers in one region $(32 - 27 = 5)$, is the same as the distance in another region $(74 - 69 = 5)$. For example, temperature
Nominal	Numerical values are assigned to categories. There is no inherent order, nor is there any indication of the importance of the different classes. For example, male = 1, female = 2 or died = 0, survived = 1
Ordinal	Numerical values are assigned to a scale of responses, which is classified such that it implies a distinct order. For example, in a questionnaire you may see possible answers classified as 1 = very satisfactory, 2 = satisfactory, 3 = neither satisfactory nor unsatisfactory, 4 = unsatisfactory and 5 = very unsatisfactory
Ratio	Data that have a true zero point. For example, weight, height or income, as in each case it is meaningful to speak of one value being so many times greater than another value

The type of scale and therefore the type of data in the trial help to determine the types of statistical tests one can perform on the results obtained from the clinical trial. *See* **Baseline; Endpoint; Hierarchy of evidence; Interim analysis; Outcome; Qualitative analysis; Quantitative analysis; Statistical test diagram**.

Sensitivity

The sensitivity is one of two standard measures that are used to evaluate the accuracy of a test (the other one being the specificity).

Sensitivity is a measure of how many patients have the disease and test positive. More generally, it is a measure of how effective the test is in detecting those individuals who are truly diseased or who have some condition of interest.

For example, Qanadli and colleagues reported on the diagnostic accuracy of dual-section helical computed tomography versus selective pulmonary arteriography in patients with suspected acute pulmonary embolism.

Suppose that, as requested, the patient gives you a 10-mL sample of urine. You send this sample to the high-volume laboratory for testing, and 4 days later the test results are encrypted and emailed to your surgery. No test is 100% accurate, but you want to know how well the test can detect disease in individuals who have that disease.

Table 58 Sensitivity

| Test result | True condition of the person tested | | Total |
	Has the adverse medical condition	Does not have the adverse medical condition	
Positive	a (100)	b (200)	a + b (300)
Negative	c (300)	d (400)	c + d (700)
Total	a + c (400)	b + d (600)	a + b + c + d (1000)

In Table 58 the sensitivity (Sen) is calculated as follows:

$$\text{Sen} = \frac{a}{a + c}$$

Using the values in Table 58 above as an example, the sensitivity is:

$$\text{Sen} = \frac{100}{100 + 300} = 0.25$$

Thus the test will identify only 25% of the patients with the disease.

In terms of searching and retrieving literature, the term 'sensitivity' has been used to refer to the likelihood of retrieving relevant material. Naturally one would wish to include as much relevant material as possible in any search (e.g. in a systematic review).

Sensitivity is sometimes called the true-positive rate. *See* **Specificity; Systematic review**.

○ Qanadli SD, Hajjam EL, Mesurolle B *et al.* (2000) Pulmonary embolism detection: prospective evaluation of dual-section helical computed tomography versus selective pulmonary arteriography in 157 patients. *Radiology.* **217**: 447–55.

Sensitivity analysis

This involves methods of calculating how responsive results are to changes in the underlying variables or assumptions.

For example, sensitivity analysis can be performed on the following:

• how a patient fares if they are given different doses of a drug

• how many patients would be eligible to enter a trial if the entry and exclusion criteria were changed in some way

• how the conclusions change if one more piece of evidence is added.

See **Assumptions; Cumulative meta-analysis; Dose–response trial; Take-up rate; Threshold-point analysis; Titration.**

Sequential trial

A sequential trial is a clinical trial that continues until:

- a clear benefit is found of one intervention over another *or*

- it becomes clear that no significant difference between the interventions will emerge.

In a sequential trial, the data are analysed as soon as they become available from each patient.

As the results are continuously monitored and the trial is stopped according to a predefined stopping rule, sequential trials require:

- outcomes to be well defined

- outcomes to appear relatively quickly

- clear, explicit and predefined trial stopping rules.

See **Adaptive–adoptive trial; Clinical trial steering committee; Closed sequential design; Cross-over trial; Data-monitoring committee; Early stopping rule; Factorial trial; Interim analysis; Open sequential trial; Protocol; Random-effects trial; Stopping rules; Zelen consent design.**

Side-effect

A side-effect is a result of an intervention that is not the primary effect of interest. It may or may not be beneficial. *See* **Adverse event; Adverse reaction; Primary outcome; Unanticipated beneficial effects; Unanticipated harmful effects.**

Significance

Significance means importance. *See* **Analytic perspective; Clinical significance; Significance level; Statistical power; Statistical significance.**

Significance level

The significance level is the probability of a type 1 error – that is, the probability of rejecting the null hypothesis when it is in fact true. A level of 5% is usually chosen, but there is no firm theoretical reason for choosing that value. However, there are some good practical reasons for choosing 5%, including the fact that it is generally understandable and most journals accept it as a reasonable marker. Better still, one can report the significance level found in the study (e.g. 4.6%, 5.3%) and cite the exact numbers.

Mathematically, the significance (Sig) level is:

$$\text{Sig} = P(\text{type I error}) = \alpha \text{ (alpha)}$$

See **Clinical significance; Duhem's irrefutability theory; Falsificationism; Power; Power of a test;** *P*-value; **Significance; Statistical significance; Type 1 error.**

○ Sterne JAC and Smith GD (2001) Sifting the evidence – what's wrong with significance tests? *BMJ*. **322**: 226–31.

Simple random sample

A simple random sample is a method of selecting study subjects by the use of random numbers. There is no other sophistication involved in selecting the sample. *See* **Blind; Random; Random number table; Sampling strategies.**

Single-blind trial

A single-blind trial is generally a clinical trial in which the person receiving the intervention (e.g. a medicine) is not told and does not know what the intervention is. Some trials have used the doctor as the single-blind entity. Therefore it is useful to find out who is actually blind in the single-blind trial. Some trials cannot involve blinding. (Can you think why?) *See* **Bias; Blind; Compliance; Data-monitoring committee; Double-blind trial; Institutional review board; Protocol; Quadruple-blind trial; Triple-blind trial.**

Single-site trial

This is a clinical trial that takes place in one setting. For example, using a children's hospital in Leicester as the single site, Wesseldine and colleagues addressed the question of whether or not a structured discharge package given by a nurse reduced the rates of hospital readmission and reattendance. *See* **Local research ethics committee; Medical Research Council Guidelines for Good Practice in Clinical Trials; Multi-centre trial; Research governance in the NHS.**

○ Wesseldine LJ, McCarthy P and Silverman M (1999) Structured discharge procedure for children admitted to hospital with acute asthma: a randomised controlled trial of nursing practice. *Arch Dis Child.* **80**: 110–14.

Specificity

The specificity is one of two standard measures that are used to evaluate the accuracy of a test (the other being the sensitivity).

Specificity is a measure of how many patients are correctly identified as not having the disease.

For instance, Qanadli and colleagues reported on the diagnostic accuracy of dual-section helical computed tomography versus selective pulmonary arteriography in patients with suspected acute pulmonary embolism.

Suppose that you take a blood sample and send it to the laboratory for testing. No test is 100% accurate. Two days later the laboratory emails you the following data (*see* Table 59).

Table 59 Specificity

| Test result | True condition of the person tested | | Total |
	Has the condition	Does not have the condition	
Positive	a (100)	b (200)	a + b (300)
Negative	c (300)	d (400)	c + d (700)
Total	a + c (400)	b + d (600)	a + b + c + d (1000)

The specificity (Sp) can be calculated as follows:

$$Sp = \frac{d}{b + d}$$

Thus, from Table 54 we have:

$$Sp = \frac{400}{200 + 400} = 0.67$$

This suggests that 67% of the patients are correctly identified as being without the disease.

With regard to searching and retrieving literature, the term specificity has been used to denote the likelihood of excluding irrelevant material. Naturally one would wish to exclude as much irrelevant material as possible in any search (e.g. in a systematic review).

Specificity is sometimes called the true-negative rate. *See* **Sensitivity; Systematic review**.

○ Qanadli SD, Hajjam EL, Mesurolle B *et al.* (2000) Pulmonary embolism detection: prospective evaluation of dual-section helical computed tomography versus selective pulmonary arteriography in 157 patients. *Radiology.* **217**: 447–55.

Split-half method of analysis

The split-half method of analysis is a method of assessing the consistency of results and relationships in a clinical trial.

It works as follows:

- Divide the full set of results into two equal parts, A and B.
- Analyse the data in subset A.
- Analyse the data in subset B.
- Compare the results.

Figure 43 illustrates this method.

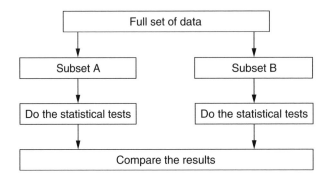

Figure 43 Split-half method.

See **Baseline; Cross-validation; Statistical test diagram**.

Sponsor
This is a person or organisation responsible for the financing of a clinical trial.

For example, if the Medical Research Council sponsors a trial, it is responsible for the finance of that trial, and the principal investigator is responsible for the management of the trial. *See* **Clinical trial steering committee; Data-monitoring committee; Principal investigator; Questions to ask before getting involved in a clinical trial**.

Statistical power
A clinical trial is said to have sufficient statistical power if it is large enough to detect a statistically significant difference if one exists. By 'large enough', we usually mean in terms of the number of patients who are involved in the trial.

We can look at this in another way. Suppose you have a theory that there is no clinical advantage of one particular product over another for a certain group of patients. Let us call this the null hypothesis.

The statistical power is the probability that the null hypothesis will be rejected if it is false.

The statistical power is determined by factors such as the following:

- the number of participants involved
- the outcome
- the number of events (e.g. myocardial infarctions)
- the confidence interval that we wish to use (e.g. 95%).

See **Clinical significance; Null hypothesis; Power; Statistical significance.**

○ Moher D, Dulberg CS and Wells GA (1994) Statistical power, sample size and their reporting in randomized controlled trials. *JAMA.* **272**: 122–4.

Statistical significance

If a result is said to be statistically significant at, say, the 5% level, this means that you are 95% confident that the result did not occur by chance.

You could use any level of significance (e.g. 1%, 3%, 10%), but the custom now is to use the 5% level.

A result that is statistically significant is not necessarily clinically significant. *See* **Clinical significance; Confidence interval;** *P***-value; Significance; Statistical test diagram.**

Statistical test diagram

Although this book is not about statistics, they do play an important part in clinical research. The best place to learn statistics is by practice alongside a mentor who knows about the subject.

What is offered here is a simple diagram (*see* Figure 44) to help you to see the different issues and tests that can be used to examine the results of clinical trials. The type of data, the assumptions that you can safely make, the number of categories, and the number of groups of patients all predetermine what test you should perform on the data.

You can also use Figure 44 in another way. If a trial reports results according to a particular test, you can use the statistical test diagram to check that it is an appropriate test. Furthermore, if a trial reports results according to a more obscure statistical test (e.g. one that is not listed in Figure 44), then you should ask why such an apparently exotic test was used.

With the help of Figure 44 you can now look at the results of one trial, check what statistical tests have been performed, and decide whether they are appropriate and whether they have explained their choice of test in the paper.

There are many other ways to analyse data. For example, data can be subjected to regression analysis, where one factor is tested for its dependence on a set of other factors (e.g. risk of myocardial infarction dependent on clinical variables, lifestyle and patient-specific issues, such as obesity, and diabetes).

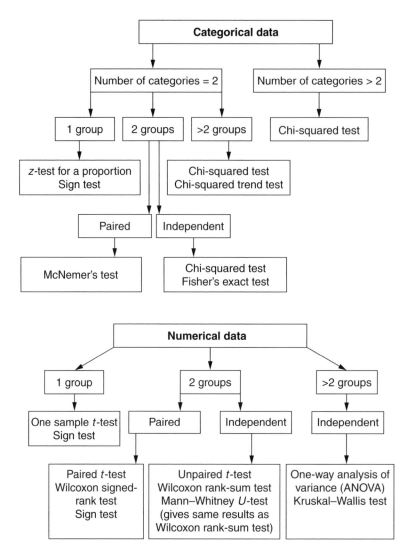

Figure 44 Statistical test diagram.

Computer software allows many tests to be performed very easily at the press of a button. The more exacting and exciting part is deciding what tests to perform and interpreting the clinical trial results.

The terms in Figure 44 are intended to be signposts, not detailed descriptions or definitions. To gain a fuller understanding of these terms, you are advised to consult a reputable medical statistician and a good medical statistics book. *See* **Algorithm; Clinical significance; Data-display format; Data types; Evidence-based medicine; Statistical significance**.

○ Altman D (1997) *Practical Statistics for Medical Research.* Chapman and Hall, London.

○ Bowers D (1996) *Statistics from Scratch: an introduction for healthcare professionals.* John Wiley & Sons, Chichester.

○ Bowers D (1996) *Further Statistics from Scratch: an introduction for healthcare professionals.* John Wiley & Sons, Chichester.

○ Greenhalgh T (1997) Statistics for the non-statistician. 1 Different types of data need different statistical tests. *BMJ.* **315**: 363–6.

○ Pereira-Maxwell F (1998). *A–Z of Medical Statistics: a companion for critical appraisal.* Edward Arnold, London.

○ Petrie A and Sabin C (2000) *Medical Statistics at a Glance.* Blackwell Science, Oxford.

Statistical tests: ten ways to cheat with statistical tests

Trish Greenhalgh's second paper on 'statistics for the non-statisticians', on significant relations and their pitfalls, presents a table listing ten ways to cheat with statistical tests when writing up results. The table is reproduced here to act as a salutary reminder that creativity or deception is the darker side of some statistical enterprises. Table 60 also suggests some of the issues to look out for when interpreting someone else's research or results.

Table 60 Ten ways to cheat with statistical tests

1 Throw all your data into a computer and report as significant any relationship where $P < 0.05$.

2 If baseline differences between the groups favour the intervention group, remember not to adjust for them.

3 Do not test your data to see whether they are normally distributed. If you do, you might get stuck with some non-parametric tests, which are not so much fun.

4 Ignore all withdrawals (dropouts) and non-responders, so the analysis only concerns subjects who fully complied with treatment.

5 Always assume that you can plot one set of data against another and calculate an '*r*' value (the Pearson correlation coefficient), and assume that a significant '*r*' value proves causation.

6 If outliers (points which lie a long way from others on your graph) are messing up your calculations, just rub them out. However, if outliers are helping your case, even if they seem to be spurious results, then leave them in.

7 If the confidence intervals of your results overlap zero difference between the groups, leave them out of your report. Better still, mention them briefly in the text but do not plot them on the graph – and ignore them when drawing your conclusions.

8 If the difference between two groups becomes significant four and a half months into your 6-month trial, stop the trial and start writing it up.

9 If your results prove uninteresting, ask the computer to go back and see if any particular subgroups behaved differently. You might find that your intervention worked after all in a particular ethnic group aged 52–61 years.

10 If analysing your data in the way you had planned does not give the results that you wanted, run the data through a selection of other tests.

Medical care increasingly relies on statistics to help to reveal what to do, what not to do, and how well something works. At best, medical statistics can aid decision making, but decisions in clinical practice should never rely solely on medical statistics.

See **CONSORT; Due process; Statistical test diagram; Statisticians' checklist (*BMJ* recommended); Transparency.**

○ Bland M (1995) *An Introduction to Medical Statistics* (3e). Oxford University Press, Oxford.

○ Campbell MJ and Machin D (1999) *Medical Statistics: a common sense approach* (3e). John Wiley & Sons Ltd, Chichester.

○ Collins R and MacMahon S (2001) Reliable assessment of the effects of treatment on mortality and major morbidity. I. Clinical trials. *Lancet.* **357**: 373–80.

○ Greenhalgh T (1997) How to read a paper: statistics for the non-statisticians. I. Different types of data need different statistical tests. *BMJ.* **315**: 364–6.

○ Greenhalgh T (1997) How to read a paper: statistics for the non-statisticians. II. Significant relations and their pitfalls. *BMJ.* **315**: 422–5.

Statisticians' checklist (*BMJ* recommended)

The *British Medical Journal* (*BMJ*) produces a checklist for statisticians (*see* Table 61). Whilst other checklists do exist, this one offers a good starting point for opening discussion and debate about what should and should not be included in such a list. More fundamentally, it raises the issue of the need for such a checklist.

Randomised controlled trials must conform to the CONSORT statement and the following checklist.

Table 62 shows the *BMJ*'s *general* statistical checklist.

See **Qualitative analysis; Quantitative analysis; Statistical significance; Statistical test diagram; Statistical tests: ten ways to cheat with statistical tests.**

Stopping rules

Stopping rules are procedures to be followed for stopping a clinical trial, or for preventing a patient, investigator or physician from continuing in a trial.

For example we may:

• prevent a patient from continuing in a clinical trial if they have not followed the trial protocol

• stop a doctor recruiting into a trial if they do not follow explicit recruitment procedures, or if they fail to provide robust answers to detailed audits of their trial data records

• stop an analyst studying the data if they or their family have recently bought shares in the company whose product is under trial

• stop new recruitment into a trial until emerging adverse events in current participants have been better explored and explained

Table 61 Statisticians' checklist (*BMJ* recommended)

Design features
 1 Is the objective of the trial adequately described?
 2 Is there a satisfactory statement of diagnostic criteria for entry to the trial?
 3 Is there a satisfactory statement of the source of participants?
 4 Are concurrent (not historical) controls used?
 5 Are the interventions well defined?
 6 Is random allocation to intervention used?
 7 Is the method of randomisation described?
 8 Is there an acceptably short delay from allocation to the start of intervention?
 9 Is a potential degree of blindness used?
10 Is there a satisfactory statement of criteria for outcome measures?
11 Are the outcome measures appropriate?
12 Is the pre-study calculation of sample size reported?
13 Is the duration of post-intervention follow-up stated?

Conduct of trial
14 Are the intervention and control groups comparable in relevant measures?
15 Is a high proportion of participants followed up?
16 Did a high proportion of participants complete the intervention?
17 Were participants who dropped out from the intervention and control groups described adequately?
18 Are the adverse effects of the intervention reported?

Analysis and presentation
19 Are all statistical procedures adequately described or referenced?
20 Are the statistical analyses appropriate?
21 Are the prognostic factors adequately considered?
22 Is the presentation of statistical material satisfactory?
23 Are confidence intervals given for the main results?
24 Are the conclusions that are drawn from the statistical analysis justified?

Recommendation on paper
25 Is the paper of an acceptable statistical standard for publication?
26 If not, could it become acceptable?

- stop a trial if the benefits are unequivocally in favour of one regimen over another
- stop a trial if a certain number of fatalities occurs
- stop a trial due to the emergence or incidence of non-fatal adverse events
- stop a trial if no significant benefit arises between options
- stop a trial if the evidence shows superiority of one regimen over another.

Table 62 General statistical checklist of the *BMJ*

Design features
1 Was the objective of the study adequately described?
2 Was an appropriate study design used to achieve the objective?
3 Was there a satisfactory statement given about the source of subjects?
4 Was a pre-study calculation of the required sample size reported?

Conduct of study
5 Was a satisfactory response rate achieved?

Analysis and presentation
6 Was there a statement adequately describing or referencing all of the statistical procedures that were used?
7 Were the statistical analyses that were used appropriate?
8 Was the presentation of statistical material satisfactory?
9 Were the confidence intervals given for the main results?
10 Was the conclusion drawn from the statistical analysis justified?

Recommendation on paper
11 Is the paper of an acceptable statistical standard for publication?
12 If not, could it become acceptable with suitable revision?

See **Clinical trial steering committee; Data-display formats; Data-monitoring committee; Institutional review board; Interim analysis; Protocol; Research governance in the NHS; Sequential trial.**

○ Elting LS, Martin CG, Cantor SB and Rubenstein EB (1999) Influence of data-display formats on physician investigators' decisions to stop clinical trials: perspective trial with repeated measures. *BMJ.* **318**: 1527–31.

○ Meinert CL (1998) Clinical trials and treatment effects monitoring. *Control Clin Trials.* **19**: 515–22.

Stratified randomisation
Stratified randomisation is the random selection of patients from groups or strata of the population.
For example:

• stratified randomisation was used to select subgroups of premenopausal and post-menopausal patients with breast cancer

• a group of patients on methadone treatment was stratified into those who had a dual diagnosis of schizophrenia and drug addiction, and those who were not diagnosed with schizophrenia

• elderly people were stratified according to their risk of entering a nursing home.

Stratification can get quite complicated quite quickly. For example, we may wish to extend the stratification of the cancer trial to consider tumour size, and then the extent of node involvement, as well as menopausal status.

In general, the more strata we use the larger the number of patients we need to enter the trial. *See* **Block randomisation; Mega-trial; Multilevel modelling; Randomisation; Sample size; Stratification; Stratified sampling**.

○ Stuck AE, Minder CE, Peter-Wuest I *et al.* (2000) A randomized trial of in-home disability prevention in community-dwelling older people at low and high risk for nursing home admission. *Arch Intern Med.* **160**: 977–86.

Stratified sampling
Stratified sampling is sampling within groups of a population. For example, the clinical trial at the hospital may sample only:

• from those over 60 years of age

• women aged between 35 and 55 years

• paediatric asthmatics who have recently been prescribed CFC inhalers with spacers.

Stratified sampling is not necessarily the same as stratified randomisation, as the former can include non-randomisation. *See* **Sampling strategies; Stratified randomisation; Subgroup analysis**.

Subgroup analysis
Subgroup analysis occurs when some but not all of the patients in a clinical trial are subject to further assessment.

Examples of subgroups include the following:

• age bands of patients

• gender

• ethnicity

• socio-economic status (in testing links between smoking, exercise, alcohol intake and stroke)

• comorbidity

• dual diagnosis

• outcome (e.g. looking in detail at the patients who had a myocardial infarction).

Subgroup analysis can be used to find positive results in a trial with no overall gain. This is good news in fact, because it shows that the trial worked for a particular group of people and not for the wider group in the study.

For example, in a systematic review of the use of ACE inhibitors in the early treatment of acute myocardial infarction, subgroup analysis showed a greater proportional survival benefit for:

- patients aged 55–74 years

- patients with a baseline heart rate of $\geqslant$100 beats/minute

- patients with evidence of anterior myocardial infarction.

Whenever you encounter subgroup analysis, it is important to find out the overall result of the trial. See **A posteriori**; **Data dredging**; **Data fishing**; **Protocol**; **Statistical test diagram**.

○ ACE Inhibitor Myocardial Infarction Collaborative Group (1998) Indications for ACE inhibitors in the early treatment of acute myocardial infarction: systematic overview of individual data from 100 000 patients in randomized trials. *Circulation*. **97**: 2202–12.

○ Bennett JC (1993) Inclusion of women in clinical trials – policies for populations and subgroups. *NEJM*. **329**: 288–92.

○ Oxman AD and Guyatt GH (1992) A consumer's guide to subgroup analysis. *Ann Intern Med*. **116**: 78–84.

○ Yusuf S, Wittes J, Probstfield J and Tyroler HA (1991) Analysis and interpretation of treatment effects in subgroups of patients in randomised clinical trials. *JAMA*. **266**: 93–8.

Subject

This is an impersonal term for the patient or healthy volunteer in a clinical trial.

If the trial involves cultures, genes, materials or tissue, then 'subject' may be an appropriate and palatable term to use. See **Participants**; **Principal investigator**; **Sponsor**.

Superiority trial

The primary objective of a superiority trial is to show that one regimen is superior to another. It is designed to detect a difference.

In a superiority trial, the null hypothesis is that one regimen is superior to another. Pre-definition of a trial as a superiority trial is necessary to:

- define the relevant hypothesis

- ensure that the superiority criteria are pre-defined and justified

- ensure that the comparator treatments, doses, patient populations and endpoints are appropriate

- set up appropriate statistical tests

- allow proper power calculations to be performed

- ensure that the quality of the trial matches its objectives

- design relevant invitations to enter the trial.

Key issues with regard to superiority trials include the following.

- On what dimensions is one regimen thought to be superior to another?
- Just how superior is one regimen?
- What is the regimen being compared with?
- What happens if the test of superiority fails to reach the level of significance?
- Is the superiority clinically significant?

See **Clinical significance; Clinical trial; Data dredging; Data fishing; Dose comparison trial; Equivalence trial; Non-inferiority trial; Null hypothesis; Primary outcome; Research governance in the NHS; Statistical significance; Statistical test diagram.**

○ European Agency for the Evaluation of Medicinal Products (1999) *Committee for Proprietary Medical Products (CPMP) points to consider on biostatistical/methodological issues arising from recent CPMP discussions on licensing applications: superiority, non-inferiority and equivalence.* EMEA, London.

○ The Symphony Investigators (2000) Comparison of sibrafiban with aspirin for prevention of cardiovascular events after acute coronary syndromes: a randomised trial. *Lancet.* **355**: 337–45.

Surrogate endpoint

A surrogate endpoint in a clinical trial is an observation marker that is believed to relate to the primary endpoint of interest.

Surrogate endpoints can be clinical, physiological, chemical or biological identifiers. For example, the following surrogate endpoints may be used in clinical trials:

- bone mineral density for fractured neck of femur
- cholesterol levels for cardiovascular mortality
- lipid levels for arteriosclerosis
- p53, cytomorphometric indices, ploidy, PNCA, erbB-2, erbB-3, EGF receptor, TGF-alpha tumour-associated glycoprotein-72, fatty acid synthetase and Lewis Y antigen for prostate cancer malignancy
- relapse time in multiple sclerosis
- cancer cell growth for survival time
- viral load in HIV patients.

Surrogate endpoints should be:

- reasonably easy to identify

- identified relatively quickly

- good proxies or true predictors of the final outcome of interest.

Surrogate endpoints are sometimes also called proxy endpoints. *See* **Outcome; Outcomes pyramid; Primary outcome**.

○ Greenhalgh T (1997) Papers that report drug trials. *BMJ*. **315**: 480–3.

Synergy

Synergy occurs when the total exceeds the sum of the individual parts. For example:

- if streptomycin and sodium aminosalicylate are used together to treat tuberculosis, their combined effects exceed each drug's individual effect

- if two brain surgeons work together in a multicentre brain cancer clinical trial, they may provide a higher quality of clinical services and complete a greater number of successful cases than they could individually.

See **Additive effect; Multiplicative effect.**

Systematic review

This is an approach that involves capturing and assessing the evidence by some systematic method, where all the components of the approach and the assessment are made explicit and documented.

Some examples of these components include the following:

- a clear research question

- where the researchers looked for information (e.g. Medline, Controlled Trials, Embase, NHS National Research Register)

- the criteria they used to select the evidence

- the criteria they used to discard particular pieces of evidence

- the way in which the evidence was collated

- the way in which the key messages were derived.

Systematic reviews are based on the following premises.

- Large amounts of information must be reduced to smaller quantities for consumption.

- Such reviews integrate critical pieces of available information.

- A review is usually quicker to complete and less expensive than a new study.

- The generalisability of the evidence can be established.

- The consistency of relationships can be established.

- Inconsistencies in the evidence can be determined.

- Gaps in the evidence can be identified.

- Increases in the statistical power of studies can be achieved.

See **Accountability; Due process; Funnel plot; Grey literature; L'Abbe plot; Meta-analysis; National Institute for Clinical Excellence; Pooled analysis; Research question; Transparency; Triangulation**.

○ Chalmers I and Altman D (eds) (1995) *Systematic Reviews*. BMJ Books, London.

○ Earl-Slater A (2001) Critical appraisal of clinical trials: critical appraisal and hierarchies of the evidence. *J Clin Govern*. **6**: 59–63.

T

Take-up rate

The take-up rate is the number of people who take up a service compared with the total number who are eligible to take up the service. Suppose that in a clinical trial 1000 women in their menopause are eligible for a new procedure in cancer screening but, for various reasons, only 750 women go and have the screening. The take-up rate in this trial would then be 0.75 (750/1000).

As another example, Tod and colleagues reported on a qualitative study of barriers to uptake of services for coronary heart disease.

Estimates of the take-up rate are important in clinical trials and clinical practice with regard to the following:

- planning of the trial

- running of the trial

- resources required

- cost

- analysis.

See **Causes of delay and failure to complete a clinical trial; Ethical issues; Fate of research studies; Feasibility trial; Local research ethics committee; Mega-trial; Multicentre trial; Reasons given by the investigator for a study being abandoned or in abeyance; Reasons given by the investigator for a study never being started; Research governance in the NHS; Statistical tests: ten ways to cheat with statistical tests.**

○ Tod AM, Read C, Lacey A and Abbot J (2001) Barriers to uptake of services for coronary heart disease: qualitative study. *BMJ.* **323**: 214.

Threshold point analysis

Threshold point analysis is a method of finding the point above which success lies and below which failure lies. *See* **Boundary approach; Dose comparison trial; Interim analysis; *P*-value; Sensitivity analysis; Superiority trial.**

Titration

During the course of a trial, the process of changing the strength, amount or frequency of a particular intervention is called titration.

Recently published examples of titration in trials include the following:

- titrating metoprolol in the trial reported by Hjalmarson and colleagues

- titrating imipramine from 50 mg/day to 100 mg/day by day 5 in the trial reported by Philipp and colleagues

- titrating glyburide from 2.5 mg to 20 mg 'as needed' and insulin up 'as needed' in the trial reported by Langer and colleagues.

In general, titration can include, for example:

- changing the dose strength of a medicine

- changing the amount (e.g. volume)

- changing the frequency of administration

- changing the dose of radiation

- changing the dose of chemotherapy.

See **Dose comparison trial; Titration trial.**

○ Hjalmarson A, Goldstein S, Fagerberger B *et al.* for the MERIT-HF Study Group (2000) Effects of controlled-release metoprolol on total mortality, hospitalizations and well-being in patients with heart failure: the Metoprolol CR/XL Randomized Intervention Trial in Congestive Heart Failure (MERIT-HF). *JAMA.* **283**: 1295–302.

○ Langer O, Conway DL, Berkus MD *et al.* (2000) A comparison of glyburide and insulin in women with gestational diabetes mellitus. *NEJM.* **343**: 1134–8.

○ Philipp M, Kohnen R and Hiller KO (1999) *Hypericum* extract versus imipramine or placebo in patients with moderate depression: randomised multicentre study of treatment for eight weeks. *BMJ.* **319**: 1534–9.

Titration trial

A titration clinical trial is a trial in which study subjects receive different doses of a drug during the period of the trial.

For example, if a patient fails to respond to 10 mg once-a-day medication in the trial, they may be given 15 mg once a day.

Titration may be used:

- to raise the dose

- to lower the dose

- to raise and lower the dose over the full course of the trial (e.g. to find the appropriate dosage range).

There are generally two types of titration trial.

- In a *forced titration trial*, titration occurs at a predefined point of time in the trial (e.g. week 3).

- In an *open titration trial*, titration occurs in the light of the patient's response, or lack of it, to the intervention.

Some examples are given above in the entry on **titration**.

Another example is provided by Wetter and colleagues, who reported on titration in a randomised controlled trial to address the question of whether pergolide was effective in improving symptoms and sleep in patients with idiopathic restless leg syndrome. This is quite a complex trial including, for example, open titration, then doses held constant for 2 weeks, 1-week of down-titration, then placebo for 1 week, and a 1-week washout period before crossing to the other arm of the trial. *See* **Dose comparison trial; Sensitivity analysis; Titration; Washout period**.

○ Wetter TC, Stiansny K, Winkelmann L *et al.* (1999) A randomised controlled study of pergolide in patients with restless legs syndrome. *Neurology.* **52**: 944–50.

Trade-off

A trade-off is said to exist if there are two apparently incompatible options.

There may be a trade-off between:

- the volume and quality of healthcare

- the feasibility of a trial based on strong entry and exclusion criteria, and the wider patient population that may receive the product of interest.

A trade-off exists between the absolute number of lives saved by thrombolytic therapy and the time from the onset of symptoms to administration of treatment in patients with ST-segment elevation or bundle branch block in cardiovascular disease. Figure 45 shows that the longer the time between the onset of symptoms and the administration of treatment, the fewer the number of patients' lives that will be saved. Conversely, more patients' lives will be saved if treatment is administered quickly.

See **Primary outcome; Protocol; Value-for-money table**.

○ NHS Centre for Reviews and Dissemination (1995) *Relationship Between Volume and Quality of Health Care: a review of the literature.* NHS Centre for Reviews and Dissemination, York.

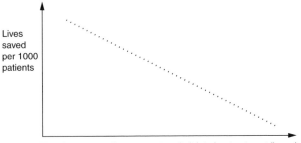

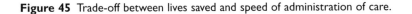

Time from onset of symptoms to administering treatment (hours)

Figure 45 Trade-off between lives saved and speed of administration of care.

Transparency

Transparency is another term for clarity, visibility or openness.
Some examples are listed below.

- How transparent was the method of allocation in a particular trial?

- Did the authors report on why people dropped out of the trial?

- Did the authors report on all outcome measures in the trial, regardless of how well the patients fared on all outcomes?

- Why was the trial protocol not put on the Internet for all to see?

- Why did an ethics committee refuse to allow a certain trial to go ahead?

See **Accountability; Data-monitoring committee; Ethics committee; Multicentre research ethics committee; Questions to ask before getting involved in a clinical trial; Research governance in the NHS; Systematic review.**

Treatment effect

A treatment effect is a consequence of treatment. *See* **Association; Causal relationship; Placebo effect; Primary outcome; Side-effect.**

Treatment group: experimental

The experimental treatment group is generally considered to consist of those patients who are given the experimental intervention of interest in the clinical trial (e.g. a new drug).
Recently published examples of trials have included experimental groups such as:

- those on donepezil in an Alzheimer's dementia trial

- those on pramipexole in a Parkinson's disease trial
- those on bupropion in a smoking cessation trial
- those on orlistat in an obesity trial
- those on sildenafil in a male erectile dysfunction trial
- those on zaleplon in an insomnia trial.

In a clinical trial it is sometimes safer to classify those individuals in the experimental treatment group as the cases. *See* **Case group; Clinical trial; Control group; Research questions and research methods**.

Trial site

A trial site is the location where the actual trial activity takes place. If it is a multicentre trial, there will be more than one trial site. *See* **Multicentre trial**.

Trial steering committee

This is another term for a clinical trial steering committee. *See* **Clinical trial steering committee; Data-monitoring committee; Institutional review board; Local research ethics committee; Research governance in the NHS**.

Triangulation

In triangulation, the basic idea is to take information from one source and see whether it is corroborated by information from other sources or other methods of data collection. Similar findings from various sources provide at best corroboration or reassurance.

The data may come from various areas (e.g. clinical trials, cohort studies, case–control studies, observational analysis, interview transcripts, medical records, computerised databases). For example, in a study of triple-vaccination mumps–measles–rubella (MMR) practice, you can obtain information from database analysis, case studies, medical records and interview transcripts. You could also obtain information from clinical trials where these are available.

Triangulation is a term that is commonly encountered in qualitative research. It also has a growing application in quantitative analysis, and is often used outside clinical trials and clinical practice (e.g. in courts of law).

Key issues in triangulation include the following:

- the research question that you want answered
- what sources of information to search
- what information to include

- how to rate its quality

- whether different weights should be attached to information from different sources

- how to integrate the portfolio of information.

As Hammersley and Atkinson have warned, 'one should not adopt a naively optimistic view that the aggregation of data from different sources will unproblematically add up to produce a more complete picture', and Fielding and Fielding have argued that 'rarely does the inaccuracy of one approach to the data complement the accuracies of another'. *See* **Meta-analysis; Qualitative analysis; Systematic review.**

○ Barbour RS (2001) Checklists for improving rigour in qualitative research: a case of the tail wagging the dog? *BMJ*. **322**: 1115–17.

○ Fielding N and Fielding J (1986) *Linking Data: qualitative research methods.* Sage Publishing, London.

○ Jick T (1979) Mixing qualitative and quantitative methods: triangulation in action. *Admin Sci Quart.* **24**: 602–11.

○ Pope C and Mays N (2000) *Qualitative Research in Health Care* (2e). BMJ Books, London.

Triple-blind trial

A triple-blind trial is a clinical trial in which the patient, clinician and outcome assessor do not know what option (e.g. a medicine) a patient has received in the trial.

Triple-blind experiments need close attention because the 'blindness' implies a degree of ignorance in the trial. Some trials cannot be triple-blinded (e.g. surgery). *See* **Blind; Blind trial; Data-monitoring committee; Double-blind trial; Quadruple-blind trial; Single-blind trial; Unblinded.**

Truncated data

Truncated data are data for which some values are not used in analysis. For example, numbers greater than X or less than Y may not be used in an analysis of a clinical trial. *See* **Available case analysis; Censoring; Data-monitoring committee; Statistical tests: ten ways to cheat with statistical tests.**

Two-armed bandit allocation

The two-armed bandit allocation is a method of allocating patients to interventions in a clinical trial where the probability of any one patient being assigned to a particular arm of the trial is a function of the observed difference in outcomes of patients who are already in the trial (*see* Figure 46).

The aim is to minimise the number of patients in the less rewarding arm of the trial.

The main difficulty is that relevant outcomes may take some time to be seen and confirmed. *See* **Allocation; Clinical trial; Play-the-winner rule; Protocol; Random allocation; Statistical test diagram; Surrogate endpoints.**

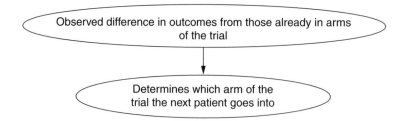

Figure 46 Two-armed bandit allocation.

Two-stage sampling

Two-stage sampling involves methods of selecting a sample, and then selecting a further sample from that sample.

It has been used:

- in quality assurance of manufacturing drugs

- to select patients on a particular medication and then to select types of patients from that sample for a clinical trial

- to select patients with a particular disease and then to select patients of a specific age in that group.

Figure 47 illustrates this.

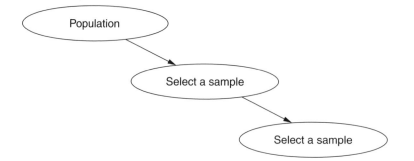

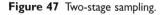

Figure 47 Two-stage sampling.

Two-tailed test

A two-tailed test is a test in which the direction of the effect is not specified in advance.

For example:

- in women with breast cancer in remission, does the level of satisfaction with health service delivery differ when follow-up is conducted in a primary care setting rather than in a specialist-care hospital outreach setting?

- in women with heavy menstrual bleeding, how does transcervical resection of the endometrium compared with medical management perform in terms of affecting menstrual symptoms in the long term?

- in postmenopausal women who are receiving tamoxifen for breast cancer, does clonidine change the incidence of hot flushes?

- in patients who need long-term oral anticoagulation treatment, how does self-management compare with specialist anticoagulation clinic management in terms of effectiveness?

- in patients with severe congestive heart failure caused by systolic left ventricular dysfunction, does spironolactone combined with usual care have any discernible effect on all-cause mortality?

- in clinically obese children, does dietary advice alone have any impact on the level of obesity after one year?

- do the smoking quit rates of men differ from those of women under alternative interventions for quitting?

The reason for using the two-tailed tests is that we have not stated whether the results from one regimen are better or worse than those from another. For instance, in the smoking quit rate study, men may have a higher or lower quit rate than women. Therefore we use a two-sided test to allow for any eventuality, as we are uncertain of the direction of any difference. *See* **Alternative hypothesis; One-tailed test; Statistical test diagram.**

Type I error

A type 1 error occurs when we reject, or do not accept, something that is true.

For example, if the null hypothesis is of no difference between one drug and another, then a type 1 error would occur if we concluded that the drugs produced different effects when in fact there was no such difference.

A type 1 error is generally regarded as failing to accept the null hypothesis when the latter is true. *See* **Acceptance area; Bias; Null hypothesis; Type 2 error.**

Type 2 error

A type 2 error occurs when we accept something that is false.

For example, if the null hypothesis is of no difference between one drug and another, then a type 2 error would occur if we concluded that there was no difference between the two drugs when in fact they produced different effects.

A type 2 error is generally regarded as the probability of failing to reject the null hypothesis when the latter is in fact false. The larger the type 2 error, the weaker the power of the study. A type 2 error is often the result of a sample size being too small. *See* **Acceptance area; Bias; Power; Type 1 error.**

Types of research questions

Table 63 gives an indication of the different categories of questions that can be found in clinical research and clinical practice. It also provides examples and suggestions for improvement.

Table 63 Types of questions

Type of question	Example	Suggestions for improvement
Open	From your experience, what key messages would you offer to those planning a phase 3 double-blind placebo-controlled parallel clinical trial in primary care for the treatment of insomnia?	Check that the respondent understands the terminology in the question, obtain background information about their clinical trial experience, determine the time scale (was it a trial that they were involved in some time ago, or is it one in which they are just finishing involvement, or one that they are still heavily involved in?). Think about the individuals to whom the answer(s) will be relayed. Select a particular trial, and then ask a more specific question about its key messages. Because it is an open question, be aware that the respondent may give many answers, or they may give very few answers, and any answer that they do give could be vague with regard to the actual detail. More questions should be asked in order to tease out the respondent's key messages
Closed	What was the length of time, in minutes, between the patient with myocardial infarction arriving at the emergency unit and their receiving thrombolytic therapy?	Consider whether the patient could have received the treatment on the way to hospital (e.g. in an ambulance). Try to trace when the myocardial infarction started, who was called to attend, who attended, who diagnosed the condition, and what specific interventions were given (dose, etc.) and when
Leading	Your family doctor, who is very good at his work, has done everything possible to help you in this trial. Are you happy with your care?	Provide evidence of how good the doctor is (e.g. independent clinical audit reviews, qualifications, trial experience and testimonies), evidence of what was done, evidence of what could have been done (e.g. outside the trial), evidence of the trial protocol and standard operating procedures, and then specifically ask a series of questions relating to the care and satisfaction
Imprecise	Did you arrive at the hospital quickly after developing chest pains?	Find out when the pains started, where the person was when they started, how they got to the hospital, when they got there, and who they saw on arrival

continued opposite

Table 63 continued

Type of question	Example	Suggestions for improvement
Open to interpretation	Did the surgeon tell you what was going to happen after the trial?	Make sure that the respondent knows who the surgeon is, find out what information was provided by whom, when and in what form, find out what happened, establish the points in time, and then ask a more specific question
Composite	Did you understand and follow the clinical trial protocol completely?	Divide the question into separate parts. Did you know what the trial protocol was? Did you understand the trial protocol? Did you follow the protocol completely?
Double negative	Would you not have preferred not to be asked to join the trial?	Disentangle. Would you have preferred not to be asked to join the trial?
Presumptuous	How long have you been having unprotected sex?	Avoid making unnecessary assumptions. First ask whether or not they have had unprotected sex. Then ask relevant questions about time scales, frequency, type of sex (vaginal, anal) and number of partners

In protocol-driven ethically approved clinical trials, most of the problems associated with the questions should have been resolved before the trial started. However, all of the above examples have been seen in clinical trials, so there is no guarantee that just because a clinical trial has ethical approval to start, it will be free of problems with regard to its questions.

Therefore Table 63 has a multitude of uses.

- It shows you a range of different types of questions.

- It indicates that the type of question could predetermine the answer.

- It illustrates the point that one question could lead to a whole series of other questions.

- It makes you aware of the need to be vigilant about what questions were or are being asked (e.g. in committees, research publications, trial protocols, during patient interaction).

- It makes you think about what types of question should have been asked.

- It encourages you to think harder about your own questions before you ask them.

See **Comparing research methods; Hierarchies of the evidence; Types of study.**

Types of study

There are various types of study, and Figure 48 shows a classification system to illustrate this.

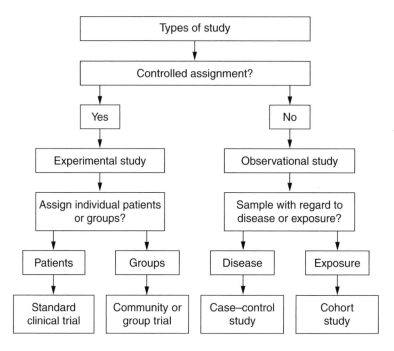

Figure 48 Types of study.

As a word of warning, Figure 48 will only give you a flavour of the different types of studies. You should read the entries that are cross-referenced below for further details. *See* **Case–control study; Clinical trial; Cohort study; Community trial; Comparing research methods; Observational study; Randomised controlled trial; Research questions and research methods; Sampling strategies.**

U

Unanticipated adverse effect

Unanticipated adverse effects are undesirable effects in a clinical trial that could not have been predicted on the basis of prior knowledge, experience or understanding. *See* **Adverse effects; Anticipated adverse effects; Anticipated beneficial effects; Phases of a clinical trial; Unanticipated beneficial effect; Yellow card scheme**.

Unanticipated beneficial effect

Unanticipated beneficial effects are desirable effects of an intervention in a clinical trial that could not have been predicted on the basis of prior knowledge, experience or understanding.

One popular example of this is as follows. In the early clinical trials of sildenafil, the drug was being tested in patients for its effects on angina. One side-effect was an improvement in some patients' erectile function. The product was then put under formal trials for the treatment of male erectile dysfunction, and it is now on the market for that condition. *See* **Anticipated adverse effects; Anticipated beneficial effects; Outcomes pyramid; Phases of a clinical trial; Side-effects; Unanticipated adverse effect; Yellow card scheme**.

Unblinded clinical trial

This is a clinical trial in which the patient, clinician, outcome assessor and statistician know what regimen is being or was given to the patient.

For example, in patients with depression, Simon and colleagues ran a randomised unblinded controlled trial with a 24-month follow-up to determine whether initial treatment with fluoxetine improves clinical, quality-of-life and economic outcomes more than desipramine or imipramine.

When you encounter a trial that is unblinded, try to find out exactly why this was so. *See* **Blind; Open-label trial; Quadruple-blind trial; Single-blind trial; Triple-blind trial**.

○ Simon GE, Heiligensein J, Revecki D *et al.* (1999) Long-term outcomes of initial antidepressant drug choice in a 'real world' randomized trial. *Arch Fam Med.* **8**: 319–25.

Validity

Four common types of validity of an instrument (e.g. a questionnaire, a scale measuring outcomes, or a patient satisfaction diagram) are face validity, content validity, construct validity and criterion validity.

We shall look at these with respect to questionnaires.

Face validity

This is usually the first test of validity of a questionnaire. Face validity is often approached as follows. On the face of it and without further investigation, do you expect the questionnaire to collect the information required accurately and effectively? This is therefore a test laden with subjectivity. It simply refers to the subjective assessment of the presentation and the relevance of the questionnaire.

For example, a study analysing customers' perceptions of the quality of service from a group of pharmacies was independently tested for face validity. Some of the questions were revised, some new questions were added, some existing questions were deleted, and the order of questions was improved in the light of the comments. This was mainly because the pharmacists writing the questionnaire were in a sense 'too close to the topic' and blinded to some of the perceptible problems in the original questionnaire.

Content validity

This is concerned with the extent to which the questionnaire covers all relevant issues. Content validity, it is claimed, has stronger theoretical foundations than face validity, and it can usually provide more systematic and less subjective impressions. Overlooking issues that are important to the respondents results in a questionnaire that lacks content validity. Exploratory interviews, discussion groups, focus groups, field notes, a review of the literature and common sense can usually yield an accurate impression of the issues to be addressed.

For example:

- in one trial the refinement of a questionnaire on diabetes home management was considerably improved after a series of discussions with diabetic patients and their families

- the primary endpoints to be included in a trial questionnaire on multiple sclerosis care were improved by exploratory interviews and discussion groups that included clinicians, patients, families and carers

- in-depth interviews with pharmacists and community nurses proved useful in refining a questionnaire in a trial designed to compare pharmacy lead care with hospital outpatient care.

Construct validity

This is the extent to which a group of questions, or even just one question, correspond to what is understood by a construct or concept.

For example, health status questionnaires on pain, anger, mobility, mood, visual acuity or quality of life need to make clear the meaning of the underlying construct (e.g. what mobility or mood means). No single observation can prove construct validity. Rather, what is required is a series of observations or a series of converging experiments to help to build up a picture of the relationships and constructs.

Criterion validity

This compares the results which have been obtained in a questionnaire against other measures of the same variable, or against some 'gold standard'. Thus it covers correlations with another measure.

For example, to test the criterion validity of a measure of lower back pain, the results of the questionnaire would be compared with the results obtained from another more commonly used measure or the 'gold standard', if one exists. The General Health Questionnaire (28-questions version, GHQ-28) was used in a study of drugs prescribed for patients aged 85 years or over living in their own homes in an area of inner London. The GHQ-28 has been extensively used to screen for anxiety and depression in different age groups. Its criterion validity is based on its results correlating with clinical diagnoses of anxiety and depression.

See **Outcomes pyramid; Primary outcome; Research questions and research methods; Scales of measurement; Secondary outcome.**

○ Bowling A (1997) *Research Methods in Health: investigating health and health services.* Open University Press, Buckingham.

○ Smith F (1997) Survey research. 2 Survey instruments, reliability and validity. *Int J Pharm Pract.* 5: 216–26.

○ Stevens A, Abrams K, Brazier J, Fitzpatrick R and Lilford R (eds) (2001) *The Advanced Handbook of Methods in Evidence-Based Healthcare.* Sage Publishing, London.

Validity checks

Validity checks are methods of assessing data to check that only allowable values or codes are recorded. *See* **Data cleaning; Data-monitoring committee; Dirty data; Interim analysis; Protocol.**

Value-for-money table

The value-for-money table is a table that summarises the relative costs and benefits of options. Table 64 gives an example.

Table 64 Value-for-money table

A	Costs less to implement than B	Costs the same to implement as B	Costs more to implement than B
Shows fewer benefits than B	4	7	9
Shows the same benefits as B	2	5	8
Shows greater benefits than B	1	3	6

For example, the options may include the following:

- conducting a trial in a pharmaceutical company, compared with conducting it in an academic laboratory
- using a local GP to relay the evidence from a new trial, compared with using another method of disseminating the evidence to the primary care group
- using one type of tissue sample refrigerator compared with another
- conducting one large trial compared with conducting five smaller-scale trials
- assessing the merits of one product compared with another.

Look at the bottom left-hand corner of the table. Cell 1 is where option A would provide more benefits and cost less than option B. Anything that falls into cells 1, 2 or 3 would be generally considered to be good value for money.

Cell 9 is where A would provide fewer benefits and actually cost more than option B. Anything that falls into cells 7, 8 or 9 would generally be considered to be poor value for money.

If the calculation shows that A and B offer the same benefits at the same cost, then we are in cell 5. Attention now has to be focused on other reasons for going ahead with either A or B.

If the results fall into in cell 4, then A costs less than B, but it also provides fewer benefits than B. The question now turns on whether the lower benefits would be acceptable at the lower cost. We can calculate the cost per unit benefit and establish other reasons for taking any one course of action (e.g. local politics, patients' preferences, budgetary limits).

If we are in cell 6, then A shows greater benefit than B, but it also costs more than B. For cell 6 an example would be as follows. McCrory and colleagues reviewed the literature to see whether there was evidence that newer technologies (e.g. thin-layer cytology, computer rescreening) improved sensitivity in detecting cervical cancer and cervical intra-epithelial neoplasia, compared with the conventional papanicolaou

(Pap) test. Cervical cancer is one of the major causes of death from cancer among women worldwide. McCrory and colleagues concluded that implementation of the newer technologies improved the sensitivity of primary cervical screening compared with the Pap test, but at a substantially increased cost. In cell 6, judgements have to be made as to whether the increased benefits are worth the increased cost, the practicalities of changing services, the take-up rates, available funds, local politics and priorities. Cell 6 is the converse of cell 4.

The value-for-money table is important in clinical trials and clinical practice for the following reasons:

- It helps to summarise the costs and merits of different courses of action.

- It helps to determine what type of trials to undertake.

- It can help to interpret the merits of strategies of implementing clinical trial evidence in practice.

- It can be used to help to show the value of current practice compared with another practice.

See **Accountability; Barriers to putting evidence into practice; Clinical trial; Due process; Economic analysis and clinical trials; Equivalence trial; Evidence-based medicine; National Institute for Clinical Excellence; Non-inferiority trial; Outcomes pyramid; Primary question; Superiority trial; Transparency.**

○ Earl-Slater A (1999) *Dictionary of Health Economics*. Radcliffe Medical Press, Oxford.

○ McCrory DC, Matchar DB, Bastian I *et al.* (1999) *Evaluation of Cervical Cytology*. Agency for Health Care Policy and Research, Rockville, MD.

Venn diagram

A Venn diagram is a picture that shows the extent to which two or more groups have mutually inclusive or mutually exclusive characteristics. Figure 49 provides an example.

In Figure 49 there is only one area where the patients have A, B and C, namely area 5. For example, ABC could be triple therapy, and it can be compared with other combinations (e.g. A and B, A and C, B and C, A alone, B alone, C alone, or nothing). *See* **Additive effect; Combination trial.**

Virement

Virement is the movement of funds from one budget heading to another. For example, it could involve moving funds:

- from one particular trial to another

- from clinical trials to teaching

- from sales to trials

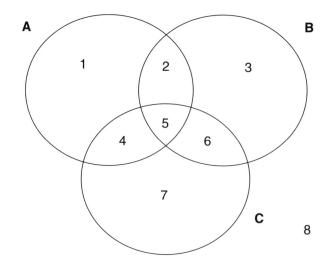

Figure 49 Venn diagram.

- from the refurbishment of a hospital outpatient ward towards treating more patients

- from primary healthcare spending to social care support for elderly patients recently discharged from hospital

- from primary care to hospital care.

See **Accountability; Research governance in the NHS; Value-for-money table.**

Volunteer

A volunteer is someone who acts of their own free will and offers their services to a study programme. For example, many phase 1 clinical trials rely on healthy volunteers as study subjects. *See* **Participant; Phase 1 clinical trial; Volunteer bias.**

Volunteer bias

Volunteer bias can arise if those who volunteer for a clinical trial have significantly different characteristics or respond differently to treatment compared with other participants. *See* **Bias; Halo effect; Hello-goodbye effect; Significance; Volunteer.**

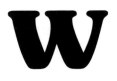

Washout period

The washout period is the time it takes for a patient's system to be completely cleared of the drug or therapy.

In terms of medicine, the washout period depends on factors such as the following:

- the half-life of the drug
- metabolic discharge
- the duration of the effects of the drug
- how long it takes for those effects to be detected
- patient-specific issues.

The main reason for building a washout period into a clinical trial is to try to eliminate any contamination of results when:

- the patient moves from current care to care in the trial
- the patient moves between regimens in the trial.

For example, Wetter and colleagues used a 1-week washout period in a randomised placebo-controlled trial of pergolide in patients with restless leg syndrome. *See* **Cross-over trial; Pharmacodynamics; Run-in period**.

- Wetter TC, Stiansy K, Winkelmann J *et al.* (1999) A randomized controlled study of pergolide in patients with restless legs syndrome. *Neurology.* **52**: 944–50.

Ways of presenting results

There are various ways of presenting results from clinical research, each of which has its own strengths and weakness.

The way in which results are presented can affect their interpretation, and some examples of this are described below.

- Fahey and colleagues reported on a study showing that the way in which results are presented affects the willingness to fund a programme. They gave 182 health authorities results from a randomised trial on breast cancer screening and from a systematic review of cardiac rehabilitation. The objective was to determine whether the way in which results were presented affected the health authorities' inclination to purchase. All four sets of data summarised the same results, namely relative risk reduction, absolute risk reduction, percentage of event-free patients, and numbers needed to treat. Presenting results in terms of relative risk reduction produced a significantly stronger inclination to purchase, followed by numbers needed to treat. Only three out of 140 respondents said that they understood that all four formats summarised the same results.

- Naylor and colleagues compared clinicians' ratings of therapeutic effectiveness when the results were presented in different ways. They randomly allocated questionnaires among doctors at a teaching hospital. Data were presented in terms of the absolute risk reduction, relative risk reduction and numbers needed to treat. The doctors were asked to use a scoring system to rate the results (such that the higher the score, the greater their perception of clinical effectiveness). Naylor and colleagues found that the doctors scored relative risk reduction data highest, then absolute risk reduction data, and data on numbers needed to treat were scored lowest. This means that the doctors interpreted the intervention as being more effective with regard to relative risk reduction data than in relation to the other ways of presenting the data, even though all of the data were derived from the same set of results. Thus the way in which the results were presented clearly mattered.

- Bobbio and colleagues studied GPs' willingness to prescribe a drug based on different presentations of the results of cardiac events and deaths. The results were presented as relative risk reduction, absolute risk reduction, numbers needed to treat, difference in event-free patients, or events reduction and mortality. The authors found that GPs' willingness to prescribe was greatest if results were presented as relative risk reduction data, and lowest if the results were presented in the form of absolute risk reduction or events reduction and mortality.

Thus several key points arise.

- The results from a clinical trial can be presented in various ways.

- The way in which they are presented can affect their interpretation.

- The way in which you yourself interpret results can be conditioned by the way in which they are presented to you.

See **Absolute risk reduction; Data-display formats; Mortality; Number needed to treat; Problems with regard to putting evidence into practice; Relative risk reduction; Take-up rate.**

○ Bobbio M, Demichelis B and Giustetto G (1994) Completeness of reporting trial results: effects on physicians' willingness to prescribe. *Lancet.* **343**: 1209–11.

○ Fahey T, Griffiths S and Peters TJ (1995) Evidence-based purchasing: understanding results of clinical trials and systematic reviews. *BMJ*. **311**: 1056–60.

○ Naylor CD, Chen E and Strauss B (1992) Measured enthusiasm: does the method of reporting trial results alter perceptions of therapeutic effectiveness? *Ann Intern Med*. **117**: 916–21.

Wennberg's design

Wennberg's design is a type of clinical trial in which some patients' preferences determine the treatment that they receive.

The Wennberg design works as follows.

- Patients are randomised to either the preference group or the non-preference group.

- Those who are allocated to the preference group receive the treatment of their choice.

- Those who are allocated to the non-preference group are randomised to receive whatever treatment options are available in that arm of the trial.

Figure 50 gives an example of this.

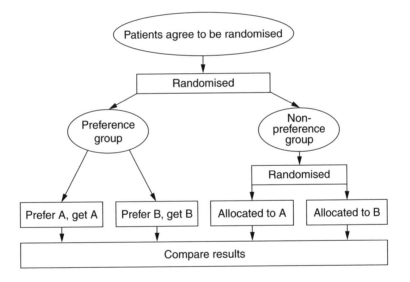

Figure 50 Wennberg's design.

See **Belmont Report; Comprehensive cohort design; Consent; Declaration of Helsinki; Ethical issues; Informed consent; Institutional review board; Preference trials; Zelen consent design.**

○ Awad MA, Shapiro SH, Lund JP and Feine JS (2000) Determinants of patients' treatment preferences in a clinical trial. *Commun Dental Oral Epidemiol*. **2**: 119–25.

○ Jadad A (1998) *Randomised controlled trial*. BMJ Books, London.

○ Lambert MF and Wood J (2000) Incorporating patient preferences into randomised trials. *J Clin Epidemiol.* **53**: 163–6.

○ Silverman WA and Altman D (1996) Patient's preferences and randomised trials. *Lancet.* **347**: 171–4.

William's agreement measure

William's agreement is an assessment of the level of agreement of individuals compared with the rest of the group.

If we have 10 individuals (A, B, C…J), then we can conduct a William's agreement measure for J with respect to the rest of the group.

William's agreement measure (WA) is calculated as follows:

$$WA = \frac{\text{percentage agreement of J with rest of group}}{\substack{\text{average percentage agreement between all pairs of raters} \\ \text{in the rest of the group (e.g. pairs AB, AC, AD, DE…FG…)}}}$$

How do you interpret the result? In general, the higher the William's agreement (WA) measure the better.

So far, you may be thinking that all of this seems rather abstract. At first glance it does seem so. However, William's agreement-type measures are being used all the time – you have just not formally recognised this until now. The interest in William's agreement is not just for assessing agreement in clinical trials, but it can also be used to assess how a person's views, impressions and statements about the evidence from a clinical trial compare with other people's views, impressions and statements.

For example:

- when a consultant presented a case for using a new product, William's agreement measure was used to establish how that consultant's views compared with those of her peers

- when a health authority pharmaceutical adviser argues in favour of one product, William's agreement measure can show how the arguments rate in relation to other advisers' views

- William's agreement measure can be used to see how many hospitals agree to pay for a newly launched, expensive but effective first-line breast cancer drug and their reasons for agreeing to pay for it

- it can be used to see what practitioners in the primary care group believe is the best way to implement the evidence from a recently published trial.

It should be noted that just because a group of people agree, as seen in a high William's measure, they may not be right! For example, last year a group of psychogeriatricians agreed on an issue related to Alzheimer's dementia, but others, especially drug purchasers, were more sceptical about the issue. Therefore you should not just slavishly accept a high measure as a sure basis for making a decision – do not be lulled into a false sense of security or complacency when you see high agreement. Ask and analyse the issue under consideration. Find out what others think. Bear in mind the perspective and vested interests of the individuals in the measure. If it is not wide enough, can you widen it to include other people's views? *See* **Analytic perspective; Bias; Research governance in the NHS**.

Withdrawal

Withdrawal is the act of withdrawing. Patients who are removed from the research before it ends are considered withdrawals. Withdrawals in research studies can occur, for example, because of protocol violation, medical, ethical or personal reasons. Trial managers generally remove certain patients who then become classified as the 'withdrawals'. A withdrawal may, with care, be replaced in the study by another patient. Data on withdrawals from a study should not be ignored in the subsequent analysis of the research. *See* **Dropout; Early stopping rule; Interim analysis; Last observation carried forward; Missing values**.

Yellow card scheme

The yellow card scheme, as it operates in the UK, is a system that enables healthcare professionals to report unwanted and unexpected adverse drug reactions to the Committee on Safety of Medicines (CSM).

The CSM receives around 20 000 reports per year. This is a significant number, but we have to remember that:

- not all unwanted and unexpected adverse drug reactions are actually reported

- not all of those that are reported will be serious or fatal

- the total number of prescriptions dispensed in the community is now more than 530 000 000 per year in England.

In contrast, the body that holds the market licence for the product (a pharmaceutical company) is subject to statutory obligations. By law, the holder of a product licence has a statutory obligation to maintain a record of reports, of which they are aware, of adverse effects in one or more human beings or animals associated with the use of any medicinal product to which the licence relates. These records must be available for inspection by anyone who is 'authorised to inspect the records'.

The yellow card scheme is designed to operate only for medicines that are already on the market. It does not automatically cover medicines under clinical trial. Any adverse event in a clinical trial must be reported to the principal investigator, who must then act on the evidence and requirements under the trial protocol. For example, they may pass on the information and advice to the trial sponsors, the Medicines Control Agency, other trial site managers and the appropriate local or multicentre research ethics committees. The rights, safety and well-being of the trial participants – the patients – are the most important consideration, and should prevail over the interests of science, society, trial sponsors and the careers of those who are running the trial.

The yellow card system does not cover non-medical interventions (e.g. technology, surgery). The UK government announced in mid-2000 that it was seeking to design and develop a system to record, act upon and learn from critical incidents in healthcare more generally.

The yellow cards have a standard reporting format and are available inside prescription pads, at the back of the *British National Formulary*, in the Association of the

British Pharmaceutical Industry's publication, *Data Sheets and Summaries of Products' Characteristics*, or from the Medicines Control Agency, Committee on Safety of Medicines, Freepost, London SW8 5BR. *See* **Adverse effects; Audit; Committee on Safety of Medicines; Medicines Control Agency; Outcomes; Post-marketing surveillance; Transparency.**

Zelen's consent design

In a Zelen's consent design trial, patients are randomised before being asked to consent. Zelen's consent design has been used in clinical trials of the following:

- extracorporeal membrane oxygenation and conventional medical therapy in neonates with persistent pulmonary hypertension
- osteoporosis screening
- faecal-occult-blood screening for colorectal cancer
- hip replacements.

Since Zelen's initial publication, variations on and interpretations of the theme have emerged. Two of the more common versions of Zelen's consent design trials are described here.

In Zelen's *double-consent design*:

- all those randomised are asked if they want the regimen to which they have been assigned
- if they want it (i.e. consent), they can receive it
- if they do not want it, they receive another regimen.

Figure 51 illustrates Zelen's double-consent design.

In Zelen's *single-consent design*:

- only those randomised to the experimental regimen are asked to consent
- if they want that regimen (i.e. consent), they receive it
- if they do not want it, they receive another regimen.

What happens to those individuals in the non-experimental group varies depending on the exact study, but usually they receive the regimen they have been allocated, and in some cases have not even been made aware of the existence of the experimental treatment.

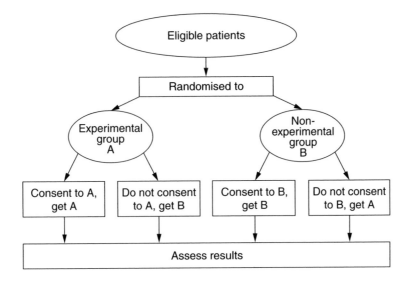

Figure 51 Zelen's double-consent design.

Figure 52 illustrates Zelen's single-consent design.

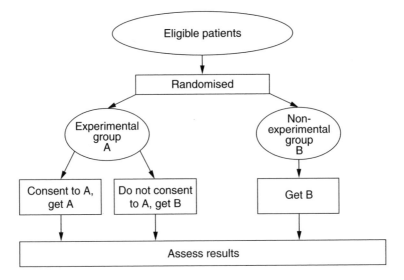

Figure 52 Zelen's single-consent design.

In the light of the serious issues surrounding consent, or the lack of it, trials where people are randomised before they are asked for consent are less likely to be regarded favourably by sponsors or ethical committees. Whether it is right or wrong, it seems that the strengths of Zelen designs are being overshadowed by political, practical, legal, regulatory, moral and ethical concerns about when to get consent.

However, some ongoing UK trials and overseas trials may involve Zelen design, and it is important to remember this. Finally, Zelen design does not necessarily agree with the way in which the initial design has been subsequently interpreted. *See* **Belmont Report; Comprehensive cohort design; Consent; Declaration of Helsinki; Deferred consent; Ethical issues; Informed consent; Institutional review board; Preference trial; Randomised controlled trial; Research governance in the NHS; Wennberg's design**.

○ Awad MA, Shapiro SH, Lund JP and Feine JS (2000) Determinants of patients' treatment preferences in a clinical trial. *Commun Dental Oral Epidemiol.* **2**: 119–25.

○ Edwards SJL, Lilford RJ, Jackson JC *et al.* (1998) The ethics of randomised controlled trials: a systematic review. *Health Technol Assess.* **2**: 1–128.

○ Lambert MF and Wood J (2000) Incorporating patient preferences into randomised trials. *J Clin Epidemiol.* **53**: 163–6.

○ Silverman WA and Altman DG (1996) Patients' preferences and randomised trials. *Lancet.* **347**: 171–4.

○ Snowdon C, Elbourne D and Garcia J (1999) Zelen randomisation. Attitudes of parents participating in a neonatal trial. *Control Clin Trials.* **20**: 149–71.

○ Torgerson DJ and Roland M (1998) What is Zelen's design? *BMJ.* **316**: 606.

○ Zelen M (1979) A new design for randomised trials. *NEJM.* **300**: 1242–5.

○ Zelen M (1990) Randomised consent designs for clinical trials: an update. *Stat Med.* **9**: 1242–5.